The Essence of
Liu Feng-wu's
Gynecology

The Essence
of Liu Feng-wu's
Gynecology

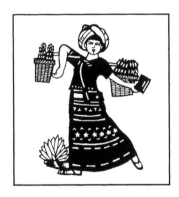

by Liu Feng-wu

translated by
Shuai Xue-zhong
and Bob Flaws

BLUE POPPY PRESS, INC.
Boulder, Colorado

Published by:
BLUE POPPY PRESS
A Division of Blue Poppy Enterprises, Inc.
5441 Western Ave., Suite 2
BOULDER, CO 80301

First Edition, February, 1998
Second Printing, October, 2005
Third Printing, February, 2007
Fourth Printing, August, 2008

ISBN 0-936185-88-0
ISBN 978-0-936185-88-0
LC 97-77996

COMP Designation: Functional translation using a standard translational terminology

Cover caligraphy by Michael Sullivan (Seiho)

The cover picture is of the divine doctor, Qi Bo. It has been lent to us by the kind permission of Signor L. Paroli of GMT 2000, Laverno, Italy, publisher of the Italian Journal, *Yi Dao*.

10 9 8 7 6 5 4

Printed at Fidlar Doubleday, Kalamazoo, MI on recycled paper and soy inks.

Editor's Preface

This book is a partial translation of *Liu Feng Wu Fu Ke Jing Yan (Liu Feng-wu's Experiences in Gynecology)* compiled by the Beijing College of Chinese Medicine and the Beijing Municipal Academy of Chinese Medicine and published by the People's Health & Hygiene Press and the Sichuan New China Publishing Company in 1982. Judging from the Chinese editor's preface in the source text, this book was originally compiled in 1976 while Liu Feng-wu was still alive. At that time, he was credited with having over 40 years of clinical experience in Chinese medical gynecology.

At the time this book was compiled, China was still in the throes of the Cultural Revolution. Therefore, the Chinese editor's preface begins with Mao Ze-dong's famous quote:

> Chinese medicine and medicinals are a great treasure house. Efforts should be made to explore these and take them to a higher level.

Likewise, in the preface, there is mention of the "needs of the peasants" and no authors' names are given on the cover or title page, only the authors' *dan wei* or work units, thus stressing communal effort. Similarly, nothing is said about Liu Feng-wu's personal biography. Therefore, this book might be dismissed by some as typical "TCM Maoist medicine." Although it does contain a few obligatory lines which are allusions to Communist rhetoric, this book also contains some very valuable and high quality Chinese medicine. This underscores that what has come to be called TCM (for Traditional Chinese Medicine) in the West is not some bowdlerized or truncated version of Chinese medicine. It is merely a standardized and systematized version built upon the bedrock of the full 2,000 years of Chinese medical literature.

As the reader will see, Liu Feng-wu was a highly educated practitioner who was well conversant with all the major historic theories of Chinese medicine. He then filtered these theories through the lens of his more than 40 years of clinical experience and arrived at a masterful distillation of the essence of Chinese medical gynecology. He threw out what had not worked for him in clinical practice and consistently searched for new, more effective treatments. In this sense, Liu Feng-wu was a direct descendant of the great eighteenth century Chinese gynecologist, Fu Qing-zhu, who also created new approaches to gynecological problems based on his personal, first-hand experience. Thus we have titled this version of Dr. Liu's work simply *The Essence of Liu Feng-wu's Gynecology*.

The Chinese source text appears to have been compiled from several sources. First there are medical essays which seem to have been written by Dr. Liu himself. Secondly, there are case histories which speak of Dr. Liu in the third person. These were most probably compiled and edited by Dr. Liu's students from their personal clinic notes. In the People's Republic of China, patients typically carry around their own medical records. However, Dr. Liu undoubtedly had students sitting with him in clinic who wrote down each case in their own notebooks. It is not uncommon in China for such students to compile, edit, and publish a selection of these as a way to honor and promote their teacher. And third, there is a section on Dr. Liu's experiential formulas and his ideas about 98 key medicinals. In total, there are 16 formulas which Dr. Liu created himself. Although these are typically based on standard formulas, they are modifications based on Dr. Liu's personal experience.

This present book is a functional translation of selections from all three sections of *Liu Feng Wu Fu Ke Jing Yan*. In actual fact, the selections in the first two sections attempt to be a denotative translation, while the third section is only a functional translation in that only what we have taken to be the most important and useful parts for Western readers have been included without necessarily noting each abbreviation or omission. Our standard for all Chinese medical technical terms is Nigel

Wiseman's *English-Chinese Chinese-English Dictionary of Chinese Medicine* published by the Hunan Science & Technology Press in Changsha in 1995. Medicinal identifications were based first on Bensky and Gamble's *Chinese Herbal Medicine: Materia Medica*, Eastland Press, Seattle, 1993. If a medicinal does not appear in that source, we then looked in Hong-yen Hsu's *Oriental Materia Medica: A Concise Guide* published by Oriental Healing Arts Institute, Long Beach, CA, 1986. If this source does not give an identification for the medicinal, we next looked in the *Zhong Yao Da Ci Dian (Dictionary of Chinese Medicinals)* published by the Shanghai Science & Technology Press, Shanghai, 1991. This methodology is based on the fact that the first materia medica is the most commonly used English language *ben cao* in the West. However, the second English language materia medica does include medicinals not included in Bensky and Gamble. If neither of these two English language materia medica contained a specific Chinese medicinal, then we went to a definitive Chinese language dictionary of materia medica. Since most Chinese herbal purveyors and pharmacies in the West use some version of the Latinate names found in Bensky and Gamble or Hong-yen Hsu *et al.*, we feel this methodology will enable practitioners to not only identify but prescribe and/or purchase these ingredients.

In addition, ingredients in formulas are given first in Latinate pharmacological nomenclature followed by Pinyin in parentheses. The first word is typically the part or piece used. This is given in nominative case and is followed by the name of the species and subspecies in genitive or possessive case. Therefore, Semen Cuscutae Chinensis means the seeds of Chinese Cuscuta. However, once those identifications have been made in any given section or case history, then we have typically used a single common English name, such as Dandelion, or the nominative cases of the species name, such as Mentha. If more than one part or piece of a species is commonly used in Chinese medicine, then we have kept a simplified version of the Latinate pharmacological nomenclature after its first full introduction, for instance, Cortex Cinnamomi instead of Cortex Cinnamomi Cassiae and in contradistinction to Cinnamon Twigs. Since the vast majority of Western practitioners refer to Radix Angelicae Sinensis by its Chinese name, Dang Gui, except when it is a listed ingredient in a formula with dosage, we have simply referred to it as Dang Gui. Thus we hope that identifications in formulas are precise and unambiguous, while discussions read more like Western practitioners talk amongst themselves.

Material in brackets [ ] has been added by the translators in order to clarify the meaning of a passage while still identifying what the Chinese actually says. All translations are a balancing act between saying what the text says and saying what the translator thinks that means. Sometimes it is possible to do both at the same time, but sometimes this is not possible. This is especially the case when translating from Chinese into English due to the vast dissimilarity between these two languages. Most translators make either a conscious or unconscious choice between these two methods of translation—translating the words or translating the meaning. The house standard of Blue Poppy Press is to translate the words as closely as possible and then, if that fails to convey the meaning in easily understandable English, to add words in brackets which are not in the source text or to provide explanations of the meaning in footnotes or other such commentaries. Because books such as this on Chinese medicine attempt to convey information which is meant to be put into real-life clinical practice, we believe that the precision necessary in the transmission of instructional information is much different from and far higher than for translations which are merely meant to entertain. Hopefully, using our standard glossary, readers knowledgeable in Chinese can put this work back into Chinese and arrive at something very close to the original. Material in parentheses ( ), other than those used for Chinese medicinal and formula identifications and acupuncture point identifications, are parenthetical additions made by the Chinese authors or editors and appear in the source text.

Book One, the medical essays of Liu Feng-wu, contains some extremely interesting and important reading. The first essay on the spleen and stomach should, in my opinion, be required reading for all English language Chinese medical students and is obviously based on an elaboration of Li Dong-yuan's ideas in the *Pi Wei Lun (Treatise on the Spleen & Stomach)*. In addition, there are essays on the role of the liver and kidneys in Chinese gynecology, these three viscera—the liver, spleen, and kidneys—being what Dr. Liu considered the three most important in gynecology. There is an enlightening essay on the *chong* and *ren* and how they relate to the qi and blood on the one hand and the liver, spleen, and kidneys on the other. The essay on "heat entering the blood chamber" clarifies an issue which has been an enigma for anyone familiar with Chinese gynecology since Zhang Zhong-jing introduced this concept in his *Jin Gui Yao Lue (Essentials of the Golden Cabinet)* in the second century CE. And there are very useful essays on *Chan Hou Sheng Hua Tang* (Postpartum Engendering & Transforming Decoction), Radix Bupleuri (*Chai Hu*), *Qin Lian Si Wu Tang* (Scutellaria & Coptis Four Materials Decoction) and uterine myomas, and the Chinese pattern discrimination of menstrual irregularities of which, in my opinion, no one attempting to practice Chinese gynecology can afford to be ignorant.

Book Two contains a number of case histories showing how Dr. Liu applied the theories contained in these medical essays in everyday clinical practice. Each of these case histories is then followed by an analysis of the case and why Dr. Liu did what he did. Since case histories are records of the treatment of real-life patients, they typically contain more complicated pattern discriminations than those met with in beginner's textbooks on treatment based on pattern discrimination. As such, case histories are the necessary next step in a practitioner's study of Chinese medicine. Unfortunately, till now, few examples of high quality Chinese case histories have been available in English. Frequently, beginners lament that their patients do not look like the simple patterns listed in their textbooks. However, many of the patients described in these case histories do look like the complex patients in my gynecology clinic. The case histories are arranged in this book in a roughly longitudinal order, beginning with premenstrual tension and ending with climacteric syndrome.

Book Three is a description of the composition, functions, and indications of 16 experiential formulas created and used by Dr. Liu. These descriptions also contain commentaries on the analysis and rationale for each formula. Each of these formulas was created by Dr. Liu in response to some clinical situation which he felt was not adequately addressed by an already existing standard Chinese formula. After explaining the main disease mechanisms at work in the disease under discussion, the authors, presumably Dr. Liu's students, then go on to explain why Dr. Liu felt that the already existing formulas were insufficient and the rationale behind his new formula. These discussions are very reminiscent of those in *Fu Qing Zhu Nu Ke (Fu Qing-zhu's Gynecology)* in which Fu Qing-zhu introduces a disease, says what everyone else thinks and does, and then gives his thoughts, experiences, and new formulas for that disease. For anyone specializing in Chinese medical gynecology, these formulas are a gold mine. Personally, I have found a number of them to be very useful in clinical practice with my Western patients. For instance, Dr. Liu's concern for damp heat and transformative heat is very germane to Western gynecological patients.

Readers will find that Dr. Liu liked to use certain medicinals, such as Herba Dianthi (*Qu Mai*) and Cortex Cedrelae (*Chun Gen Bai Pi*), which are not that frequently met in the standard textbook Chinese medical literature. Thus this book containing Dr. Liu's personal approach to Chinese gynecology is bound to cause pause for thought even in experienced practitioners who are otherwise familiar with the already existing English language literature on Chinese gynecology. While working on the editing and translation of this book, I have found it to be an important addition to my own understanding of Chinese gynecology, and I would like to extend my sincere thanks to Prof. Shuai Xue-zhong of the Hunan College of Chinese Medicine in Changsha for suggesting that Blue Poppy Press publish an English language version of it and for making such an English language version available.

Those who would like to compare Liu Feng-wu's gynecology with a more standard or introductory level of Chinese medical gynecology should see *A Handbook of Traditional Chinese Gynecology*. Those interested in learning more about Chinese menstrual diseases in particular should see my *Handbook of Menstrual Diseases in Chinese Medicine*. And those who would like to compare Liu Feng-wu's masterful 20th century approach to Chinese gynecology to a masterful 18th century approach should see *Fu Qing-zhu's Gynecology*. All three of these other books on Chinese gynecology are also available from Blue Poppy Press.

Bob Flaws
Boulder, CO

Table of Contents

Book Three: Experiential Formulas

BOOK ONE
MEDICAL ESSAYS

1
The Clinical Significance of the Spleen & Stomach's Upbearing & Downbearing

The spleen and stomach are connected to each other by a membrane and are located in the abdomen. One is a viscus, while the other is a bowel. They have an exterior-interior relationship and are the pivots of the qi transformation's upbearing and downbearing. The spleen governs movement and transformation, while the stomach rules reception and absorption. The spleen moves fluids and humors for the stomach, upbears the clear, downbears the turbid, and transports the finest essence of water and grains. It is the origin of the engenderment and transformation of qi and blood. If the stomach is strong and the spleen is fortified, water and grain qi is exuberant, essence is sufficient, and the spirit is effulgent. The qi mechanism flows smoothly and is harmonious. Thus the former heaven obtains nourishment, while the latter heaven obtains assistance. In addition, the spleen also has the important actions of boosting the qi, containing the blood, governing the muscles and flesh, and governing the four limbs. The spleen and stomach are also capable of conducting and abducting, transporting and transforming the dregs and the bowel qi via the large intestine, thus transforming the turbidity within the bowels and discharging toxic heat. Therefore, they are called "the latter heaven root."

I. The close functional relationship of the spleen & stomach's upbearing & downbearing

The spleen and stomach exist in a functional interrelationship *vis à vis* the dispersion and transformation [*i.e.*, digestion] of water and grains and the assimilation and transportation of fluids and humors. The spleen resides in the central islet [*i.e.*, the middle burner] in the interior which is categorized as yin. It stores and does not discharge. Therefore, the spleen is a yin viscus. However, its nature is to govern upbearing, and upbearing is yang. In order to upbear, it necessarily depends on yang qi. This is what transports fluids and humors upward. If the spleen does not upbear, it is of no use [*i.e.*, it does not function], while if there is no yang, it cannot upbear. The spleen governs movement and transformation and produces stirring [*i.e.*, activity]. Stirring is yang. Therefore, the spleen is yin in substance but yang in function. The stomach is categorized as a yang bowel. It discharges and does not store. Its nature is mainly downbearing. Downbearing is yin. Water and grains enter the stomach and obtain movement downward. All this depends on the stomach bowel's function of descending and downbearing. If there is no yin, there is no downbearing. If there is no downbearing, the bowel qi does not flow freely and the dregs are not descended. Hence, toxic, turbid substances are not transformed. Therefore, the stomach is yang in form but yin in function.

The spleen likes dryness and is averse to dampness, while the stomach likes moisture but is averse to dryness. Dampness is a yin evil. If damp evils are excessive, spleen yang suffers encumbrance and is not able to upbear. This then leads to the spleen's movement losing its command. If the stomach obtains dampness and moistening, it is able to descend and downbear. Dryness is a yang evil. If dry qi is excessively exuberant, this necessarily leads to yin qi being damaged. If yin qi is damaged, then it will lose its function of moistening and descending [or precipitating]. Therefore, in the *Ye Tian Shi Yi An (Ye Tian-shi's Medical Records)* it says:

> If the spleen appropriately upbears, this leads to fortification, while if the stomach appropriately downbears, this leads to harmonization. When *tai yin* damp earth obtains yang , it can move. When *yang ming* dry earth obtains yin, it is quiet.

The spleen likes dryness, and the stomach likes moisture. However, this cannot be too excessive. If dry qi is excessive, this results in damaging the spleen's yang qi and consumes fluids and humors. If damp evils are excessive, this results in damaging the stomach's yang qi. Dryness and dampness are mutually antagonistic yet mutually co-productive, while functions of upbearing and downbearing are necessarily interdependent.

II. The relationship between the spleen & stomach's upbearing & downbearing and the other viscera

A. The liver & spleen

In "The Pulse Signs of the Viscera & Bowels, Channels & Network Vessels, and Former & Latter [Heaven] Diseases" in the *Jin Gui Yao Lue* (*Essentials of the Golden Cabinet*), it says:

> When liver disease appears, know that the liver will conduct [the disease] to the spleen. Therefore, first replete [*i.e.*, supplement or fortify] the spleen.

This is what is meant by reinstating the function of the spleen and stomach and secondarily treating liver disease. In order to treat the spleen, one should upbear. In order to treat the stomach, one should downbear. If the liver qi is depressed and bound, it may counterflow horizontally and first damage the spleen. Liver effulgence leads to gallbladder fire depression and binding. If this combines with the stomach qi, it leads to upward counterflow. Counterflow produces disease. It leads to the appearance of nausea, vomiting, a bitter [taste] in the mouth, and other such conditions. At the time of treatment, one should course the liver and resolve depression, orderly reach [*i.e.*, free the flow of] the qi mechanism, and clear liver-gallbladder fire while also descending and downbearing the stomach qi and upbearing the spleen qi. Thus all such conditions can be eliminated. This is what is meant by treating the liver and secondarily treating the spleen.

Another example is liver effulgence and spleen vacuity. This results in the spleen qi not upbearing. [In that case,] necessarily there must be painful diarrhea. At the time of treatment, one should restrain the liver and fortify the spleen. The formula to use is *Tong Xie Yao Fang* (Painful Diarrhea Essential Formula). Within this, Radix Albus Paeoniaé Lactiflorae (*Bai Shao*) harmonizes and restrains the liver. Radix Ledebouriellae Divaricatae (*Fang Feng*) courses the liver and upbears spleen yang. Rhizoma Atractylodis Macrocephalae (*Bai Zhu*) fortifies the spleen and supplements the qi. And Pericarpium Citri Reticulatae (*Chen Pi*) harmonizes the stomach. Thus liver depression is coursed and resolved, spleen qi obtains upbearing, and painful diarrhea is stopped automatically.

B. The heart & spleen

The heart stores the spirit, while the spleen governs thinking. Excessive thinking and worrying damage both the heart and spleen. If spleen qi depression endures, it leads to qi binding and non-obtaint of upbearing. If the heart qi becomes debilitated, the spleen qi easily suffers detriment and the muscles and flesh become emaciated. In gynecology, one commonly uses *Gui Pi Tang* (Restore the Spleen Decoction) in order to nourish the blood and supplement the heart, upbear the spleen and boost the qi. When the heart qi is nourished, it is able to resolve depression and binding. When depression and binding are resolved, spleen yang is upborne and flows smoothly. The qi is effulgent and blood is automatically engendered.

C. The lungs & spleen

The spleen governs the scattering [*i.e.*, distribution] of essence which is upwardly transported to the lungs. If the spleen qi is effulgent and exuberant, the lung qi is full and sufficient. If the spleen qi is insufficient, the lung qi must be vacuous. Therefore, in order to treat the lungs, it is necessary to treat the spleen. The lungs govern the management and regulation and diffusion of fluids and humors. If the lung qi does not diffuse, it will be difficult for the spleen qi to upbear smoothly. Hence, within *Si Jun Zi Tang* (Four Gentlemen Decoction), Radix Panacis Ginseng (*Ren Shen*) supplements the lung qi, Rhizoma Atractylodis Macrocephalae (*Bai Zu*) supplements the spleen qi, and Sclerotium Poriae Cocos (*Fu Ling*) assists Atractylodes by fortifying the spleen and percolating dampness, while Radix Glycyrrhizae (*Gan Cao*) boosts the qi and supplements the center. Thus the spleen is fortified, the stomach is nourished, yang is upborne, and the qi is supplemented. If the lung qi is vacuous or there is lung consumption, vacuity detriment, or other such conditions, yin fluids may be insufficient and eating and drinking may be reduced and scanty. Then essence blood will be insufficient, and, in women, there will be blocked menstruation [*i.e.,* amenorrhea]. Typically, this can be rapidly treated by supplementing both the lungs and spleen.

D. The spleen & kidneys

The kidneys are the viscera which store essence and are "the former heaven root." They are located in the lower burner. Therefore they are ultimate yin within yin. They store not only true yin but also true yang. The spleen [on the other hand] is the source of qi and blood and fluid and humor transformation and engenderment. It supplies the material basis for the continuous enrichment and engenderment of kidney yin and kidney yang. If kidney yang is insufficient, it may not be able to stir spleen yang. Hence spleen qi is not easily and smoothly upborne. If the spleen qi is weak, movement and transformation lose their duty and are not able to transport essence to the kidneys. This then results in kidney qi insufficiency. Thus the spleen and kidneys mutually enrich and assist one another. For example, *Si Shen Wan* (Four Spirits Pills) are said to mainly treat kidney diarrhea. However, within them, Fructus Psoraleae Corylifoliae (*Bu Gu Zhi*) supplements the fire of the gate of life; Fructus Evodiae Rutecarpae (*Wu Zhu Yu*) warms the center and dispels cold;

Fructus Myristicae Fragrantis (*Rou Dou Kou*) moves the qi and disperses food, warms the center and rectifies the intestines; Fructus Schisandrae Chinensis (*Wu Wei Zi*) astringes yin and boosts the qi, secures and astringes and stops diarrhea; uncooked Rhizoma Zingiberis (*Sheng Jiang*) warms the center; and Fructus Zizyphi Jujubae (*Da Zao*) fortifies the spleen. Therefore, this formula warms the kidneys *and* warms the spleen, secures the intestines and stops diarrhea. The spleen and kidneys are both treated even though the treatment of the kidneys is the main [focus].

III. The clinical significance of the spleen & stomach's upbearing & downbearing

A. The internal link between the treatment of the spleen & the treatment of the stomach

The spleen and stomach have an interior-exterior relationship. If the spleen is diseased, the stomach is not able by itself to move fluids and humors. If the stomach is diseased, the spleen loses the place from which it receives its endowment. Therefore, diseases of the spleen and stomach are mutually interrelated. In clinic, one may see stomach disease accompanied by symptoms and signs of spleen disease. While if the spleen is diseased, one will see simultaneous signs of stomach disease. If [disease] manifests simply as spleen vacuity, the spleen can be heavily [*i.e.*, greatly] supplemented. The formulas used are: *Sheng Ling Bai Zhu San* (Ginseng, Poria & Atractylodes Powder), *Bu Zhong Yi Qi Tang* (Supplement the Center & Boost the Qi Decoction), etc. [However,] sometimes, the external manifestations seem to be due to spleen vacuity, yet their source is stomach disease. For instance, what looks like spleen vacuity diarrhea may be due to stomach stagnation downwardly disinhibiting the spleen qi. [In such cases,] heavy emphasis [on supplementation alone] is not able to treat the spleen. Instead, one should disperse food and abduct stagnation. When stagnation is removed, disinhibition will be stopped and the spleen qi will be able to obtain recovery. On the contrary, if scanty intake of food, dry mouth, heart fluster [*i.e.*, palpitations], and shortness of breath are due to stomach stagnation torpid intake, then only using dispersing and abducting formulas will not be able to achieve the [desired therapeutic] effect. [In this case,] one should use *Xiang Sha Liu Jun Zi Tang* (Auklandia & Amomum Six Gentlemen Decoction), *Wu Wei Yi Gong San* (Five Flavors Special Effect Powder), etc. to mainly supplement the spleen. Then one will be able to affect a cure. Hence, it is very hard to separate fortifying the spleen from harmonizing of the stomach. What is necessary is to clearly divide the main from the secondary. Then stress should be laid accordingly so that one treats the root.

B. The dialectical relationship between upbearing yang & enriching yin

The relationship between upbearing yang and enriching yin is nothing other than the concrete measures adopted in clinic based on the inherent characteristics of the spleen's liking dryness and the stomach's liking moisture. It is also an apposite and united principle that suits the upbearing of spleen qi and downbearing of stomach qi. If the spleen is vacuous and the spleen qi does not upbear, then movement and transformation have no authority [*i.e.*, power]. This then results in the appearance of venter chill and abdominal distention. Food enters but moves slowly and there is a preference for warm drinks. The stools are loose and the urination is clear and uninhibited. Women's menstruation is irregular or there may be flooding and leaking and abnormal vaginal discharge. If severe, qi vacuity may fall downward and the four limbs may lack strength. [There may be] shortness of breath, disinclination to speak, prolapse of the anus, etc. In that case, *Wan Dai Tang* (End Vaginal Discharge Decoction) is often used for treating women's spleen vacuity and damp stagnation, lassitude of the spirit, poor appetite, loose stools, swollen feet, and ceaseless vaginal discharge. Within this formula, Radix Codonopsitis Pilosulae (*Dang Shen*), Rhizoma Atractylodis

Macrocephalae (*Bai Zhu*), Rhizoma Atractylodis (*Cang Zhu*), Pericarpium Citri Reticulatae (*Chen Pi*), and Radix Glycyrrhizae (*Gan Cao*) supplement the spleen and boost the qi, upbear yang and dry dampness, with upbearing of yang being the aspect that is stressed. At the same time, Radix Bupleuri (*Chai Hu*) and Herba Seu Flos Schizonepetae Tenuifoliae (*Jing Jie Sui*) are used to strengthen the action of upbearing yang and scattering dampness. Radix Albus Paeoniae Lactiflorae (*Bai Shao*) and Radix Dioscoreae Oppositae   (*Shan Yao*) are used to enrich yin, harmonize the liver, and supplement the spleen. Semen Plantaginis (*Che Qian Zi*) disinhibits water and eliminates dampness. Thus, as a whole, this formula supplements and scatters (upbears), disperses (dries dampness) and upbears (yang), and supplements vacuity without stagnating evils. The dialectic relationship between upbearing yang and enriching yin should be dealt with correctly so as to make yang upbear and yin grow, yin engender and yang grow, and balance yin and yang.

As another example, for spleen vacuity accompanied by dampness and flooding and leaking downward bleeding [*i.e.*, uterine bleeding], *Sheng Yang Yi Wei Tang* (Upbear Yang & Boost the Stomach Decoction) with additions and subtractions is often used. This boosts the stomach. When it is replete, it fortifies the spleen. Within this formula, *Liu Jun Zi* (Six Gentlemen [Decoction]) strengthens yang and boosts the stomach. To this is added uncooked Radix Astragali Membranacei (*Huang Qi*) in order to increase and strengthen the function of supplementing the qi and upbearing yang. Radix Bupleuri (*Chai Hu*) and Radix Et Rhizoma Notopterygii (*Qiang Huo*) upbear yang and scatter dampness. ([Dr. Liu] never gave up using them because they emit sweat and resolve the exterior.) These stress the aspect of upbearing yang. Radix Albus Paeoniae Lactiflorae (*Bai Shao*) restrains yin in order to harmonize the constructive. While Sclerotium Poriae Cocos (*Fu Ling*) and Rhizoma Alismatis (*Ze Xie*) disinhibit dampness and downbear turbidity. A small amount of Rhizoma Coptidis Chinensis (*Huang Lian*) is added to discharge and downbear vacuity fire. The above-mentioned formula and medicinals are the best examples of correctly dealing with the relationship between upbearing yang and enriching yin in association with the characteristics of upbearing the spleen and downbearing the stomach.

The stomach likes moisture but is averse to dryness and its nature is mainly downbearing. If there is dry heat in the stomach and yin fluids are insufficient, the throat will be dry and the mouth will be thirsty. Stomach grasping [*i.e.*, the intake of food] will be devitalized. [In that case,] treatment should mainly clear (stomach) heat and nourish yin. For instance, in *Sha Shen Mai Dong Tang* (Glehnia & Ophiopogon Decoction), Radix Glehniae Littoralis (*Sha Shen*), Tuber Ophiopogonis Japonici (*Mai Dong*), Rhizoma Polygonati Odorati (*Yu Zhu*), and Radix Trichosanthis Kirlowii (*Tian Hua Fen*) are ingredients which clear heat and moisten dryness, engender fluids and nourish yin, heavily moistening and downbearing. These are combined with Semen Dolichoris Lablab (*Bian Dou*) and Radix Glycyrrhizae (*Gan Cao*), which boost the qi and harmonize the center, and Folium Mori Albi (*Sang Ye*), which lightly diffuses, upbears, and scatters, in order to upbear, diffuse, and strengthen the spleen.

As another example, due to dry evils damaging yin, a woman's menstruation may become blocked because her blood is vacuous and her fluids are debilitated. [In that case,] it is OK to use *San He Tang* (Triple Combination Decoction, *i.e.*, the combination of *Tiao Wei Cheng Qi Tang* , Regulate the Stomach & Order the Qi Decoction, *Liang Ge San*, Cool the Diaphragm Powder, and *Si Wu Tang*, Four Materials Decoction). When dry heat obtains clearing, yin fluids will recover. When the stomach obtains downbearing, spleen qi obtains upbearing. The *chong* [penetrating] and *ren* [conception or controlling] vessels and pathways become freely flowing and uninhibited, and the menstrual water becomes self-regulated.

11

Yet another example from gynecology is that, during a warm heat disease, there may sometimes appear a bowel repletion condition. Internally, heat accumulates and is exuberant. [In that case,] one should use *Da Cheng Qi Tang* (Major Order the Qi Decoction) with additions and subtractions to urgently precipitate. This will free the flow and downbear dryness and heat. The result will be the engenderment of fluids and the preservation of yin. Sometimes there may be blood vacuity blocked menstruation. [In that case,] one should use *Gui Pi Tang* (Restore the Spleen Decoction) to treat it. Wishing to downbear, first upbear. Wishing to free the flow, first supplement. When yang is upborne and the blood is sufficient, the *chong* and *ren* will be full and exuberant, and hence the menstrual blood will automatically be free-flowing. Thus, the aim lies in correctly dealing with the dialectic relationship between upbearing yang and enriching yin no matter whether urgently precipitating to preserve yin, using sweet, moistening [medicinals] to increase fluids or upbearing yang and boosting the qi. When yang is upborne, yin grows.

Therefore, the medical experts who have discussed [and based treatment on] the spleen and stomach are very many. Their experiential knowledge based on clinical practice can be summarized thus: The spleen and stomach have an interior-exterior relationship. One is yin and one is yang; one upbears and one downbears; and they function interdependently. The spleen is a yin viscus but its function is yang. Without upbearing, yang cannot function. [Therefore,] for yang to function, one must upbear. The stomach is a yang bowel but its function is yin. Yin governs downbearing. If there is no downbearing, yin cannot function. Thus, in treating the spleen, one must know how to promote upbearing, while in treating the stomach, one must know how to promote downbearing. Only if one observes yin and yang, knows upbearing and downbearing, and is clear about supplementing and discharging is one able to grasp the key point of spleen and stomach function.

2
A Talk on the Kidneys

The kidneys store essence. They govern the growth, development, and reproductive function of the human body. In addition, they govern the water fluid metabolism. Therefore, they are called "the former heaven root." The essence stored in the kidneys includes the essence originated from food and drink and the essence of the kidneys themselves (the reproductive essence). Their production and storage are governed by the kidney qi. Thus, the kidneys contain kidney essence and kidney qi. These can also be divided into the two parts [or aspects] of kidney yin and kidney yang. The kidney essence is the material basis of the kidney qi, while kidney qi is the functional manifestation of kidney essence. The functions of both of these are interdependent. The physiological functions and pathological changes of the kidneys are closely related to a woman's growth and development, as are all the conditions of the fetus, birthing, menstruation, and abnormal vaginal discharge. Besides those which are described in other chapters, there are these additional points [concerning the kidneys and gynecology].

I. The kidneys govern opening & closing

In "The Treatise on the Images of the Six Nodal [*i.e.*, Pivotally Important] Viscera" in the *Su Wen (Simple Questions)*, it says, "The kidneys govern hibernation [*i.e.,* dormancy] and sealing [*i.e.,* closing] and are the root of storing essence." In "The Treatise on the True Speech from the Golden Cabinet" in the *Su Wen (Simple Questions)*, it says, "The kidneys open and close the two yin, storing essence in the kidneys." So-called "opening the portals" and "sealing and storing" include not only water and fluid metabolism but also the growth and development of the urogenital and excretory organs. Categorically speaking, this is what is referred to as the opening and closing function of the kidneys. If kidney qi is full and exuberant, opening and closing are disciplined. When opening is appropriate, there is opening, and, when closing is appropriate, there is closing. When the kidney qi opens, the two excretions are automatically regulated, the menstruation arrives at its proper time, and the discharge of essence and blood and fluids and humors are in their proper degree. Sexual desire is normal and, when the two essences mutually combine, one is able to have babies [i.e., conceive]. If kidney qi opens but does not close, then one will see diarrhea, frequent urination, flooding and leaking, fetal leakage, sexual desire frenetically stirring, etc. If kidney qi closes but does not open, this leads to intestinal dryness constipation, forceless discharge of stools, dribbling urinary block, and sparse [or rare, i.e., infrequent] emission of the menses which is scanty in amount. If severe, there will be blocked menstruation. Essence and blood and fluids and humors will be withered and exhausted and the sexual desire will be reduced. The external genitalia will be dry and withered and the vaginal meatus will lose its flourishing. If severe, it will be blocked and locked [i.e., impenetrable]. In that case, intercourse will be difficult and there will be infertility due to weak ova or inability to form the fetus. Therefore, in treating the above conditions in clinical practice, one should treat the kidneys in order to treat their root. Stress should be laid on enriching and supplementing kidney essence so as to boost detriment or on filling and nourishing the kidney qi to promote its function of opening and closing. For example, when Ding Jing Tang (Stabilize the Menses Decoction) is often used to regulate and rectify menstruation, Shou Tai Yin (Fetal Longevity Drink) is used to treat flooding and leaking, or when experiential formulas and medicinals are used for treating habitual miscarriage, climacteric syndrome, and infertility, all of these are mainly used to supplement the kidneys or are combined with medicinals to supplement the kidneys. These make the kidney qi full and abundant and thus opening and closing are automatically in compliance.

II. The kidneys communicate with the brain

In "The Treatise on the Bone Hollows" in the *Su Wen (Simple Questions)*, it says:

> The governing vessel arises from the center of the bone below the lower abdomen. In women, it enters into and connects with the perineum and its network vessel runs along the yin [*i.e.*, genital] organ... It joins the *shao yin* [channel]. Then it ascends to the posterior medial aspect of the thigh, penetrates through the spine, and homes to the kidneys.

This clearly explains that foot *shao yin* kidney vessel and the governing vessel mutually link. The governing arises from the uterus and descends to exit at *Hui Yin* (CV 1). Then it ascends along the spinal column and passes through *Feng Fu* (GV 16), where a network vessel enters the brain. It arrives at the vertex and traverses the point *Bai Hui* (GV 20). Then it travels down the forehead and bridge of the nose to unite with the conception vessel at the point *Ren Zhong* (GV 26). Therefore, kidney qi penetrates and flows freely to the brain via the governing vessel. If kidney essence is full and exuberant, then the power of the brain will also be full and abundant. [Conversely,] the brain governs thinking. If the mind and emotions are smoothly and easily flowing, then this can also promote the function of the kidney qi. In Chinese medicine, it is held that the kidneys are the former heaven root upon which the *tian gui* depends for its enrichment and nourishment. If the kidneys are vacuous, the *tian gui* will be exhausted and the menstruation will be blocked and stop. There will be lumbar soreness and flaccidity [*i.e.*, weakness] of the legs. Sexual desire will be reduced and the facial complexion will be dark and dull. The whole body will lack strength and the essence spirit will be listless and fatigued while the memory will be impaired [*i.e.*, decreased]. From the Western medical point of view, whether menstruation is normal or not depends upon the balanced and regular function between the cerebral cortex, hypothalamus, hypophysis [*i.e.*, pituitary], ovaries, and uterus. The occurrence of disease in any of these may lead to menstrual irregularity.

Take, for instance, Sheehan's syndrome.[1] In addition to blocked menstruation, this manifests as atrophy of the genital organs, decreased secretion of milk, falling of genital and axillary hair, decreased sexual desire, emaciation, an ashen white facial complexion, decreased memory power, essence spirit listlessness, extreme susceptibility to overtaxation, decreased muscular tension and strength, decreased basic metabolism, hypotension, hypoglycemia, etc. If this is clinically treated with *Si Er Wu He Fang* (Four , Two, Five Combined Formula, an experiential formula), certain therapeutic effect will be obtained. Within this formula, *Wu Zi Yan Zong Wan* (Five Seeds Increase Progeny Pills) are used to supplement the kidney qi. Rhizoma Curculiginis Orchioidis (*Xian Mao*) and Herba Epimedii (*Xian Ling Pi*) supplement kidney yang. *Si Wu Tang* (Four Materials Decoction) nourishes the blood and supplements the essence. Thus treatment is based via the kidneys. Based on clinical experience, [this formula] not only improves the symptoms and enables the menstruation to flow freely, but examination also shows that it gradually recuperates genital organ atrophy and improves endocrine function. Hence, in terms of the pathological changes of this disease described above, there exists a common point between Chinese and Western medicines which is worthy of further research.

III. The lungs & kidneys are mutually related

In "The Chapter on the Channels & Vessels" in the *Ling Shu (Spiritual Pivot)*, it is said:

> The kidney foot *shao yin* vessel...penetrates the spine, homes to the kidneys, and networks with the urinary bladder. A vertical branch ascends from the kidneys to penetrate through the liver and diaphragm.

---

[1] Sheehan's syndrome is the result of pituitary necrosis from hypovolemia and shock in the immediate peripartum period. In this case, lactation may not develop postpartum, the patient may complain of fatigue, and there may be loss of axillary and pubic hair.

It enters the lungs, runs along the throat, and comes to the root of the tongue.

This clearly explains that the lungs and kidneys mutually connect with each other via the channels and network vessels. In terms of water and fluid metabolism, the lungs govern the free flow and regulation of the water passageways. Thus they are the upper source of water. The kidneys govern opening and closing. Therefore, they are the lower source of water. In terms of respiration, the lungs' respiratory function depends upon the kidney's absorption of the qi. Hence, the lungs govern the exhalation of the qi, while the kidneys govern the absorption of the qi. The lungs are the florid canopy and are located in the upper burner, in the highest position of the human body, while the kidneys are located in the lower burner, the most yin place. The upper one and the lower one are quite distant from each other. Superficially, they do not seem to be connected. But when the body is viewed as an integrated whole, the lungs and kidneys are most definitely connected. This connection is that the lungs govern the transportation and distribution of essence. Whether the lung qi is vacuous or replete is dependent on the kidney qi. The kidneys receive qi from the lungs but are also the root of the lungs. Therefore, both [viscera] mutually subsidize each other. In "The Treatise on Channel & Vessel Divergences" in the Su Wen (Simple Questions), it says:

Drink enters the stomach and produces essence qi. This is transported upward by the spleen. The spleen qi scatters the essence, and it gathers above in the lungs. [The lungs] free the flow and regulate the water passageways and transport [water fluids] downward to the urinary bladder. [Thus] water essence is spread to the four [corners] and also moves to the five channels...

The foot tai yang bladder channel and the foot shao yin kidney have an interior-exterior relationship. Therefore, the bladder is the tai yang bowel, and the tai yang governs the exterior qi (skin and hair) of the

17

entire body. The lungs also govern the skin and hair. Hence the relationship between the bladder and the lungs in terms of the qi transformation of the triple burner is that between bowel qi and exterior qi. If the skin and hair are affected by cold, the interstices become blocked and obstructed. The bladder qi cannot open and the kidney qi's function of opening and closing suffers limitation. If one desires to open the kidney qi and disinhibit the bladder, one must diffuse the lung qi via the skin and hair. This will then get an effect. For instance, within *Wu Ling San* (Five [Ingredients] Poria Powder), Ramulus Cinnamomi Cassiae (*Gui Zhi*, which enters the *tai yang* channel) warms and frees the flow of the skin and hair and opens the exterior of the *tai yang*. Thus the kidney qi is boosted and obtains opening, while the bladder qi transforms and obtains movement. Hence, dribbling urinary block obtains free flow. Some patients with postpartum urinary retention are categorized according to this type of pattern. It can be seen [in such cases] that the lungs, kidneys, and bladder are extremely closely related.

In terms of the internal relationship of these two viscera, the foot *shao yin* kidney channel vessel penetrates the spine and homes to the kidneys, networks with the urinary bladder, upwardly penetrates through the liver and diaphragm, and enters into the lungs. The essence flourishing of the lungs can directly enter into the kidneys to nourish kidney qi. Lung vacuity leads to the kidneys' loss of nourishment, while kidney vacuity can also affect the lungs. For example, *Hei Xi Dan* (Black Lead Elixir) is used to treat lung-kidney insufficiency, [in the case of] kidneys not absorbing the qi vacuity panting. [This formula] uses Galenitum (*Hei Xi*) and Sulfur (*Liu Huang*) to warm and supplement the kidneys in order that they may absorb the lung qi and thus level [or calm] panting [*i.e.*, asthma]. As another example, Radix Panacis Ginseng (*Ren Shen*) and Radix Astragali Membranacei (*Huang Qi*) originally were supplementing the lungs and boosting the qi medicinals. Yet Li Shi-zhen said that Astragalus governs vacuity panting and treats kidney vacuity deafness. In terms of his viewpoint on Ginseng, he cited Zhu Dan-xi's words, "If lung-kidney vacuity is extreme, *Du Shen Tang* (Solitary

Ginseng Decoction) rules this." It can thus be seen that medicinals which supplement the lungs can be used to boost the kidneys. In the *Yao Xing Fu (Prose Poem on Medicinal Natures)*, it says, "Fructus Schisandrae Chinensis (*Wu Wei Zi*) can stop coughing and phlegm and enrich kidney water." This clearly shows that Schisandra was originally a lung medicinal which is able to supplement the lung qi so that it is able to enter the kidneys.

In commonly seen gynecological diseases, those that are directly related to the lungs are relatively few, while many are related directly to the kidneys. [However, even in such cases,] sometimes, when treating the kidneys, it is advantageous to assist this by supplementing the lung qi, and this gets a higher [*i.e.*, better] therapeutic effect. For instance, for profuse sweating in emergency hemorrhagic conditions of flooding downward [*i.e.*, uterine bleeding], qi may be vacuous and on the verge of desertion. One should urgently use *Du Shen Tang* (Solitary Ginseng Decoction) in order to stem desertion. If only the kidneys are supplemented, the movement of water will not be resolved and will be on the verge of exhaustion. [In such cases,] one will not be able to save the emergency condition. In recent years, [the author] has used *Si Er Wu He Fang* (Four, Two, Five Combination Formula, an experiential formula) to treat Sheehan's syndrome and the therapeutic effects have been good. Afterwards, [I] added Ginseng and Astragalus and the therapeutic effect was even better. Gradually it has become clear that the reason for this is due to the relationship between the lungs and kidneys.

3
Why it is Said That "The Liver is the Thief of the Five Viscera & Six Bowels"
Plus a Discussion of Eight Methods for Treating the Liver in Gynecology

In clinic, there is always someone who says, "The liver is the thief of the five viscera and six bowels," (while others say it is the thief of the five viscera [only]). What does this mean? Truly this [saying] is worthy of further research.

I. The physiological functions of the liver

In order to clarify the meaning of the [above] sentence, one must first understand the physiological functions of the liver. The liver stores the blood and is the root of the importance of movement. This means that [the liver] stores blood and fluids and regulates and disciplines the volume of blood so that the body can tolerate fatigue and taxation and resist external evils. [The liver] is the root of the sinews and has its flourishing in the fingernails. It opens into the portals of the eyes and its fluid is the tears. [The liver] governs coursing and discharging and orderly reaching. Life's activities in humans depends upon the integrated physiological function consisting of the close connection between the viscera and bowels. The liver is closely related to other viscera and bowels, organs, and channels and network vessels. These are interconnected, interdependent, interinhibiting, and interpromoting. This makes clear the point that the liver is able to engender and nourish the viscera and bowels.

The saying that, "The liver is the thief of the five viscera and six bowels," must necessarily involve the relationship between the liver and the five viscera and six bowels and particularly the relationship between the five viscera.

The liver & kidneys

The liver and kidneys share a common source. They enrich and nourish each other. The liver's functions of coursing and discharging and orderly spreading and of regulating and disciplining the volume of blood depend upon the enrichment and invigoration of kidney yin, while the storage of yin (essence) material in the kidneys is carried on by the coursing and discharging function of the liver.

The liver & spleen

The spleen's movement and transformation is necessarily carried on by the coursing and discharging of the liver. Conversely, if the spleen loses its fortification and movement, this must affect the liver's coursing and discharging.

The liver & lungs

The lungs govern the regulation and rectification of the qi of the entire body. The liver governs the regulation and discipline of the blood of the entire body. The liver's transportation of blood over the whole body depends upon the lungs' depurative downbearing. If the liver loses its orderly spreading, the qi becomes congested, depressed, and stagnant. This in turn can also affect the lungs' depurative downbearing.

The liver & heart

Their relationship is mainly that between blood circulation and the regulation and disciplining of the volume of the blood. If heart blood is insufficient, this will affect the regulation and disciplining of the liver. If the liver blood is insufficient, this will affect heart function. The heart governs the essence spirit and consciousness, while the liver governs coursing and discharging and orderly spreading (the ease and smooth flow of the emotions). The essence spirit and the emotions also mutually influence each other.

In addition, the liver and the two vessels of the *chong* and *ren* are connected via the channels and network vessels. The liver is the viscus of the storage of the blood. The *chong* is the sea of blood. The *ren* governs the uterus. If liver function is normal and liver blood is sufficient and full, the sea of blood will be full and exuberant and the menses will be able to periodically descend. In terms of its relationship with the six bowels, the organs, and the channels and network vessels, all of these have an interior-exterior relationship with the five viscera and, therefore, either directly or indirectly mutually affect each other.

In sum, the liver is the blood viscus. Its function is to store, regulate, and discipline the volume of blood of the whole body. The five viscera and six bowels, the four extremities and hundreds of joints, and the various organs and tissues depend for their nourishment upon the blood. The liver is also able to course and regulate the qi mechanism. This makes the qi and blood flow smoothly, the channels and network vessels to course and mount, the viscera and bowel function harmonious and regulated, the four extremities and the joints fortified and uninhibited, and the opening and closing of the portals normal. Thus the integrated physiological function is fortified and strong. The essence power is full and abundant. The emotions are comfortable and smoothly flowing. One can tolerate fatigue and taxation and can resist external evils. Thus, the liver is able to engender and nourish the five viscera and six bowels. This is the most beneficial aspect of the liver in terms of the five viscera and six bowels.

II. The pathology of the liver

Yin blood is what the liver governs, but qi is what makes it function. Its body is yin, but its function is yang. Its nature likes tenderness and is averse to firmness. If the liver qi is either excessive or does not reach, both can result in disease. Mainly [its disease] manifests as liver qi, liver fire, liver wind, and liver cold.

Liver qi

Liver qi is normal when it is orderly reaching and coursing smoothly. If this becomes excessive or it does not reach, either can transform into pathological liver qi. If it does not reach, the qi mechanism will be inhibited. The secretion of bile will be insufficient and the spleen and stomach's function of movement and transformation will be reduced. The blood supply to the viscera and bowels and channels and network vessels will be insufficient. The sinews and bones, muscles and flesh will lose their nourishment. The ears and eyes will not be able to hear or see. The hands will not be able to grasp. The feet will not be able to step. The whole body will tend to decline and degenerate. Therefore, [the liver] is called "the root of ultimate cessation."

If it is excessive, the qi mechanism will be congested, blocked, depressed, stagnant, and not smoothly flowing. If the qi mechanism is not smoothly flowing, the channels and vessels will not be freely flowing. If mild, this manifests as wandering pain in the limbs and body, the joints, and muscles and flesh. This is referred to as "liver qi wandering pain." If severe, vexation and tension, chest oppression, suffocated qi, bilateral rib-side distention and pain, and horizontal counterflow which attacks the spleen and stomach, resulting in burping and acid swallowing [i.e., regurgitation], may appear. [There may also be] upward counterflow of stomach qi, internally engendered spleen dampness, and damp heat brewing which, if severe, may manifest as jaundice. Thus it is said, "The ten thousands of diseases do not go beyond depression, and all depression pertains to the liver." This is definitely true.

Liver fire

That caused externally usually manifests as liver fire and gallbladder heat upbearing and soaring, red eyes with profuse eye discharge, dry mouth, a bitter [taste in the] mouth, oral thirst, a red tongue with yellow fur, possibly dry stools or reddish urination, and blisters arising on the skin [*i.e.,* herpes] with local redness, swelling, and burning pain. If liver-gallbladder fire and heat pours downward, this results in testicular or vaginal area swelling and pain and difficulty walking. That due to internal causes is mostly due to qi depression transforming fire. If depressive fire is relatively moderate, vexation and agitation, chest oppression, a dry mouth, parched throat or low-grade fever are mostly seen. In addition, this can also be caused by excessive anger damaging the liver (liver results in the qi ascending). If liver qi surges and counterflows, the blood will follow the qi upward. If severe, this will lead to heat becoming depressed and binding with a tendency to stir wind. As "The Treatise on the Engenderment & Free Flow of Qi" in the *Su Wen (Simple Questions)* says, "Great anger results in the formal qi being severed and the blood winding its way upward." This manifests as spitting of blood, nosebleed, wind stroke, bleeding, and shifted [*i.e.,* vicarious] menstruation, etc.

Liver wind

"The Great Treatise on the True Essentials" in the *Su Wen (Simple Questions)* states, "All wind [results in] falling [*i.e.,* syncope] and vertigo and all pertain to the liver." Liver wind can be divided into internal, external, vacuity, and repletion [types]. Liver wind arising due to external causes is usually associated with liver-gallbladder heat exuberance which stirs wind. The conditions seen [in this case] are fright inversion, tremors and contractions. This is also called extreme heat engendering wind (or heat tetany wind). Liver wind arising due to internal causes may be due to extreme anger damaging the liver. Liver wind stirs internally and wind and fire mutually fan each other. The conditions seen are dizziness and vertigo, headache as if going to split,

25

neck traction and stiffness, tremors, incoherent speech, and tetany reversal. In case of replete fire wind stroke, one may see severe head pain, tremors and contractions, etc. If due to liver yin insufficiency with ascendant hyperactivity of liver yang, liver wind may harass above. In that case one will see headache, dizziness, insomnia, and numb extremities. This is categorized as vacuity wind. In the later stages of a heat disease, yin and blood may be greatly damaged. This can lead to the arising of blood vacuity wind stirring. This is [also] categorized as vacuity wind.

Liver cold

If liver yang is insufficient, vacuity cold may follow the channel and move downward. Then one may see cold mounting [*i.e., shan* or "hernia"]. In women, this mostly manifests as lower abdominal bilateral and lumbosacral region cold pain.

The above is a description of the pathology of the liver itself. As to the influence of liver qi, liver fire, liver wind, and liver cold upon the various viscera as well as their combinations resulting in disease, the scope is even wider.

The liver & kidneys

If liver yin is insufficient, liver yang may become hyperactive above. Since the liver and kidneys have a common source, kidney yin insufficiency may lead to liver yin vacuity and this can also lead to the production of liver qi, liver fire, and liver wind. It may also make the nature of the disease more severe. If both the liver and kidney yin are vacuous, then one can see both simultaneously. If liver fire is effulgent and exuberant, coursing and discharging will be excessive. This then can lead to the kidneys not blocking and storing.

The liver & lungs

Liver fire may scorch the lungs. In that case, one can see coughing and coughing of blood. If liver qi becomes depressed and stagnant, this can affect the lungs' depurative downbearing thus resulting in itchy throat, cough, and bilateral rib-side spastic pain or plum pit qi.

The liver & spleen-stomach

If the spleen loses command over movement, dampness may stagnate in the middle burner. This may then affect the liver's coursing and discharging. If spleen dampness and liver depression endure for [many] days, this may engender wind. Liver qi may counterflow horizontally and invade and attack the spleen and stomach. This may also lead to the arising of the spleen's loss of upbearing and lifting and the stomach's loss of harmony and downbearing.

The liver & heart

Insufficient heart blood can lead to liver blood insufficiency. Liver blood insufficiency may affect heart function. Liver fire flaring upward can lead to stirring of heart fire, while liver wind internally stirring must necessarily harass the heart spirit.

To sum up the above, if the liver's physiological function is normal, the qi mechanism will reach orderly. The channels and network vessels will be smoothly and freely flowing. The qi and blood will be harmonious and regulated. The function of the five viscera and six bowels will be able to maintain their normalcy. Therefore, it is said that the liver is able to engender and nourish the five viscera and six bowels. If liver function loses its normalcy, this may give rise to the engenderment of liver qi, liver fire, liver wind, or liver cold and the five viscera and six bowels must then necessarily incur harm. Therefore, it is said, "The liver is the thief of the five viscera and six bowels."

III. Eight methods for treating the liver in commonly seen gynecological diseases

In terms of the treatment principles pertaining to the liver, "The Treatise on Visceral Qi Methods & Times" in the *Su Wen (Simple Questions)* says, "If the liver is tense, eating sweets can relax tension." [It is also said:]

> The liver desires scattering, and eating acrid scatters tension. Use acrid to supplement and sour to drain.

This clearly explains that, since the liver is the blood viscus, blood dryness leads to bitterness [*i.e.*, suffering] and tension. Its nature likes to orderly reach. Therefore, it desires scattering. Hence scattering is supplementing, while constraining is draining. In clinical practice it is said, "There is no method to supplement the liver." This is a basic rule formulated in accordance with the physiological characteristics of the liver. However, when dealing with the clinical specialty of gynecology, the contents [*i.e.*, the treatment principles pertaining to the liver] are much richer.

In terms of the commonly seen diseases in the gynecology department and the treatment of the majority of such diseases, one can sum up eight methods for treating the liver. [These are] soothing the liver and regulating the qi, clearing the liver and discharging fire, clearing heat and leveling [or calming] the liver, repressing the liver and subduing yang, settling the liver and extinguishing wind, nourishing the blood and emolliating the liver, transforming yin and relaxing the liver, and warming the liver and warming the channels [or menses]. These are respectively described as follows:

1. Soothing the liver & regulating the qi (including soothing the liver & coursing the liver)

This is a method for coursing and freeing the flow and soothing and rectifying liver qi depression and binding. It makes the liver qi orderly reach so as to regulate and rectify the qi mechanism of the entire body. It is mainly used to treat liver qi disease. Soothing the liver and coursing the liver are somewhat similar but also somewhat different. Soothing the liver mainly refers to soothing and rectifying orderly reaching up and down. It stresses the upbearing and downbearing of the qi mechanism. Coursing the liver means coursing and freeing the flow and horizontally scattering. It stresses the opening and closing of the qi mechanism and the coursing and mounting of the qi and blood of the channels and network vessels. To soothe the liver, one commonly uses Radix Bupleuri (*Chai Hu*), Herba Seu Flos Schizonepetae Tenuifoliae (*Jing Jie Sui*), and Rhizoma Cyperi Rotundi (*Xiang Fu*). To course the liver, one commonly uses Pericarpium Citri Reticulatae Viride (*Qing Pi*), Tuber Curcumae (*Yu Jin*), Fructus Citri Aurantii (*Zhi Ke*), Fructus Amomi (*Sha Ren*), Radix Auklandiae Lappae (*Mu Xiang*), Fructus Trichosanthis Kirlowii (*Gua Lou*), and even Squama Manitis Pentadactylis (*Shan Jia*), Semen Vaccariae Segetalis (*Wang Bu Liu Xing*), and Herba Rhapontici Seu Echinposis (*Lou Lu*). Sometimes these are used together. The commonly used formulas [alternate reading: the formulas I commonly use] are *Xiao Yao San* (Rambling Powder) and *De Sheng Dan* (Obtaining Birth Elixir).

.

2. Clearing the liver & discharging fire (including clearing the liver & discharging the liver)

This is a method using bitter, cold, draining fire medicinals to clear liver heat and discharge liver fire. It results in liver heat obtaining clearing and liver fire obtaining discharge. It is mainly used to treat liver heat surging counterflow and liver fire bearing upward conditions. If liver heat is relatively mild, heat is levelled [or calmed]. If liver fire is relatively severe, it must be expelled and discharged without its pouring back in. Fire and heat are different in the degree of their intensity. Therefore, clearing the liver and discharging the liver are different even though somewhat similar. For clearing the liver, one commonly uses Radix Scutellariae Baicalensis (*Huang Qin*), Rhizoma Coptidis Chinensis (*Huang Lian*), Fructus Gardeniae Jasminoidis (*Zhi Zi*), and Spica Prunellae Vulgaris (*Xia Ku Cao*). For discharging the liver, one commonly uses Radix Gentianae Scabrae (*Dan Cao*), Herba Alois (*Lu Hui*), Radix Et Rhizoma Rhei (*Da Huang*), etc. Sometimes these are used simultaneously. The commonly used formulas [alternate reading: the formulas I commonly use] are *Long Dan Xie Gan Tang* (Gentian Drain the Liver Decoction) and *Dang Gui Lu Hui Wan* (Dang Gui & Aloe Pills).

3. Clearing heat & levelling the liver

This is a treatment method for the purpose of treating liver fire harassing above or ascendant hyperactivity of liver yang. The commonly used medicinals are Folium Mori Albi (*Sang Ye*), Flos Chrysanthemi Morifolii (*Ju Hua*), etc., not extremely bitter, cold medicinals. If liver heat is severe, one can combine these with some medicinals which clear the liver and discharge heat, such as Radix Scutellariae Baicalensis (*Huang Qin*) and Fructus Gardeniae Jasminoidis (*Zhi Zi*). If liver yang is hyperactive above due to yin vacuity, one can commonly combine these with nourishing yin and levelling the liver medicinals, such as Fructus Ligustri Lucidi (*Nu Zhen Zi*), Herba Ecliptae Prostratae (*Han Lian Cao*), Fructus Lycii Chinensis (*Gou Qi Zi*), etc. Commonly used formulas [alternate reading: the formula I commonly use] includes *Qing Xuan Ping Gan Tang* (Clear Vertigo & Level the Liver Decoction, an experiential formula).

4. Repressing the liver & subduing yang

This is a method for treating yin vacuity with ascendant hyperactivity of liver yang. On the one hand, it nourishes the liver and fosters yin. On the other, it levels and represses liver yang. The commonly used medicinals for nourishing liver yin are Fructus Ligustri Lucidi (*Nu Zen Zi*), Herba Ecliptae Prostratae (*Han Lian Cao*), uncooked Radix Rehmanniae (*Sheng Di*), Fructus Corni Officinalis (*Shan Yu Rou*), Fructus Lycii Chinensis (*Gou Qi Zi*), Plastrum Testudinis (*Gui Ban*), Gelatinum Corii Asini (*E Jiao*), etc. Medicinals for levelling and repressing liver yang are Ramulus Uncariae Cum Uncis (*Gou Teng*), Flos Chrysanthemi Morifolii (*Ju Hua*), Bombyx Batryticatus (*Jiang Can*), etc. A commonly used formula [alternate reading: a formula I commonly use] is *Qing Xuan Ping Gan Tang* (Clear Dizziness & Level the Liver Decoction) with added flavors.

5. Settling the liver & extinguishing wind

This is a method for treating liver wind. If there is heat tetany wind, use a heavy dose of clearing heat and extinguishing wind medicinals, such as Cornu Antelopis Saiga-tatarici (*Ling Yang*),[2] Flos Chrysanthemi Morifolii (*Ju Hua*), Ramulus Uncariae Cum Uncis (*Gou Teng*), and Bombyx Batryticatus (*Jiang Can*). If there is yin vacuity wind stirring, use nourishing liver yin medicinals or use settling the liver medicinals, such as uncooked Dens Draconis (*Long Chi*), uncooked Concha Ostreae (*Mu Li*), uncooked Concha Haliotidis (*Shi Jue Ming*), and Cinnabar (*Zhu Sha*). Commonly used formulas [alternate reading: the formulas I commonly use] include *Ling Jiao Gou Teng Tang* (Antelope Horn & Uncaria Decoction) and *Zhen Gan Xi Feng Tang* (Settle the Liver & Extinguish Wind Decoction).

6. Nourishing the blood & emolliating the liver

This includes nourishing the liver and softening the liver. The meaning of these two are the same. They are methods for treating liver blood vacuity. The liver is the indomitable viscus which depends on the blood to nourish it. So-called nourishing and softening the liver actually means to nourish liver blood. The commonly used medicinals are Radix Angelicae Sinensis (*Dang Gui*), Radix Albus Paeoniae Lactiflorae (*Bai Shao*), cooked Radix Rehmanniae (*Shu Di*), Radix Ligustici Wallichii (*Chuan Xiong*), Radix Polygoni Multiflori (*He Shou Wu*), etc. The commonly used formulas [alternate reading: the formulas I commonly use] are *Yi Guan Jian* (One Link Decoction) and *Si Wu Tang* (Four Materials Decoction) with added flavors.

---

[2] This medicinal is from an endangered species. Cornu Caprae (*Shan Yang Jiao*), goat horn, can and should be used instead.

31

7. Transforming yin & relaxing the liver

This is a method for treating liver yin vacuity using sour, sweet, yin-transforming medicinals. These indirectly nourish liver yin and relax liver tension. This is because the sour [flavor] is able to restrain liver yin and drain liver yang, while the sweet [flavor] is able to nourish liver yin and relax liver tension. The origin of these principles is based on the saying, "Sweet is relaxing; sour is draining." The commonly used medicinals are Radix Glycyrrhizae (*Gan Cao*), Radix Albus Paeoniae Lactiflorae (*Bai Shao*), Semen Zizyphi Spinosae (*Suan Zao Ren*), Fructus Levis Tritici Aestivi (*Fu Xiao Mai*), Bulbus Lilii (*Bai He*), uncooked Radix Rehmaanniae (*Sheng Di*), Tuber Ophiopogonis Japonici (*Mai Dong*), etc. The commonly used formulas [alternate reading: the formulas I commonly use] are *Gan Mai Da Zao Tang* (Licorice, Wheat & Red Date Decoction) and *Shao Yao Gan Cao Tang* (Peony & Licorice Decoction).

8. Warming the liver & warming the channels [and/or menses]

This is a method for treating liver cold blood stagnation and channels and vessels [or menstrual vessels] which have suffered blockage. It mainly uses warming the channels, scattering cold, and warming the liver medicinals such as Fructus Evodiae Rutecarpae (*Wu Zhu Yu*), Fructus Foeniculi Vulgaris (*Xiao Hui Xiang*), Semen Litchi Chinensis (*Li Zhi He*), and Semen Citri Reticulatae (*Ju He*). Sometimes these are combined with blood-quickening, stasis-transforming, network vessel-freeing the flow medicinals, such as Flos Carthami Tinctorii (*Hong Hua*), Semen Pruni Persicae (*Tao Ren*), Rhizoma Sparganii (*San Leng*), Herba Leonuri Heterophylli (*Yi Mu Cao*), and Radix Achyranthis Bidentatae (*Niu Xi*). Commonly used formulas [alternate reading: the formulas I commonly use] include *Nuan Gong Ding Tong Tang* (Warm the Uterus & Stabilize Pain Decoction) and *Ju He Wan* (Orange Seed Pills).

Based on practical experience, the liver is one of the most important organs in the human body. The sayings that, "The kidneys are the former heaven root" and "The spleen is the latter heaven root," explain that the spleen and kidneys are the origin of the material basis of organic function. However, in terms of the maintenance and regulation and disciplining of this function and in terms of the course of birth, aging, disease, and death, it is the liver viscus which is the pivot of regulation and discipline which guarantees the regulation and harmony of qi and blood of the body and the balance of yin and yang. For this reason, it is essential that one not only recognize the harmful aspect that, "The liver is the thief of the five viscera and six bowels," but also the beneficial aspect that it is [the liver] which is able to engender and nourish the five viscera and six bowels. The saying that, "The liver is the thief of the five viscera and six bowels," only clarifies the general significance of the liver's harmful [relationship] to the human body, resulting in disease. Nevertheless, because so many of the commonly seen diseases in gynecology are identified as liver diseases, it is good to sum up a series of principles for treating the liver. Through incessant practice and understanding, more practice and more understanding, step-by-step upon this basis, theory may be elevated.

4
A Discussion [of the Saying], "The *Chong* & *Ren* Cannot Move by Themselves"

In gynecology, the treatment of menstrual, abnormal vaginal discharge, pregnancy, and miscellaneous diseases commonly makes use of the principles of quieting the *chong*, securing the *chong*, regulating and rectifying the *chong* and *ren*, regulating and supplementing the *chong* and *ren*, downbearing *chong* counterflow, etc. However, in materia medica books, one cannot find medicinals which enter the *chong mai*, enter the *ren mai*, or enter the *chong* and *ren*. Nor are the medicinals which treat the *chong* and *ren* said to enter the two vessels of the *chong* and *ren*. This is because the *chong* and *ren* are two of the eight extraordinary vessels. They are not regular channels.[3] Therefore, it is important that the viscera to which the two vessels of the *chong* and *ren* home and their relationship with the regular channels be clearly understood.

The major portion of the medicinals used in clinical practice which regulate and treat the *chong* and *ren* have the functions of supplementing the kidneys, rectifying the spleen, and harmonizing the liver. Hence, it can be seen that the two vessels of the *chong* and *ren* cannot be regarded as independent channels and network vessels but rather as two miscellaneous vessels networking to the liver, spleen, and kidneys.

---

[3] To understand the logic inherent in this statement, one must know that the term for a medicinal's entering a channel is *gui jing*, to gather in a channel, not in a *mai* or vessel. In Chinese materia medica books, *gui jing* correspondences are only given for the 12 regular channels. This is because, although the word channel is used, this theory of Chinese medicinal categorization and function was derived from inferences concerning medicinals' effects on the viscera and bowels, not on the channels *per se*.

Therefore, it is said, "The *chong* and *ren* cannot move by themselves." In addition, the 12 regular channels mutually communicate directly with the five viscera and six bowels, while the eight extraordinary vessels do not. The constructive and defensive, qi and blood, and fluids and humors are transported to the eight extraordinary vessels via the 12 regular channels. If disease changes occur in the viscera and bowels, then gradually these will be passed on to the regular channels and thence to the extraordinary channels. Hence, during treatment, one must first treat the viscera and bowels. If disease occurs in the external location of the extraordinary channels, it must necessarily involve the regular channels or be due to the viscera and bowels via the regular channels. Therefore, in clinical practice, one mainly treats the viscera and bowels and the regular channels. The truth of [the saying that], "The *chong* and *ren* cannot move by themselves," can be explained from the following three perspectives.

I. The courses of the two vessels of the *chong* & *ren* and their physiological functions

The main branch of the *chong mai* arises from the uterus, descends to emerge at *Hui Yin* (CV 1), joins the foot *shao yin* kidney channel in the groin area (*Qi Jie*, St 30), traverses alongside the navel, enters the chest, continues to ascend to reach the throat area, and then encircles the mouth and lips. Another branch starts from within the uterus, passes through the spine, and runs over the upper back region. The *chong mai* is the "sea of the 12 channel vessels" and is also called the sea of blood. It is able to regulate and adjust the qi and blood of the 12 channels. The main diseases with which it is associated are menstrual irregularities, flooding and leaking, abnormal vaginal discharge, and other such gynecological diseases as well as lower abdominal pain and qi ascending and surging [or penetrating] the heart.

The *ren mai* arises from the lower abdominal region. It moves downward to *Hui Yin* (CV 1) from where it runs forward and ascends along the internal abdomen to the point *Guan Yuan* (CV 4). Again it ascends to reach the throat. Then it encircles the mouth and lips, passes through the face, and enters under the eye. The *ren mai*, being "the sea of yin vessels," it meets the three yin channels of the foot (the three channels of the liver, spleen, and kidneys) at *Qu Gu* (CV 2), *Zhong Ji* (CV 3), and *Guan Yuan* (CV 4). Both the yin linking vessel and the *chong mai* also meet it on the abdomen. Hence, the *ren mai* has the function of regulating and adjusting the yin channels of the human body and is related to menstruation, pregnancy, and birth. Therefore, it is said that, "The *ren mai* governs the uterus and the fetus." Its main diseases in men are mounting qi [*i.e.*, hernia], while, in women, are menstrual irregularities, abnormal vaginal discharge, infertility, concretions and conglomerations, and urinary incontinence.

The beginnings, endings, and courses of the two vessels of the *chong* and *ren*, fully elucidate that the two vessels of the *chong* and *ren* and the foot *shao yin*, foot *jue yin*, and foot *tai yin* mutually communicate. If the *chong mai* is full and exuberant and the *ren mai* is freely and smoothly flowing, then the menses descend [or are precipitated] periodically since these two mutually enrich and invigorate each other. Thus it is said in "The Essential Tricks of the Trade & Heart Methods of Gynecology" in the *Yi Zong Jin Jian (Golden Mirror of Ancestral Medicine)*:

> The former heaven *tian gui* comes from the joining of the father and mother. The latter heaven essence and blood are engendered from water and grains. In women, at two [times] seven, the *tian gui* arrives. The *ren* is freely flowing, the *chong* is exuberant, and the menses move.

II. "The *chong* & *ren* cannot move by themselves" as seen from their relationship with the three viscera of the liver, spleen, and kidneys

Although the two vessels of the *chong* and *ren* do not directly communicate with the viscera and bowels, they do indirectly communicate with the three viscera of the liver, spleen, and kidneys. In other words, the liver, spleen, and kidneys home to channels and vessels which are linked with the *chong* and *ren* (and the *dai mai*). Therefore, it can be said that the physiological functions of the two vessels of the *chong* and *ren* are the manifestations of the functions of the three viscera of the liver, spleen, and kidneys, and their signs and symptoms are also those of the liver, spleen and kidneys.

1. The relationship between the liver and the two vessels of the *chong* & *ren*

The foot *jue yin* liver channel networks with the yin [*i.e.*, genital] organ and mutually communicates with the two vessels of the *chong* and *ren*. The liver governs the storage and regulation and discipline of the blood and fluids. After the blood and fluids are transformed and engendered, besides constructing and nourishing all around the body, they are also stored in the liver. If the liver blood has a surplus, it flows downward to the sea of blood where it is transformed into the menstruation. The liver likes orderly reaching. If the liver qi becomes depressed and stagnant, the menstrual blood will not flow smoothly [or easily]. If liver qi counterflows upward, the menstrual blood may follow the *chong* qi and also counterflow upward, thus resulting in shifted [*i.e.*, vicarious] menstruation. If liver depression transforms fire and internally scorches the fluids and humors, yin blood may be consumed and exhausted. This then results in desiccated blood and possible blocked menstruation [*i.e.*, amenorrhea]. Therefore, in clinical practice, there is the saying, "First regulate the liver, for by coursing the liver, the menses are automatically regulated."

2. The relationship between the kidneys and the two vessels of the *chong* & *ren*

The *chong mai* emerges from *Hui Yin* (CV 1), arrives at *Qi Jie* (St 30), and then moves upward with the foot *shao yin* kidney channel. The *ren mai* is the sea of yin vessels and meets the foot *shao yin* kidney channel in the abdominal region. Therefore, the two vessels of the *chong* and *ren* communicate with the kidneys. The kidneys govern the two yin [*i.e.*, the

anus and vaginal meatus *cum* urethra in women]. If kidney qi is
exuberant, the *ren mai* is freely flowing, the *tai chong mai* is exuberant,
and the menses are able to descend periodically. Thus one is able to
conceive and give birth to children. If the kidney qi is debilitated, the *ren
mai* will also be vacuous and debilitated, the *tai chong mai* will be
degenerated and scanty, and the earth passageways will not be free-
flowing. Hence one will not be able to conceive and will have no
children. If the kidneys lose their blocking and storing or their opening
and closing lose their command, this can result in flooding and leaking
and abnormal vaginal discharge. If the kidneys do not tie up the fetus,
then there will be fetal leakage or no children.

3. The relationship between the spleen-stomach and the two vessels of the *chong* & *ren*

Since the foot *tai yin* spleen channel and the foot *yang ming* stomach
channel communicate with the two vessels of the *chong* and *ren* at *Qi Jie*
(St 30) in the lower abdominal region and the three venter points [*i.e.,*
Shang Wan, CV 13, *Zhong Wan*, CV 12, and *Xia Wan*, CV 10], there is a
saying that, "The *tai chong mai* homes to the *yang ming*." Hence, the two
vessels of the *chong* and *ren* indirectly communicate with the spleen and
stomach. The spleen and stomach are the source of the engenderment
and transformation of the qi and blood and are the root of menstruation.
As was said by Xue Li-zai:

> The blood is the essence qi of water and grains which is harmonized and
> regulated by the five viscera and distributed over the six bowels. In
> women, it ascends to become the milk and descends to become the
> menstruation.

If the essence qi of the spleen and stomach are full and exuberant, the
chong mai is exuberant, the sea of blood is exuberant, and the
menstruation descends periodically. If the spleen and stomach are
vacuous and weak, there is no source for the engenderment and
transformation of qi and blood. Therefore, the menstrual blood is sparse
and scanty or there is blocked menstruation [*i.e.,* amenorrhea]. If spleen

39

vacuity is not able to restrain the blood, there will be menstrual blood dribbling and dripping without cease or downward flooding of blood. Therefore, in clinical practice there is the saying, "To treat the blood, first treat the spleen."

In gathering the above together, the *chong* is the sea of blood, while the source and production of the blood depend upon the engenderment and transformation of the spleen and stomach and the liver's regulation and adjustment. The storage and discharge of the blood depend upon the closing and storing of the kidneys and the restraining and containing of the spleen. If the spleen does not engender and transform, the menstrual blood will have no source. If the liver does not store the blood, the sea of blood will be exuberant or depleted without limit. If the spleen does not restrain the blood or the kidneys lose their closing and storing, then the menstrual blood will spill over externally and lose its control. The *ren mai* governs the uterus and fetus. However, it is the spleen and stomach's engenderment and transformation which are the source for all the qi and blood, fluids and humors, and yin essence. Therefore, the spleen is the source of conception and birth. The ability to conceive and tie the fetus also depends on the exuberance and decline of the kidney qi. Therefore, the kidneys are the root of conception and birth. All the diseases of the *chong* and *ren* are caused by the three viscera of the liver, spleen, and kidneys, while the physiological and pathological manifestations of the two vessels of the *chong* and *ren* are all also those of the three viscera of the liver, spleen, and kidneys. That is the reason why "The *chong* and *ren* cannot move by themselves."

III. "The *chong* and *ren* cannot move by themselves" seen from the point of view of the formulas and medicinals used in clinical treatment

The most commonly seen diseases of the *chong* and *ren* are menstrual diseases, abnormal vaginal discharge diseases, and diseases of pregnancy, while the selection of formulas and the use of medicinals in most cases are mainly governed by regulating and rectifying the three viscera of the liver, spleen, and kidneys. For instance, in menstrual diseases, for menstruation ahead of schedule or excessive in amount or for downward flooding and leaking of blood categorized as blood heat damaging the channels and forcing the blood to move too early or too excessively, *Qing Jing Tang* (Clear the Menses Decoction) with additions and subtractions is the main formula I choose. Within this formula, Cortex Radicis Moutan (*Dan Pi*), Cortex Radicis Lycii Chinensis (*Di Gu Pi*), Cortex Phellodendri (*Huang Bai*), and Radix Albus Paeoniae Lactiflorae (*Bai Shao*) cool the blood and harmonize the liver. Herba Artemisiae Apiaceae (*Qing Hao*) nourishes yin and clears liver heat. Sclerotium Poriae Cocos (*Fu Ling*) fortifies the spleen and calms the heart. And cooked Radix Rehmanniae (*Shu Di*) supplements the kidneys and quiets the *chong*. This treatment approach's rationale can be summed up as cooling the blood and clearing liver heat, fortifying the spleen and supplementing the kidneys which then result in quieting the *chong*.

If [these same conditions] are categorized as spleen vacuity, then mostly I select *Gui Pi Tang* (Restore the Spleen Decoction) as the treatment. Within this formula, *Si Jun Zi Tang* (Four Gentlemen Decoction) and Radix Astragali Membranacei (*Huang Qi*) are the main components for fortifying the spleen and supplementing the qi. If the spleen qi is full and sufficient, it will be able to restrain the blood. The combination of Radix Polygalae Tenuifoliae (*Yuan Zhi*), Semen Zizyphi Spinosae (*Suan Zao Ren*), and Arillus Euphoriae Longanae (*Long Yan Rou*) nourish the heart. Sometimes Radix Dipscai (*Chuan Duan*) and cooked Radix Rehmanniae (*Shu Di*) are added based on the disease condition in order to supplement the kidneys. Thus the therapeutic actions of securing, containing, and quieting the *chong* are achieved via fortifying the spleen, nourishing the heart, and supplementing the kidneys.

Menstruation which is [sometimes] early, [sometimes] late, and [comes] at no fixed schedule is mainly caused by qi and blood not being regulated and dysfunction of the *chong* and *ren*. However, the origin of this arising is liver depression and dual vacuity of the spleen and kidneys. Therefore, in treatment, I mostly choose *Ding Jing Tang*

41

(Stabilize the Menses Decoction) to govern this. Within this [formula], Radix Bupleuri (*Chai Hu*) and Herba Seu Flos Schizonepetae Tenuifoliae (*Jing Jie Sui*) soothe the liver. Radix Dioscoreae Oppositae (*Shan Yao*) and Sclerotium Poriae Cocos (*Fu Ling*) fortify the spleen. Cooked Radix Rehmanniae (*Shu Di*) and Semen Cuscutae Chinensis (*Tu Si Zi*) are the main medicinals for supplementing the kidneys. These are assisted by Radix Angelicae Sinensis (*Dang Gui*) and Radix Albus Paeoniae Lactiflorae (*Bai Shao*) which nourish the blood and harmonize the liver. This further clearly shows how the actions of regulating and rectifying the *chong* and *ren* can be achieved via regulating and supplementing the liver, spleen, and kidneys.

Other [formulas] such as *De Sheng Dan* (Obtaining Birth Elixir) and *Xiao Yao San* (Rambling Powder) are also used to regulate the liver and course the qi, nourish the blood and harmonize the liver and, [therefore,] to simultaneously regulate and rectify the *chong* and *ren*. Or take Zhang Xi-chun's *chong*-securing formula, *Gu Chong Tang* (Secure the *Chong* Decoction), as an example. From the point of view of signs and symptoms, it is for spleen vacuity and debility not able to contain the blood. This then results in the *chong* and *ren* not securing [or being secured] and thus in flooding and leaking. The main medicinals within this formula are uncooked Radix Astragali Membranacei (*Huang Qi*) and Rhizoma Atractylodis Macrocephalae (*Bai Zhu*) which fortify the spleen and boost the qi. When spleen qi is sufficient, it is able to restrain and contain. Fructus Corni Officinalis (*Shan Zhu Rou*) and Radix Albus Paeoniae Lactiflorae (*Bai Shao*) supplement liver-kidney yin and blood. These are assisted by calcined Os Draconis (*Long Gu*), Concha Ostreae (*Mu Li*), Os Sepiae Seu Sepiellae (*Hai Piao Xiao*), carbonized Fibra Stipulae Trachycarpi (*Zong Lu Tan*), and Galla Rhois (*Wu Bei Zi*) which astringe and stop bleeding. Of the astringing, securing the *chong*, stop-bleeding medicinals in this [formula], Rhus enters the lungs, kidneys, and large intestine; calcined Dragon Bone enters the heart, liver, and kidney channels; Oyster Shell enters the liver, gallbladder, and kidney channels; Cuttlefish Bone enters the liver and kidney channels; and carbonized Trachycarpus enters the lung, liver, and large intestine channels. None of these enter the *chong* or *ren*. [Taken as] a whole, this formula results in securing the *chong* by way of fortifying the spleen and boosting the qi, cooling the liver and stopping bleeding.

In terms of treating abnormal vaginal discharge, the formula I commonly use is *Wan Dai Tang* (End Vaginal Discharge Decoction). Within this formula, Radix Codonpsitis Pilosulae (*Dang Shen*), Rhizoma Atractylodis Macrocephalae (*Bai Zhu*), and Radix Dioscoreae Oppositae (*Shan Yao*) are the main medicinals for fortifying the spleen and drying dampness. These are combined with Pericarpium Citri Reticulatae (*Chen Pi*) in order to harmonize the stomach and rectify the spleen qi. Radix Bupleuri (*Chai Hu*) and Herba Seu Flos Schizonepetae Tenuifoliae (*Jing Jie Sui*) soothe the liver and scatter dampness. And Semen Plantaginis (*Che Qian Zi*) discharges damp turbidity from within the kidneys and supplements the function of the kidneys. Hence drying dampness and stopping abnormal vaginal discharge are approached from the point of view of regulating the liver and rectifying the spleen.

In terms of treating diseases of pregnancy, nausea during pregnancy is commonly seen. This is due to the *chong mai* homing to the *yang ming*. The *chong* qi counterflows upward because it does not obtain downward discharge [with menstruation]. This then leads to the arising of nausea and vomiting. *An Wei Yin* (Quiet the Stomach Drink) and *Wen Dan Tang* (Warm the Gallbladder Decoction) the formulas I commonly use [for this malady] and, within these, in addition to medicinals which clear the liver and clear the stomach, the commonly used medicinals are Rhizoma Pinelliae Ternatae (*Ban Xia*), Cortex Magnoliae Officinalis (*Hou Po*), and Caulis Perillae Frutescentis (*Su Geng*) which downbear the stomach qi and hence downbear the counterflowing qi of the *chong mai*.

For other diseases of pregnancy, such as infertility and miscarriage, the kidneys are taken as the commander of the *chong* and *ren*, while the spleen is the latter heaven root. When treating these [conditions], mostly the methods consist of supplementing the kidneys, fortifying the spleen, and nourishing the blood. One formula I commonly use is *Wu Zi Yan*

Zong Wan (Five Seeds Increase Progeny Pills). Within this [formula], Fructus Lycii Chinensis (*Gou Qi Zi*), Semen Cuscutae Chinensis (*Tu Si Zi*), Fructus Rubi Chingii (*Fu Pen Zi*), and Fructus Schisandrae Chinensis (*Wu Wei Zi*) mainly supplement the kidneys and boost the essence. There is also Zang Xi-chun's *Shou Tai Wan* (Longevity Fetus Pills). Within this formula, Radix Dipsaci (*Chuan Duan*) and Semen Cuscutae Chinensis (*Tu Si Zi*) mainly supplement the kidneys. *Tai Shan Pan Shi Tang* (Mt. Tai Bedrock Decoction)[4] is *Ba Zhen Tang* (Eight Pearls Decoction) minus Sclerotium Poriae Cocos (*Fu Ling*) and plus Radix Dipsaci (*Chuan Duan*), uncooked Radix Astragali Membranacei (*Huang Qi*), Radix Scutellariae Baicalensis (*Huang Qin*), Fructus Amomi (*Sha Ren*), and Semen Oryzae Glutinosae (*Nuo Mi*). It approaches securing the *chong* and quieting the fetus by way of fortifying the spleen and boosting the qi, supplementing the kidneys and nourishing the blood.

Therefore, when viewed from the perspective of the clinically commonly used formulas and medicinals for treating *chong* and *ren* diseases, treating the liver, spleen, and kidneys results in quieting the *chong*, securing the *chong*, regulating and rectifying the *chong* and *ren*, and regulating and supplementing the *chong* and *ren*.

In a word, the relationship between the courses of the two vessels of the *chong* and *ren* and the other channels and vessels; the relationship between the three viscera of the liver, spleen, and kidneys; and the commonly used formulas and medicinals for clinically treating diseases of the two vessels of the *chong* and *ren* fully elucidate that the physiological functions of the two vessels of the *chong* and *ren* are, in fact, [nothing other than] the manifestations of the physiological functions of the three viscera of the liver, spleen, and kidneys. Therefore, in terms of diseases of the two vessels of the *chong* and *ren*, treating the liver, spleen, and kidneys secondarily results in treating the *chong* and *ren*. Thus it is said, "The *chong* and *ren* cannot move by themselves."

---

[4] The implication of this formula's name is that it makes the fetus as secure in the womb as the bedrock upon which Mt. Tai rests.

5
The Theory & Treatment of Blood Patterns in Gynecology as Learned Through Practice

"Blood patterns" in gynecology can be said to be commonly seen and account for the onset of many disease conditions. Therefore, the methods of treating the blood are comparatively wide in their application. In order to explore the foundation of the theory and treatment of blood patterns in gynecology, I would like to speak on my personal shallow views.[5]

I. The production & physiological function of the blood

Blood is the material basis for constructing and nourishing the whole body. When blood is exuberant, the formal body is exuberant. When blood is debilitated, the formal body is debilitated. The origin of the blood is the finest essence of water and grains. As it is said in "The Chapter on Secrets of Qi" in the *Ling Shu (Spiritual Axis)*, "The juice of qi that is received in the middle burner which is transformed and becomes red is called the blood." In "The Chapter on Evil Guests" in the *Ling Shu (Spiritual Axis)* it says:

> The constructive qi secretes the fluids and humors, pours into the vessels, and is transformed into blood. It constructs the four extremities and internally pours into the five viscera and six bowels.

In other words, after the finest essence of water and grains is absorbed from the middle burner, the constructive qi is formed by the action of

---

[5] Such self-deprecation of one's own knowledge is a common Asian custom. It should be remembered that the author had more than 40 years of clinical experience when this book was written.

qi transformation. The constructive qi then secretes the fluids and humors. These enter the heart and are turned red and made into blood. This pours into the blood vessels in order to construct and nourish the whole body. This is what is meant when it is said:

> That which transforms into qi is yang. That which transforms into blood is yin. That which ascends and floats is yang, while that which descends and congeals is yin. The yang one is qi, while the yin one is blood.

The production, circulation, and regulation of the blood are closely related to the functions of the three viscera of the heart, liver, and spleen. The heart engenders the blood and governs the blood vessels, the spleen restrains the blood, and the liver stores the blood. The main function of the blood is to construct and nourish the whole body. All tissues and organs, such as the skin and hair, sinews and bones, channels and network vessels, and viscera and bowels can only fully display their physiological function based on the constructing and nourishing of the blood. Therefore, it says in "The Chapter on Five Viscera Production" in the *Su Wen (Simple Questions)*:

> If the liver receives blood, it enables vision. If the feet receives blood, they are able to step. If the palms receive blood, they are able to grasp. If the fingers receive blood, they are able to contain.

There is no part of the human body that is not reached by the blood, and the circulation of blood is without cease and is not able to stop. This is what is said in "The Chapter on the Root Viscera" in the *Ling Shu (Spiritual Axis)*:

> If the blood is harmonious, the channels and vessels flow and move. The constructive revolves through yin and yang. The sinews and bones are strong and firm.

Viewed from the origin of the production of blood, on the one hand, the middle burner "receives the qi" and, on the other, it "takes up the juice." The constructive qi must also secrete fluids and humors into the heart which turns these red and pours them into the vessels. Therefore, "blood" can be regarded as actual blood *and* the qi within the blood. The former is a material substance, while the latter is [merely] function. The blood can carry on its physiological functions only on condition that the qi commands it and that it circulates. Otherwise, blood which does not flow and stir (dead blood) is useless and [in fact] harmful. If this point is not clearly understood, then one cannot understand the principles and know how to use certain qi within the blood medicinals (those that enter the blood division and are able to move the blood, such as Radix Ligustici Wallichii, *Chuan Xiong*).

II. The relationship between the qi & blood

On the one hand, "qi" refers to the constructing and nourishing finest essence material substance that flows and stirs inside the body. Concretely speaking, it refers to physiological functional activities of the viscera and bowels. On the other hand, blood is produced from the finest essence material substance after water and grains are dispersed and transformed [*i.e.*, digested] by the movement and transformation of the spleen and stomach. This then pours upward into the lungs and mutually combines with the lung qi. The heart function turns this red and it becomes blood. Therefore, the origin of the blood cannot be separated from the qi. After the blood is produced, it is restrained and commanded downward to circulate through the channels and vessels. The heart's stirring of the blood vessels, the liver's regulation and adjustment of the volume of the blood, and the spleen's restraining and containing of blood and fluids are all the action of the "qi" of the viscera and bowels. Therefore,

The qi is the commander of the blood. If the qi moves the blood moves.

Not only can the qi move the blood, it is also able to contain the blood.

However, the qi also depends on the ability of the blood for its function. Blood contains within it fluids and humors. If these obtain yang, they

47

are able to transform qi. Therefore it is said, "Blood is the mother of qi" and "Qi governs warming, while blood governs moistening." Qi is categorized as yang which governs stirring. Blood is categorized as yin which governs stillness. Yin and yang are mutually rooted in one another. If there is blood without qi, then the blood cannot move. The reason why the blood can endlessly circulate through and enrich and nourish the whole body is entirely due to the promotion and stirring of the qi. If there is qi without blood, then the qi has no place to depend on and attach to. Thus qi and blood are mutually combined and one cannot exist without the other. This is the meaning of the saying:

> Without yang, yin cannot be engendered. Without yin, yang cannot grow.

A human body must have qi and must have blood in order to live. Isolated yin cannot engender, while solitary yang cannot grow. This interdependence of qi and blood is not only able to promote the life activities of the organism but, at the same time, is responsible for the function of resistance to external evils. If the qi and blood are effulgent and exuberant and the constructive and defensive are regulated and harmonious, external evils cannot enter and harass. If the qi and blood are insufficient, the constructive and defensive are not harmonious, and viscera and bowel function loses its regulation, then this allows easy invasion of external evils.

III. The pathology of the blood & gynecological blood patterns

Blood diseases are closely related to the "qi" and the loss of regulation of the function of the three viscera of the heart, liver, and spleen. In addition, if the blood gets cold, it leads to congelation and gathering. If it gets warm, its flow is freed. If it gets hot, it moves frenetically. Based on the clinical practice of gynecology, these may be summed up as the following patterns.

A. Blood stasis

This includes relaxed, slow movement of blood; stagnation, blockage, and lack of free flow; and congelation, accumulation, gathering, and binding which are different conditions. There are many causes leading to the arising of blood stasis. The first is qi stagnation. Since the qi commands the movement of the blood, if the qi's movement becomes stagnant and relaxed, the blood flow must necessarily become astringent. If the movement of qi is obstructed, the blood necessarily must not be freely flowing. [In this case,] the degree of blood stasis is dependent on the degree of qi stagnation. In addition, blood vacuity may also lead to the arising of blood stasis. If the blood is vacuous, it is not able to fill and make exuberant the vessel passageways. Not only can it not construct and nourish the viscera and bowels, the four extremities, and the hundreds of joints, it also cannot construct and nourish the vessel of the entire body. [Further,] it can make the qi within the blood debilitated and scanty. This will cause the vessels to become astringent and the blood movement to become relaxed and slow. If severe, stasis may obstruct the vessel passageways and result in blood stasis. Therefore, in clinical practice, blood vacuity and blood stasis patterns are constantly encountered. Various types of external injury can also lead to various types and various degrees of blood stasis.

The main essential symptom of blood stasis is aching and pain. This pain is fixed in location and is either dull or piercing. If blood stasis endures for [many] days, it can result in brewing of heat which may then manifest as low-grade fever. If blood stasis [stops and] collects internally, new blood cannot abide [where it should] and this can lead to the arising of bleeding. If blood stasis collects internally, then new blood may [also] not be engendered. This can lead to blood vacuity. If blood stasis congeals and gathers, it can produce concretion lumps and substantial swellings. If blood stasis is located in the liver or spleen, it may lead to bilateral rib-side piercing pain (or one may see concretion lumps). If blood stasis [is located] in the uterus or *chong* and *ren*, it may lead to menstrual irregularities. Or one may see flooding and leaking or blocked menstruation. If blood stasis obstructs the network vessels, then there will be aching and pain in and numbness of the extremities and body. If there is blood stasis in the muscles and skin, then the skin will emit purple macules. [Blood stasis] is commonly seen in painful menstruation, blocked menstruation, flooding and leaking, postpartum conditions, and uterine myomas.

B. Blood heat

This generally refers to heat entering the blood division and can lead to the arising of various conditions. Externally caused heat evils or heat toxins entering the defensive, qi, constructive, or blood are categorized as species of warm disease. These can be seen in gynecology [in the case of] external contraction of wind heat or toxic heat conditions. In clinical practice, one mostly sees yin vacuity with fire stirring, qi depression transforming fire, blood stasis brewing heat, and damp heat entering the blood division resulting in various conditions. If the blood obtains heat, this leads to its frenetic movement or to its flowing and spilling over outside its vessels and network vessels. This can be seen in shifted [i.e., vicarious] menstruation, flooding and leaking, or menstruation ahead of schedule. If damp heat enters the blood division, one can see red abnormal vaginal discharge or midcycle bleeding. If blood heat endures for [many] days, burning and damaging the yin fluids within the blood, this my lead to the arising of blood dryness which may then result in yin blood desiccation and drying up and blocked menstruation.

C. Blood cold

If the blood gets cold, this leads to its congelation. The flow and movement of the blood vessels is not smooth. Typically, this mostly is caused by external contraction of cold evils, overeating chilled, uncooked foods, or yang qi vacuity weakness with yin qi excessive and exuberant. When blood is cold, the channels and vessels will become stagnant, astringent, and will not flow smoothly, and this may lead to the aching of the body and extremities which dreads chill. If there is cold congelation in the *chong* and *ren*, the menstruation may be sparsely emitted and this may gradually result in blocked menstruation. If there is cold lodged in the uterus, there will be uterine chill infertility. If, because of cold congelation, the vessels stagnate and the blood movement is not smooth, then the function of the blood will decline. Therefore, one can see blood vacuity and blood stasis patterns [simultaneously].

D. Blood vacuity

Blood vacuity includes the two types of both scantiness of substantial blood and insufficiency of the function [of the blood].

1. Scantiness of substantial blood is mostly caused by sudden loss of blood or by insufficient engenderment of the blood. For instance, if there is excessive bleeding after delivery, flooding or leaking, or dribbling and dripping of the menstrual blood without cease, it will be difficult to produce fresh blood. Insufficiency of blood engenderment mainly has to do with the viscera and bowel function of the heart, liver, and spleen. The key lies in the spleen and stomach. If their function becomes vacuous and debilitated, their movement and transformation may lose their duty. Thus there is no source for the engenderment and transformation of the finest essence of water and grains.

2. Insufficiency of the function of the blood refers to qi vacuity within the blood or the contraction of qi disease. This may then result in the blood flow not being smooth or its flow and movement being relaxed and slow. In this case, substantial blood is not scanty. However, the function of the blood is insufficient. This also manifests the signs and symptoms of blood vacuity. Therefore, blood vacuity is usually accompanied by blood stasis, blood heat, or blood cold. These may occur simultaneously or one may lead to the other. These do not usually exist in isolation. [Blood vacuity] is commonly seen in menstrual diseases and postpartum diseases.

It may also be seen with simultaneous qi vacuity, yin vacuity, blood dryness, loss of regulation of the *chong* and *ren*, or simultaneous contraction of wind, cold, damp, or heat external evils. Likewise, it may be seen simultaneously with loss of function of the viscera and bowels of the liver, spleen, and kidneys or with deficiency detriment of material substance. Thus, [blood vacuity] should be treated differently according to its different disease mechanisms and different stages of the same diseases. This is what is meant by the principle of "same disease, different treatment; different disease, same treatment." Therefore, step-by-step, one should search for the fundamental pattern on which to base their treatment of gynecological blood patterns.

IV. Eight methods for treating the blood in gynecology

Gynecological blood patterns can basically be generalized into four types, *i.e.*, blood vacuity, blood repletion (stasis), blood cold, and blood heat. Therefore, the great principles for treating blood patterns are none other than to supplement, disperse, warm, and clear [respectively]. In clinical practice, there is the saying, "Regulating the blood results in supplementing it." Here the word "regulate" means to regulate any erroneous tendency. If there is blood stasis, the blood flow must necessarily be relaxed and slow. If severe, congelation and gathering produces lumps and dead blood. Since the blood no longer moves under the command of the qi, the blood loses its physiological function. In addition, obstruction and stagnation of the channels and network vessels causes pain. Static blood may transform heat. Static blood may gather internally, and the fresh blood cannot abide. Thus one may see the signs of bleeding externally, and these may be accompanied by the symptoms of blood vacuity. If one uses the "dispersing method" to quicken the blood and dispel stasis, this results in the recovery of the blood's movement and circulation. This then will also result in the recovery of the blood's function, and this equals the supplementation of the blood.

If, due to blood heat, the blood flow may boil over and [move] pathologically too rapidly. It may surge upward or spill over downward. It may move frenetically [causing] vomiting of blood or spontaneous external bleeding [*i.e.*, nosebleed]. It may congest and stagnate into binding heat. Or it may burn and consume yin fluids, thus resulting in the fluids becoming desiccated and the humors dried up. If, due to scorching heat, the blood is not able to stay in the channels and go [or stay] in the network vessels and move, the blood is not able to fully display its constructing and nourishing functions. In addition to the above-mentioned symptoms, the accompanying symptoms of blood vacuity and blood scantiness may manifest. Because the "clearing method" cools the blood and discharges heat and leads the blood to gather in its channels, the recovery of its function is the same as supplementing the blood.

If the movement of the blood becomes stagnant and astringent due to cold congelation, cold obstructing the vessels and passageways, or congelation and gathering producing binding, then the channels and network vessels will be blocked and [static blood] will stand in the way. Thus the viscera and bowels, channels and vessels, the four limbs and the hundreds of joints will lose their nourishment. In addition, there will be cold congelation aching and pain. This will also be accompanied by the manifestation of blood vacuity, blood scantiness symptoms. Because the "warming method" scatters cold and warms the channels, it makes the flow and movement free and smooth. Therefore, the transformation and scattering of stasis and binding are the same as supplementing the blood.

Thus, the effect of dispersing stasis, cooling the blood, and warming cold is the same as supplementing the blood. The meaning of the saying, "Regulating the blood results in supplementing it," is that, by regulating and rectifying or correcting any error, one is able to recover and give full play to the function of the blood. In addition, if one wants to fill and make replete yin blood material substance via the blood supplementing method, it is necessary to do this via boosting the qi. This will increase the function of the qi within the blood and will result in yang engendering the growth of yin, thus automatically promoting the engenderment of new blood. Or one may nourish yin fluids. When yin becomes exuberant, yang will be augmented. If yin and yang are harmonious and regulated, then blood will automatically be sufficient. This also implies that, "Regulating the blood results in supplementing it." [In other words,] it is not that only a few flavors [*i.e.*, ingredients] of Chinese medicinals are able to supplement and fill depletion and vacuity of the blood and fluids. Hence the viewpoint [conveyed by] the saying, "Regulating the blood results in supplementing it," is, even [when using the supplementing method], meaningful in terms of the clinical treatment of blood patterns.

Below is a summation of the great methods [*i.e.*, main principles] of treatment and commonly used formulas and medicinals for the commonly seen blood patterns in gynecology.

A. For various types of blood stasis conditions: Mostly, one should use the principles of quickening the blood and transforming stasis, breaking stasis and scattering binding [or nodulation], and nourishing the blood and quickening the blood.

1. The method of quickening blood & transforming stasis

This is mainly used for blood stasis and qi obstruction and conditions where blood movement is stagnant and astringent. It mainly employs quickening the blood medicinals which move the qi within the blood, free and smooth the flow of the blood vessels, and course and dredge the channels and network vessels. The formulas I commonly use are *Shi Xiao San* (Loose A Smile Powder), *Chan Hou Sheng Hua Tang* (Postpartum Engendering & Transforming Decoction), and *Fo Shou San* (Buddha's Hand Powder).

2. The method of breaking stasis & scattering binding

This is mainly used for blood stasis which has endured for [many] days, congelation and gathering which has formed lumps, or obstruction and blockage of the vessels and passageways conditions. It mainly employs medicinal substances which break stasis. These may be combined with medicinals which soften the hard and scatter binding [or nodulation]; break and eliminate static blood, disperse and scatter dead blood and congealed lumps which have a [physical] form; dispel stasis and engender the new; and course and free the flow of the channels and vessels. The formulas I commonly use are *Di Dang Tang* (Resistance Decoction), *Gui Zhi Fu Ling Wan* (Cinnamon Twig & Poria Pills), and *Da Huang Zhe Chong Wan* (Rhubarb & Eupolyphaga Pills).

The above two types of therapeutic principles are based on varying degrees of blood stasis. In the former, static blood has no definite [physical] form. There may only be the manifestations of relaxed, slow movement of qi with lack of smooth and free flow. In the latter, congealed lumps may already be seen to have form. When using the methods and principles of quickening the blood and transforming stasis, it is [also] important to combine this with the use of qi-moving medicinals, since it is the movement of qi which commands the movement of the blood. If there is blood stasis tending to heat, it is necessary to combine these with medicinals which cool the blood so that the blood will stay in its channels and move without becoming frenetic. If there is simultaneous blood vacuity, one should supplement and engender the blood. When the blood is sufficient, it will be able to move. If there is the simultaneous appearance of liver depression qi stagnation, it is necessary to course the liver and regulate the qi. If blood stasis has congealed into lumps and has form or if dead blood has gathered and bound, then it is necessary to use strong, powerful medicinals which break stasis, soften the hard, and scatter binding [or nodulation]. In clinical practice, pattern discrimination should be accurate and the relationship between evil and righteous [qi] should be considered in order to prevent excessively damaging the righteous. Hence, the strength of action of quickening the blood medicinals and their appropriateness should be well grasped.

Based on clinical experience, the medicinals I commonly use for quickening the blood when blood stasis is without form (meaning there are only manifestations that the blood movement is relaxed and slow) are Radix Angelicae Sinensis (*Dang Gui*), Radix Ligustici Wallichii (*Chuan Xiong*), Herba Leonuri Heterophylli (*Yi Mu Cao*), and Flos Carthami Tinctorii (*Hong Hua*). The medicinals I commonly use for transforming stasis when static blood has yet to take obvious form are Semen Pruni Persicae (*Tao Ren*), Flos Carthami Tinctorii (*Hong Hua*), Resina Myrrhe (*Mo Yao*), Radix Angelicae Annomalae (*Liu Ji Nu*), Pollen Typhae (*Pu Huang*), and Feces Trogopterori Seu Pteromi (*Wu Ling Zhi*). If blood lumps have formed, I use Rhizoma Spaganii (*San Leng*), Rhizoma Curcumae Zedoariae (*E Zhu*), Semen Pruni Persicae (*Tao Ren*), Radix Salviae Miltiorrhizae (*Dan Shen*), Sanguis Draconis (*Xue Jie*), and Lignum Sappan (*Su Mu*). And if dead blood has formed, in order to break the blood and dispel stasis, I mostly use Hirudo (*Shui Zhi*), Tabanus (*Meng Chong*), Radix Et Rhizoma Rhei (*Da Huang*), and Eupolyphaga Seu Opisthoplatia (*Zhe Chong*).

3. The method of nourishing the blood & quickening the blood

This is mainly used for blood vacuity and empty vessels with the blood movement being astringent and relaxed. For blood vacuity, one should supplement the blood. When the blood vessels are full and exuberant, they will be able to flow and move smoothly and freely. This is what is meant by the principle, "If one desires to free the flow, one must first fill." If blood vacuity leads to the arising of blood stasis symptoms, then one can quicken the blood and transform stasis by supplementing the blood. The formula I commonly use is *Tao Hong Si Wu Tang* (Persica & Carthamus Four Materials Decoction). Within *Si Wu Tang*, cooked Radix Rehmanniae (*Shu Di*) supplements the yin blood. Radix Albus Paeoniae Lactiflorae (*Bai Shao*), sour and sweet, transforms yin and is able to supplement and fill the form of the blood (*i.e.*, the yin within the blood).

Radix Angelicae Sinensis (*Dang Gui*) and Radix Ligustici Wallichii (*Chuan Xiong*) tend to be acrid, sweet, and warm, while Ligusticum is able to move the qi within the blood. Thus they increase and strengthen the action of quickening the blood. Acrid and sweet is yang and therefore invigorates yang within the blood. This results in yang carrying yin and makes yin follow yang's shift [or transformation]. Thus one yin and one yang not only supplement and fill the blood but also increase and strengthen the function of the blood. When Persica and Carthamus are used in a small [amount] they are able to nourish the blood. When used in a large [amount] they are able to quicken the blood. If even more is used, they are able to break the blood. Therefore, the aim of quickening the blood can be based on nourishing the blood. When the blood is full, stasis is transformed.

B. For various types of blood heat conditions: Mostly one should use the methods and principles of clearing heat and cooling the blood, nourishing yin and transforming dryness.

1. The method of clearing heat & cooling the blood

This [method] is mainly used for blood heat giving rise to menstrual irregularities and insecurity of the *chong* and *ren*. For this, mainly cooling blood medicinal substances are combined with clearing heat prescriptions, cooling the blood and harmonizing the constructive, and regulating and rectifying the *chong* and *ren*. The formulas I commonly use are *Qing Jing Tang* (Clear the Menses Decoction) and *Qing Re Gu Jing Tang* (Clear Heat & Secure the Menses Decoction). If tending to damp heat brewing in the blood division, I commonly select *Qin Lian Si Wu Tang* (Scutellaria & Coptis Four Materials Decoction) or *Qing Gan Li Shi Tang* (Clear the Liver & Disinhibit Dampness Decoction).

2. The method of nourishing yin & transforming dryness

This [method] is mainly used for blood heat which has endured for [many] days, burning and consuming yin fluids and leading to the arising of disease. What is called fluid desiccation humor dryness mostly refers to stomach yin desiccation and exhaustion. [In this case,] the source of engenderment and transformation is dry and bound and yin blood is desiccated and dry. Therefore, it is essential that treatment increase fluids, nourish yin, and transform dryness. The formulas I commonly use are *Liang Di Tang* (Two *Di* Decoction), *Si Wu Tang* (Four Materials Decoction), and *Zeng Ye Tang* (Increase Humors Decoction). If there is dry heat binding internally, mostly I choose *San He Tang* (Three Harmonies Decoction, *i.e.*, *Si Wu Tang* and *Liang Ge San*, Cool the Diaphragm Powder, with additions and subtractions). The medicinals composing this are Radix Ligustici Wallichii (*Chuan Xiong*), Radix Angelicae Sinensis (*Dang Gui*), uncooked Radix Rehmanniae (*Sheng Di*), Radix Albus Paeoniae Lactiflorae (*Bai Shao*), Fructus Gardeniae Jasminoidis (*Zhi Zi*), Fructus Forsythiae Suspensae (*Lian Qiao*), Radix Et Rhizoma Rhei (*Da Huang*), refined Mirabilitum (*Yuan Ming Fen*), and Radix Glycyrrhizae (*Gan Cao*). Of these, *Si Wu Tang* nourishes yin and moistens dryness. Gardenia and Forsythia clear heat and scatter binding. Rhubarb and refined Mirabilitum drain fire and stem dryness. The experiential formula, *Gua Shi Tang* (Trichosanthes & Dendrobium Decoction), whose nourishing yin and transforming dryness are based on clinical experience and exploration, can [also] be offered as a reference.

C. For various types of blood cold patterns: Mostly one should use the methods and principles of warming the channels and scattering cold.

The method of warming the channels and scattering cold mainly is used for internal cold or external cold which has entered the blood division. [It may also be used for] cold evils congealing in the channels and vessels. It mainly uses medicinals which warm the blood and free the flow of the channels [or menstruation], scatter cold and dispel stasis. When warmth scatters and the flow is freed, when stasis is dispelled and the new is engendered, and when cold is dispelled and congelation is scattered, then the channels and network vessels are coursed and dredged. The formulas I commonly use are *Wen Jing Tang* (Warm the Channels Decoction, from either the *Jin Gui Yao Lue [Essentials of the Golden Cabinet]* or *Fu Ren Liang Fang Da Quan [Great Compendium of Fine Formulas for Women]*) and *Shao Fu Zhu Yu Tang* (Lower Abdomen Dispel Stasis Decoction).

When applying the therapeutic principles of warming the channels and scattering cold, one should combine these with medicinals which warmly supplement the qi and blood in accordance with the need of the disease condition. Since vacuity is able to engender cold, if cold is enduring, there must be vacuity. Therefore, use warm supplementation. In addition, qi stagnation leads to blood stasis and blood stasis leads to qi stagnation. Stagnation leads to yang qi not flowing freely and so cold cannot obtain removal. In that case, it is necessary to combine medicinals which move the qi and free the flow of the network vessels with those that warm, transform, and dispel stasis. For instance, *Si Wu Tang* (Four Materials Decoction) [plus] Radix Lateralis Praeparatus Aconiti Carmichaeli (*Fu Zi*), Cortex Cinnamomi Cassiae (*Rou Gui*), Ramulus Cinnamomi Cassiae (*Gui Zhi*), blast-fried Rhizoma Zingiberis (*Pao Jiang*), Rhizoma Cyperi Rotundi (*Xiang Fu*), Folium Artemisiae Argyii (*Ai Ye*), Fructus Evodiae Rutecarpae (*Wu Zhu Yu*), Rhizoma Curculiginis Orchioidis (*Xian Mao*), and Herba Epimedii (*Xian Ling Pi*).

D. For various types of blood vacuity conditions: Mainly this refers to qi and blood dual vacuity patterns.

1. The method of boosting the qi & nourishing blood

This refers to making yang engender and yin grow by boosting the qi in order to carry along the blood. When qi is sufficient, it is able to promote the function of the blood. This makes new blood effulgent and exuberant, thus accomplishing the aim of supplementing both the qi and blood. The formulas I commonly use are *Shen Qi Si Wu Tang* (Ginseng & Astragalus Four Materials Decoction), *Ba Zhen Yi Mu Wan* (Eight Pearls Leonurus Pills), *Ren Shen Yang Rong Wan* (Ginseng Nourish the

59

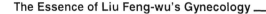

Constructive Pills), *Ba Zhen Tang* (Eight Pearls Pills), and *Shi Quan Da Bu Tang* (Ten [Ingredients] Completely & Greatly Supplementing Decoction).

2. The method of enriching yin & nourishing the blood

This [method] mainly is for yin and blood dual vacuity patterns. It aims at heavily supplementing and filling yin blood substance insufficiency. It mostly uses bloody, meaty, compassionate ingredients.[6] The formula I commonly use is *San Jiao Si Wu Tang* (Three Gelatins Four Materials Decoction). If there is a tendency to yin vacuity, I mostly use *Liang Di Tang* (Two *Di* Decoction) with additions and subtractions.

When using medicinals which boost the qi and nourish the blood, depending on the nature of the disease, it may be necessary to combine these with warming yang, upbearing yang, fortifying the spleen, or supplementing the kidneys medicinals. When using the methods and principles of enriching yin and nourishing the blood, depending on the disease nature, it may be necessary to combine these with clearing heat and transforming dryness medicinals.

To sum up the above, blood patterns can be said to be the commonly seen or most commonly seen conditions in gynecology. The methods of treating the blood are relatively many. The author has gathered and grasped these [*i.e.*, summed them up] as above in order to provide a rule for treating blood conditions based on pattern discrimination.

---

[6] This refers to medicinals made from various animal parts. The adjective bloody and meaty are self-explanatory. Compassionate in this instance means two things. First, it refers to the animal's compassion in laying down its life for the benefit of the patient (not that it had a choice!). Secondly, such animal medicinals are close in nature to the yin substance they seek to supplement. Thus they are of the same condition, the other meaning of the word *qing*, as the condition they seek to treat.

6
A Discussion of [the Author's] Understanding of "Heat Entering the Blood Chamber" Based on His Clinical Experience

Concerning the pattern of "heat entering the blood chamber", the same description exists in the *Shang Han Lun (Treatise on Damage [Due to] Cold]* and the *Jin Gui Yao Lue (Essentials from the Golden Cabinet)* where it is categorized as an externally contracted disease. As for what is called the blood chamber, experts have noted that Chinese medical books in succeeding dynasties have had different points of view [on this subject]. For instance, [it has been identified] as the *chong mai*, the liver, and the uterus. Based on [my] knowledge gained from clinical experience, [I believe] that what is called the blood chamber refers to mainly the *bao gong* (uterus) but also includes the two vessels of the *chong* and *ren* as well as the liver viscus and is a concept for the generalized function of women's menstrual physiology. Because the *chong mai* is the sea of blood and the *ren mai* governs the uterus, they are the root of women's engenderment [here meaning, however, birthing] and nourishment [here meaning lactation], while the liver vessel networks with the yin [*i.e.*, genital] organs and also is the viscus which stores the blood. Therefore, this concept of the blood chamber accords with clinical practice as long as it includes all these aspects [of women's menstrual physiology]. Otherwise, it will inevitably be limited if it is simply regarded as a substantial organ, and, [in that case,] certain symptoms [associated with the concept of the blood chamber] cannot be well explained. At the same time, [such an oversimplification] would lose [this concept's] clinical significance.

From the point of view of clinical practice, what is called "heat entering the blood chamber" mostly refers to women's suffering from contraction of wind cold or wind heat evils. If, right at the beginning of menstruation or at its end, or if postpartum there is qi and blood vacuity great damage and the sea of blood is empty and vacuous, and if external heat evils take advantage of vacuity and enter, then the righteous qi and [this evil heat] will mutually struggle, wrestling and binding in the blood chamber. This is what is called "heat entering the blood chamber." From the point of view of the type of heat, besides commonly manifesting as what the above books refer to as "continously coming cold and heat" and "malaria-like heat", it can also manifest as a non-typical heat. This refers to "occasional emission of cold and heat." From the point of view of the condition of the menstrual blood, after heat has entered the blood chamber, the menstrual water may become intermittent and the menstrual blood may not be smoothly flowing due to obstruction of the uterus. Or, heat may enter the blood division, forcing the blood to move frenetically, [in which case,] the menstrual blood may dribble and drip without cease or the blood may flood downward. It may also manifest after menstruation when the blood chamber is empty and vacuous. Evil heat binds internally and is not able to follow the menstrual blood and be resolved. This is not the same situation as stasis obstructing the uterus. Under normal conditions, if a woman has an external contraction during her menstruation, this heat can follow the blood and be resolved, thus being cured without medicinals. Yet, during the menstrual period or postpartum, when the uterus is empty and vacuous, heat may stagnate internally and evil heat and the menstrual blood may mutually wrestle, righteous and evil joined in struggle. [Hence, the external evils] are not able to be resolved externally and this can manifest as the abnormal appearance of stasis obstructing the uterus.

As for the therapeutic principles for heat entering the blood chamber, since the sea of blood is already empty and vacuous, the method of breaking the blood cannot be used recklessly no matter what heat is arresting. If heat is forcing the blood to move, one is also not able to only use clearing heat and cooling the blood. This is because heat-clearing, blood-cooling medicinals may be able to resolve heat and clear the blood, but they are not able to out-thrust evils and exit them externally.

Therefore, it is urgent to find a way to grant evil heat a way out or to enable it to be out-thrust and exited externally.

The foot *jue yin* liver channel winds around the yin organs (this can also be explained as encircling the uterus). Situated surrounding the blood chamber, one can set about out-thrusting evil heat from the blood chamber via the foot *jue yin* liver channel. Since the liver and gallbladder have a mutual interior-exterior relationship, when treating the *jue yin*, this necessarily [also] treats the *shao yang*. Thus evil heat can be resolved from the *jue yin* via the *shao yang*. On the one hand, downwardly falling evils should be out-thrust, while inwardly fallen heat should be cleared and resolved. Clearing and out-thrusting should be simultaneous. On the other hand, it is necessary to also show consideration to the righteous qi so that it is able to force the evils to exit externally.

Concerning the concrete treatment of "heat entering the blood chamber", the descriptions in the *Shang Han Lun (Treatise on Damage [Due to] Cold)* and *Jin Gui Yao Lue (Essentials of the Golden Cabinet)* are the same. Howevert, from the viewpoint of warm disease theory, they are not the same. As it was said by Ye Tian-shi:

> If the menstrual water sometimes comes and sometimes ceases [*i.e.*, comes intermittently], evils have fallen into the blood chamber and what is said of *shao yang* cold damage should be clearly understood... Even though many stirrings [*i.e.*, beats of the pulse] and cold damage are different, [Zhang] Zhong-jing prescribed *Xiao Chai Hu Tang* (Minor Bupleurum Decoction)...

This explains that, although cold damage is due to cold evils, it gradually transforms into heat as it enters the interior and heat evils are the first to sink. Therefore, the pattern that is seen is a mixture of cold and heat like malaria. In treating this, besides puncturing *Qi Men* (LI 14) (without using any medicinals), one can use *Xiao Chai Hu Tang* (Minor Bupleurum Decoction). However, the pattern of "heat entering the blood chamber" caused by inward falling of warm heat disease evils is

63

comparatively complex. Hence, one cannot mechanically adhere to the single formula of *Xiao Chai Hu Tang* but should treat this according to pattern discrimination. I have treated [this condition] with Master Tao's *Xiao Chai Hu Tang* with additions and subtractions and with *Gui Zhi Tao Hua Tang* (Cinnamom Twig & Peach Blossom Decoction) with additions and subtractions, as well as based on the principle of adding and subtracting according to the symptoms. One can say that this is a development of the treatment of "heat entering the blood chamber."

[However,] based on clinical experience, one can mainly use *Xiao Chai Hu Tang* in the treatment of heat entering the blood chamber. Within this formula, Radix Bupleuri (*Chai Hu*) and Radix Scutellariae Baicalensis (*Huang Qin*) are the main ingredients. This is because Bupleurum can soothe and resolve the liver qi and lift external evils which have fallen into the blood chamber, thus out-thrusting and exiting them. Scutellaria is bitter and cold and clears heat. It makes half-interior heat evils withdraw inward. Radix Panacis Ginseng (*Ren Shen*), Rhizoma Zingiberis (*Jiang*), and Fructus Zizyphi Jujubae (*Zao*) are ingredients for regulating and harmonizing the constructive and defensive, the aim of which is to support the righteous so as to force the evils to exit externally.

Of course, while using this [formula], additions and subtractions must be made flexibly according to the condition. Menstruation may just have begun and there is a wind cold external contraction with cold evils transforming heat. Heat [thus] enters the blood chamber. One may initially see aversion to cold and fever and then later cold and heat mixed together in a malaria-like way, and the menstrual blood may be arrested and sometimes cease. For mild cases or those accompanied by a righteous qi vacuity of the body, one can simply use *Xiao Chai Hu Tang* and it will be OK. Heat will be removed and the menstrual water will stop and start on time. If there is simultaneous blood clots or lower abdominal distention and pain, this clearly shows there is static blood obstructing internally. [In that case,] it is ok to add Herba Leonuri Heterophylli (*Yi Mu Cao*), Radix Angelicae Sinensis (*Dang Gui*), Herba

Lycopi Lucidi (*Ze Lan*), and Flos Carthami Tinctorii (*Hong Hua*) to quicken the blood and regulate the menses, course, abduct, and transform stasis. If there is an external contraction of wind heat or evil heat is relatively heavy, simultaneously one may see *chong* and *ren* irregularity and the liver not storing the blood. Heat forces the blood to move and the menstrual blood either dribbles and drips without cease or there is flooding of blood downward with a prolonged period that does not stop. In that case, it is necessary to also use heat-clearing, blood-cooling medicinals. Based on the experience handed down from my master that, "*Xiao Chai* (Minor Bupleurum), uncooked Radix Rehmanniae (*Sheng Di*), and Cortex Radicis Moutan (*Mu Dan Pi*) are able to treat flooding and leaking", it is [my] experience that this can treat heat entering the blood chamber. Therefore, I commonly use *Xiao Chai Hu Tang* plus uncooked Radix Rehmanniae (*Sheng Di*), Cortex Radicis Moutan (*Dan Pi*), Herba Artemisiae Apiaceae (*Qing Hao*), Cortex Radicis Lycii Chinensis (*Di Gu Pi*), and other such medicinals which nourish yin and clear heat. If one sees that the *chong* and *ren* are not secure [or not securing] and that bleeding is relatively profuse, one can add carbonized Rhizoma Cimicifugae (*Sheng Ma*), carbonized Radix Sanguisorbae (*Di Yu*), and carbonized Receptaculum Nelumbinis Nuciferae (*Lian Fang*) in order to secure the *chong* and *ren*. Or one may add powdered Radix Pseudoginseng (*San Qi*) to stop bleeding.

Also, if heat evils are relatively heavy and blood is arrested by this heat which is obstructing the uterus, then heat evils and static blood may wrestle and bind. If this follows the two vessels of the *chong* and *ren* and counterflows upward, it may be conducted into the *yang ming*. [In that case,] the manifestations will be a dry mouth with bitter [taste], oral thirst, headache, a red face, and vexation and agitation. If mild, one can add Rhizoma Coptidis Chinensis (*Huang Lian*) and Fructus Gardeniae Jasminoidis (*Zhi Zi*) in order to clear heat. If there is *yang ming* dryness and binding and the stools are not freely flowing, then one can add Radix Et Rhizoma Rhei (*Da Huang*) or use *Da Chai Hu Tang* (Major Bupleurum Decoction) with additions and subtractions to treat this. If the menses have already ceased or if postpartum the sea of blood is empty and vacuous but there is contraction of external evils, evil heat may bind internally and stasis may obstruct within the uterus's vacuity pattern. Then attention should be paid to the severity of the characteristics of blood vacuity and stasis obstruction, and one should use [either] *Chai Qin Si Wu Tang* (Bupleurum & Scutellaria Four Materials Decoction), *Xiao Yao San* (Rambling Powder), or *Dan Zhi Xiao Yao San* (Moutan & Gardenia Rambling Powder) with additions and subtractions to treat this. In order to explain these views, the following cases are presented below.

Case 1: Wang, female, 25 years old, a simple case in the out-patient department

Date of initial examination: November 7, 1974

She came to the hospital due to menstruation ahead of schedule with profuse volume for over one year. She had taken prescriptions to fortify the spleen and nourish the blood, secure the *chong* and stop bleeding, but the bleeding had not stopped. During this period, she suddenly suffered from a flu with fever (her body temperature was 38°C), dizziness, no desire to eat, heart vexation, nausea, desire to vomit, chest fullness and oppression, a pale tongue body, and a slippery, fine, rapid pulse.

This was discriminated as evils invading the *shao yang* with heat entering the blood chamber. Treatment was in order to harmonize and resolve the *shao yang*, clear heat and cool the blood. The formula's medicinals were as follows: Radix Bupleuri (*Chai Hu*), 1 *qian*, Radix Codonopsitis Pilosulae (*Dang Sheng*), 2 *qian*, Radix Scutellariae Baicalensis (*Huang Qin*), 2 *qian*, Rhizoma Pinelliae Ternatae (*Ban Xia*), 2 *qian*, Radix Glycyrrhizae (*Gan Cao*), 1 *qian*, uncooked Radix Rehmannia (*Sheng Di*), 4 *qian*, Cortex Radicis Moutan (*Dan Pi*), 2 *qian*, Cortex Radicis Lycii Chinensis (*Di Gu Pi*), 2 *qian*, Herba Artemisiae Apiaceae (*Qing*

Hao), 2 *qian*, Rhizoma Thalictri Foliosi (*Ma Wei Lian*),[7] 2 *qian*, uncooked Rhizoma Zingiberis (*Sheng Jiang*), 3 slices, Fructus Zizyphi Jujubae (*Da Zao*), 3 pieces, powdered Radix Pseudoginseng (*San Qi*), 8 *fen* (washed down separately).

On Nov. 9, [the patient reported that] after taking one *ji*[8] of the above formula, her vaginal bleeding had stopped and her body temperature was normal. Her cold [*i.e.,* chills] and fever were already abated and her essence spirit [*i.e.,* mood] was improved. Her intake of food had regained its flavor, but there was still dizziness and stifling qi [in her chest]. Her two excretions were self-regulated [*i.e.,* normal]. [Therefore,] Pseudoginseng was removed from the above formula. She was administered three more *ji* continuously, [at which time] all her symptoms had been eliminated.

Commentary: The patient originally had suffered from functional uterine bleeding for over one year. Her menstruation began on Oct. 26 and was very profuse in volume, was fresh red in color, and contained large blood clots. This had continued for eight days without a break. During the period when the blood in the uterus was vacuous, the patient suffered from an external contraction of external evils and heat had entered her blood chamber. This manifested as a typical pattern of evils having entered the *shao yang*. The treatment was in order to harmonize and resolve the *shao yang*, clear heat and cool the blood. The formula used was *Xiao Chai Hu Tang* (Minor Bupleurum Decoction) plus uncooked Rehmannia, Moutan, Cortex Lycii, and Sweet Wormwood to

---

[7] This medicinal, like Rhizoma Piccrorhizae (*Hu Huang Lian*), may be used as a substitute for the more expensive Rhizoma Coptidis Chinensis (*Huang Lian*), and as such, is commonly employed by Dr. Liu.

[8] The word *ji* literally means formula or prescription. However, it is also used to denote a single packet of a formula. It is not a single dose, since a single packet of medicinals is usually taken in two or three divided doses in a day. Rather, it refers typically to one day's dose when used as a numerical cipher.

nourish yin, clear heat, and cool the blood. Thalictrum when combined with Scutellaria clears and resolves depressed heat counterflowing upward. And Pseudoginseng quickens the blood and stops bleeding. Since the medicinal and the pattern mutually agreed, the therapeutic effect was very rapid.

Case 2: Han, female, 28 years old, a simple case in the out-patient department

Date of initial examination: April 19, 1975

After delivering on Dec 10, 1974, [the patient] suffered from high fever due to an external affection. However, the fever abated after treatment with Chinese medicinals. [Since then,] she had constantly suffered from insomnia, heart vexation, chaotic thinking, and sometimes there was the appearance of cold and heat [*i.e.,* fever and chills]. In the past week, her sleep at night was not replete, her dreams were choatic and confused, and she had hallucinations. There were two people before her eyes, one black and one white. At night this appeared and in the daylight this disappeared. Therefore, she did not dare to sleep after turning off the light. She also felt headache and dizziness, heart vexation, tension, and agitation. Sometimes her body felt hot and there was sweating. She had heart fluster and fright palpitations, gallbladder timidity, nausea, chest and rib-side distention and fullness, lower abdominal distention, short, yellow urination, and her menstruation had not arrived. Her tongue was red and her pulse was bowstring.

This was discriminated as postpartum external contraction but the evils had not been eliminated. Heat had entered the blood chamber and this was harassing her spirit brightness. Treatment was in order to harmonize and resolve the liver and gallbladder, clear heat and quiet the spirit. The formula's medicinals were as follows: Radix Bupleuri (*Chai Hu*), 2 *qian*, Radix Codonopsitis Pilosulae (*Dang Sheng*), 3 *qian*, Rhizoma Pinelliae (*Ban Xia*), 3 *qian*, Radix Scutellariae Baicalensis (*Huang Qin*), 3 *qian*, Radix Glycyrrhizae (*Gan Cao*), 2 *qian*, Fructus Citri Aurantii (*Zhi*

Ke), 2 *qian*, Fructus Gardeniae Jasminoidis (*Zhi Zi*), 3 *qian*, Fructus Forsythiae Suspensae (*Lian Qiao*), 3 *qian*, Radix Albus Paeoniae Lactiflorae (*Bai Shao*), 3 *qian*, uncooked Rhizoma Zingiberis (*Sheng Jiang*), 3 slices, Fructus Zizyphi Jujubae (*Da Zao*), 3 pieces, uncooked Dens Draconis (*Long Chi*), 1 *liang*, Cortex Radcis Moutan (*Dan Pi*), 2 *qian*.

On Apr. 24, after having taken three *ji* of the above formula, [the patient reported] that various of her symptoms had been alleviated and her chills and fever had been relieved. The patient could sleep after turning off the lamp and her hallucinations had disappeared. There was still dizziness, nausea, torpid intake, and chest and rib-side distention. She was administered three more *ji* continuously and all her symptoms were cured.

Commentary: This case was one of the gynecological postpartum diseases. It is usually diagnosed as neurosis in Western medicine. [However,] from the point of view of Chinese medicine, the patient's trouble was due to external affection after delivery. After being treated with Chinese medicinals, her fever had abated. However, it had not been completely eliminated. Afterwards, continuous insomnia, heart vexation, chaotic thoughts, and occasional fever and chills had been occurring for over two months. In the last week, her sleep at night was not replete, her dreams were chaotic and confused, and she was having hallucinations. Thus she did not dare to go to sleep, her body was hot, and she was sweating. This resembled the pattern described in "The Pulses, Patterns &Treatment of Gynecological Miscellaneous Diseases" in the *Jin Gui Yao Lue (Essentials from the Golden Cabinet)* when it says: "If a woman is damaged by cold and has fever, her menses come intermittently, and her mind is clear during the day, but with night comes delirious speech and seeing of ghosts, this is due to heat entering the blood chamber." Judging from its degree, [this case] was milder than that described in that book, but its disease course was longer. The remaining evils had hidden internally in her blood chamber, which is to say that they were deep-lying internally in the blood division. Because the liver channel brewed heat and this ascended and was upborne, there was headache, dizziness, heart vexation, tension, and agitation. Liver heat depression and obstruction in the chest and rib-side led to nausea, chest and rib-side distention and fullness. Liver fire had reached the heart and heart channel fire was exuberant. This fire then harassed her spirit brightness, and, therefore, there was heart fluster, fright palpitations, hallucinations, insomnia, and not daring to go to sleep. Liver fire had reached the gallbladder, and, therefore, there was nausea and gallbladder timidity. Because the *chong mai* homes to the *yang ming*, when heat hidden in the blood chamber involves the *yang ming*, generalized fever, perspiration, lower abdominal distention, short, and yellow urination may be seen. The red tongue and relaxed pulse showed that the condition was one of postpartum great damage to the yin and blood.

Hence, [this case] can be summed up and its pattern discriminated as postpartum external affection with remaining evils not eliminated and heat entering the blood chamber which was harassing the spirit brightness.

Because the course of this disease had already endured for [many] days, there was no high fever or malaria-like [symptoms]. It only manifested itself as occasional fever and chills (not high fever). This was caused by harassing of the remaining heat under the circumstance of postpartum qi and blood dual vacuity. The righteous qi was already vacuous but the remaining evils had not been eliminated. Therefore, the righteous was vacuous and evils were replete.

As the *Jin Gui Yao Lue (Essentials of the Golden Cabinet)* makes clear, this type of condition seems severe superficially but is actually not severe. It is mainly because menstruation has not yet been blocked and stopped that the evils have fallen inward deeply. Thus it is said, "If there is no invasion of the stomach qi and the upper two burners, it must necessarily heal by itself." However, in this case, [the patient's] body was vacuous postpartum and deep-lying heat had already affected the heart, liver, spleen, and stomach viscera and bowels. Although the heat was not heavy, it had already entered the blood division. Also, because the menstruation does not come during puerperium, the remaining evils cannot be removed by following the menstrual blood. So, because the righteous failed to overcome the evil, it had lasted over two months and, in the last week, the symptoms had become heavier. Thus it was impossible [for this case] to heal by itself.

In terms of the above treatment, it was necessary to consider whether to first nourish the blood and quiet the spirit, settle the heart and quiet the spirit, or soothe the liver and resolve depression. However, it was recognized by minutely inquiring about the disease history and analyzing its course that the essence of its pathology was "heat entering the blood chamber." [Therefore,] it was advisable to adopt the methods of harmonizing and resolving the liver and gallbladder, clearing heat and quieting the spirit. [Hence, I used] *Xiao Chai Hu Tang* (Minor Bupleurum Decoction) to harmonize and resolve the *shao yang* and thus out-thrust evils from the *jue yin*. Moutan and Gardenia were added to clear liver-gallbladder heat and cool the blood. Gardenia combined with Forsythia can clear heart channel heat. White Peony nourishes the blood and cools the blood. When it is combined with Codonopsis, these can boost the qi and nourish the blood in order to support the righteous. Bupleurum combined with Aurantium courses depression and clears heat. A small amount of Dragon's Teeth settles the liver, clears the heart, and quiets the spirit. Thus this formula has the functions mainly of harmonizing, resolving, and out-thrusting, cooling the blood and clearing heat. This is assisted by boosting the qi, nourishing the blood, and supporting the righteous. On the one hand, it out-thrusts evils and exits them externally, out-thrusting while clearing. On the other hand, it supports the righteous forcing evils to exit externally. Once these evils are removed, the righteous is quiet.

Based on the experience gained from treating the above two cases, it can be known that, in clinical practice, what is called "heat entering the blood chamber" is never as typical as that described in the books. Therefore, we must always start from clinical practice in order to grasp the pathological essence of "heat entering the blood chamber" and base its treatment on pattern discrimination. Thus we can more completely understand its clinical significance.

7
Experiences in the Use of *Chan Hou Sheng Hua Tang* (Postpartum Engendering & Transforming Decoction) Accompanied by a Talk about "Dispelling Stasis & Engendering the New"

*S*heng Hua Tang (Engendering & Transforming Decoction) is found in *Fu Qing Zhu Nu Ke (Fu Qing-zhu's Gynecology)*. It is composed of the medicinal flavors [*i.e.*, ingredients] of Radix Angelicae Sinensis (*Dang Gui*), 8 *qian*, Radix Ligustici Wallichii (*Chuan Xiong*), 3 *qian*, Semen Pruni Persicae (*Tao Ren*), 14 pieces with tip and skin removed, blackened Rhizoma Zingiberis (*Hei Jiang*), 5 *fen*, and mix-fried Radix Glycyrrhizae (*Gan Cao*), 5 *fen*. It is taken [orally] after being decocted half with yellow [*i.e.*, rice] wine and half with child's urine. Its functions are that it quickens the blood and transforms stasis, warms the channels and stops pain. It mainly treats a postpartum lochia that does not move [*i.e.*, come] and lower abdominal aching and pain. It is widely used in southern [China].[9] In some regions, it is even used as a routine formula postpartum. In the *Cheng Fang Bian Du (An Easy Reader of Prepared [i.e., Patent] Formulas)*, [this formula] is clearly and minutely explained. In that book, [it is thought that,] postpartum, the qi and blood are greatly vacuous. Therefore, one must bank and supplement. However, if vanquished blood is not removed, new blood cannot be engendered. This is evidenced by lower abdominal pain and other such conditions. [In that case,] one should mainly dispel stasis.

---

9   This means anything south of the Yangtze River.

73

Within this formula, Dang Gui is used in relatively large amounts. Its function is to nourish the blood. Licorice supplements the middle. Ligusticum Wallichium rectifies the qi within the blood. Persica moves stasis within the blood. Blast-fried Ginger, which is the color black, enters the constructive. It stregnthens Dang Gui and Licorice's engendering the new and assists Ligusticum Wallichium and Persica's transforming stasis. Child's urine is able to boost yin and eliminate heat. It leads vanquished blood to move downward.

Modification of this formula by additions and subtractions was already mentioned in the notes of the original book, [*i.e.*, *Fu Qing Zhu Nu Ke*]:

> If due to cold, cool food stuffs, binding lump pain is severe, add Cortex Cinnamomi Cassiae (*Rou Gui*), 8 *fen*, to *Sheng Hua Tang*. If blood clots are not dispersed, it is not ok to add Radix Panacis Ginseng (*Shen*) and Radix Astragali Membranacei (*Qi*) or the pain will not stop.

From the point of view of clinical practice, it is generally thought that this formula mainly suits postpartum contraction of cold affection with stasis and stagnation.

The *Sheng Hua Tang* routinely used in northern [China] is not Fu Qing-zhu's *Sheng Hua Tang*. It is called *Chan Hou Gong Tang* (Postpartum Official Formula) (also called *Chan Hou Sheng Hua Tang*, Postpartum Engendering & Transforming Decoction). Its medicinal composition and medicinal dosages are different from Master Fu's *Sheng Hua Tang*. After many years of use, it is relatively stable, without side effects, and its [therapeutic] effect is fully satisfactory.[10] It is composed of the medicinal flavors of Radix Ligustici Wallichii (*Chuan Xiong*), 1 *qian*, Radix Angelicae Sinensis (*Dang Gui*), 3 *qian*, Flos Carthami Tinctorii (*Hong Hua*), 1 *qian*, Herba Lonori Heterophylli (*Yi Mu Cao*), 1 *qian*, Herba Lycopi Lucidi (*Ze Lan*), 1 *qian*, Semen Pruni Persicae (*Tao Ren*), 5 *fen*,

---

[10] Although the author does not say it, the inference is that Dr. Liu is responsible for the composition of this formula.

mix-fried Radix Glycyrrhizae (*Gan Cao*), 5 *fen*, blast-fried Rhizoma Zingiberis (*Pao Jiang*), 5 *fen*, southern Fructus Crataegi (*Nan Shan Zha*), 2 *qian*, and old wine, 5 *qian*. In comparison to the *Sheng Hua Tang* in *Fu Qing Zhu Nu Ke* (*Fu Qing-zhu's Gynecology*), this one has Carthamus, Leonurus, Lycopus, and southern Crategus and the dosages of the medicinals is smaller. The amount of Dang Gui is large, but is only 3 *qian*. The amount [or dose] of most of the other medicinals is 1 *qian* or 5 *fen*. From the point of view of its composition of medicinal flavors, [this formula] is formed from the *Sheng Hua Tang* in *Fu Qing Zhu Nu Ke* but with added flavors and reduced amounts.

Compared with Master Fu's *Sheng Hua Tang*, the main characteristics of this formula are that it is comprised of more than four flavors and the medicinal amounts are less. Why can it be widely used in clinic and why does it achieve an ideal effect? [To answer these questions,] one must analyze [this formula] from the point of view of the basic concepts of blood and blood patterns. In terms of the production of the blood, "The Secrets of Qi Chapter" of the *Ling Shu (Spiritual Pivot)* says, "What is called the blood is the qi which is received and the juice which is adopted by the middle burner which is transformed and becomes red." Hence, we should not only consider the aspect [of the blood] which pertains to its material substance. More important is that aspect [of the blood] which pertains to its function. From the perspective of its production, it can be seen that this can be divided into the two parts, "the qi which is received" and "the juice which is adopted." Only if the "qi" and the "juice" are transformed red can there be blood. [However,] the human body's "blood" can only function if it continually circulates. If the movement of the blood becomes slow, ceases, or becomes stagnant, or even more severely, if it congeals and gathers and does not transform, thus producing static blood (also called dead blood), it loses its function.

Therefore, in terms of the concept of blood vacuity, in clinic, one must differentiate whether it pertains to insufficiency of the material substance or a disturbance in its function. Thus it is said, "Qi is the commander of the blood, while blood is the mother of qi." From the point of view of its circulation, "If the qi moves, the blood moves; if the qi stagnates, the blood gathers [or stops]." It is generally thought that quickening the blood can transform stasis and that dispelling stasis can engender the new. This static blood is dead blood that is not commanded [*i.e.,* moved] by the qi and, [therefore,] loses its circulating function. The aim of quickening blood is to promote the circulation of blood and fluids. This is because only if [both] the generalized and local blood circulation is normal and new blood gradually enriches and engenders can the vessels and passageways be full and exuberant. If the blood is vacuous and the vessels and passageways are not able to be full and exuberant, then the blood movement will be relaxed [*i.e.,* retarded]. Only if the qi and blood fill and make the vessels and passageways exuberant can movement be normal and constant and circulation be endless.

If the blood flow stirs normally, static blood is able to be broken, transformed, and scattered. Thus "quickening the blood and transforming stasis, dispelling stasis and engendering the new" are mutually contradictory yet also united. Only by understanding that dispelling stasis can engender the new can one see this matter from this unified perspective. The ancients said, "If you want to free the flow, one must first fill." In other words, if one wants to quicken the blood and free the flow of stasis, one must first supplement the qi and blood. By making the qi and blood full and abundant, the vessels and passageways are full and exuberant. The blood and fluids are then able to circulate smoothly and uninhibitedly and static blood is able to be coursed and freed. Therefore, the function of the blood is based on material substance. [Conversely,] if its function is effulgent and exuberant, this can also promote the engenderment of new blood.

Based on the above-mentioned view and method, it is easy to understand the meaning and characteristics of *Chan Hou Sheng Hua Tang*. Within this formula, Dang Gui is the ruling medicinal. Dang Gui is sweet, acrid, and warm. It enters the three channels of the liver, heart, and spleen. Sweetness and warmth supplement the spleen and thus boost the source of engenderment and transformation of the qi and blood. Acridity is able to free the flow of the channels. Warmth is able to transform, scatter, and free the flow of the blood. Therefore, Dang Gui is able to both supplement and quicken the blood. Its ability to supplement the blood is due to its effect of quickening the blood. Ligusticum Wallichium is acrid and warm. It quickens the blood and moves the qi within the blood. Carthamus, Leonurus, Lycopus, and Persica are all ingredients which quicken the blood and transform stasis. They are used in relatively small amounts. Using [these] in small [amounts] quickens and nourishes the blood. Using [them] in large [amounts] is able to break the blood. Southern Crataegus enters the blood division and transforms static blood. In this formula, a number of blood-quickening medicinals in small amounts are concentrated. They mutually assist each other to mainly quicken the blood and engender the new. Blast-fried Ginger, 5 *fen*, is added to strengthen the warm, freeing power. Mix-fried Licorice is the assistant which helps Dang Gui to supplement the middle and engender the qi and blood. Thus this [formula] is a manifestation of the principle that, if you want to free the flow, you must first fill. When the blood vessels are full and exuberant, the qi movement and circulation are smooth and reach [*i.e.*, spread properly]. Thus static blood is able to be transformed, scattered, and removed. The new is engendered, and secondarily, stasis is transformed.

If there is postpartum qi and blood vacuity and there is static blood which has not been eliminated from the body, it can be hard to do what is appropriate to both. That is why this [formula] was named *Chan Hou Sheng Hua Tang* (Postpartum Engendering & Transforming Decoction). It is 100% meaningful. This is the reason why it cannot be simply and directly explained that [first] it dispels stasis and then it engenders the new. To sum up the functions of *Chan Hou Sheng Hua Tang*, it nourishes the blood, quickens the blood, and transforms stasis. It is mainly appropriate for [treating those with] a postpartum lochia that has not stopped with static blood gathering internally. This then causes postpartum blood stasis which leads to the arising of abdominal pain, low-grade fever, and ceaseless bleeding from the yin passageway [*i.e.*, vaginal tract]. In addition, it can be used for abdominal pain and vaginal tract bleeding caused by retention of fetal membranes after spontaneous miscarriage and artificial abortion. In terms of its clinical effects, it can not only supplement blood and support the righteous but it also makes any remaining fetal membranes slough off and be shed. Thus, it has the effect of a medicinal uterine curettage.

When using *Chan Hou Sheng Hua Tang*, it is advisable to use the whole formula and the recommended amounts as long as there are no unusual circumstances or concomitant patterns. However, it is important that suitable additions and subtractions be made based on the disease condition. If abdominal pain is marked, it is ok to add *Shi Xiao San* (Loose a Smile Powder) to this formula. In other words, one can add Feces Trogopterori Seu Pteromi (*Wu Ling Zhi*) and Pollen Typhae (*Pu Huang*). If abdominal pain is severe and vaginal tract bleeding is profuse, use stir-fried [till] carbonized Pollen Typhae to enable it to simultaneously stop bleeding. If there is static blood and low-grade fever, omit blast-fried Ginger. If there is lumbar pain, add Radix Dipsaci (*Chuan Duan*), Cortex Eucommiae Ulmoidis (*Du Zhong*), and Ramulus Loranthi Seu Visci (*Sang Ji Sheng*). The following cases may be taken as examples to elucidate the knowledge gained through experience in clinical application.

Case 1: Chou, female, 28 years old, a simple case in the out-patient department

Date of initial examination: August 21, 1975

[The patient] had gone into spontaneous labor two months previously. [Since then,] dribbling and dripping of blood had been ceaseless for two months. The color of the blood was black, it contained clots, and its amount was sometimes profuse and sometimes scanty. There was lower abdominal pain accompanied by stomach pain. The tongue was dark red and the pulse was bowstring,[11] slippery, and relaxed.[12]

Western medical diagnosis: Incomplete postpartum uterine involution

Chinese medical pattern discrimination: Postpartum contraction of cold, static blood internally obstructing

Treatment methods: Nourish the blood and warm the center, quicken the blood and transform stasis

Formula & medicinals: Radix Angelicae Sinensis (*Dang Gui*), 3 *qian*, Radix Ligustici Wallichii (*Chuan Xiong*), 1 *qian*, Flos Carthami Tinctorii (*Hong Hua*), 1 *qian*, Herba Leonrui Heterophylli (*Yi Mu Cao*), 1 *qian*, Herba Lycopi Lucidi (*Ze Lan*), 1 *qian*, Semen Pruni Persicae (*Tao Ren*), 5 *fen*, mix-fried Radix Glycyrrhizae (*Gan Cao*), 5 *fen*, southern Fructus Crataegi (*Nan Shan Zha*), 2 *qian*, Rhizoma Alpiniae Officinari (*Gao Liang Jiang*), 2 *qian*, Fructus Amomi (*Sha Ren*), 2 *qian*, Feces Trogopeterori Seu Pteromi (*Wu Ling Zhi*), 3 *qian*

Course of treatment: After administering five *ji* of the above formula, the bleeding stopped. Afterwards, on follow-up, all her symptoms had been eliminated.

Commentary: This case was a typical postpartum one. There was bleeding from the vaginal tract which dribbled and dripped without

---

[11] Wiseman's suggested term for *xian mai* is a stringlike pulse. It replaces his wiry pulse since the Chinese lacked the technology to create metal wire at the time this character was created. However, the definition of this term is a bow or musical instrument string which is tightly strung. Stringlike does not necessarily convey this sense of tension. Therefore, we prefer bowstring to Wiseman's stringlike.

[12] The relaxed pulse, *huan mai*, may also be called the moderate pulse when it is used to describe a normal, healthy pulse. As a disease pulse image, it means a slightly slow pulse, coming at 50-60 beats per minute.

stop. This had already endured for two months, thus the disease course was relatively long. Cold congelation and blood stasis obstructed the uterus. Because this cold congelation was accompanied by qi stagnation, there was stomach pain. Hence there was both lower abdominal and stomach venter pain. *Chan Hou Sheng Hua Tang* was used in its entirety as the basic formula to which was added Alpinia Officinarus in order to warm the center and harmonize the stomach, Amomum to move the qi and stop pain, and Flying Squirrel Droppings to strengthen the action of quickening the blood and transforming stasis.

Case 2: Liu, female, 33 years old, a simple case in the out-patient department

Date of initial examination: July 4, 1975

[The patient] had had her third spontaneous miscarriage on May 25 (after a two month pregnancy). She herself was a gynecologist and thought that her fetus was completely expelled. Therefore, she had not had uterine curettage. However, after the miscarriage, there was dribbling and dripping of blood from the vaginal tract which did not cease. This had gone on already for 50 days. The amount of blood was sometimes scanty and sometimes profuse. Its color was purple and it contained clots. There was [also] lumbar soreness and pain. Her hematochrome was 10g and pregnancy antibody test was negative. After discussion, it was decided to perform a uterine curettage. [However,] the patient refused to have the operation and came to see me for an examination [*i.e.*, treatment]. Her tongue body was dark [*i.e.*, dull][13] and pale and her pulse was small and weak.

Western medical diagnosis: Incomplete miscarriage to be excluded

---

[13] Dark and pale are mutually contradictory in English. However, in Chinese pulse examination, the tongue can be pale in color and yet still be dark or dull in hue.

Chinese medical pattern discrimination: Blood vacuity and blood stasis, blood not returning to the channels

Treatment methods: Quicken the blood and transform stasis, nourish the blood and warmly free the flow

Formula & medicinals: Radix Angelicae Sinensis (*Dang Gui*), 3 *qian*, Radix Ligustici Wallichii (*Chuan Xiong*), 1 *qian*, Herba Leonuri Heterophylli (*Yi Mu Cao*,) 1 *qian*, Herba Lycopi Lucidi (*Ze Lan*), 5 *fen*, mix-fried Radix Glycyrrhizae (*Gan Cao*), 5 *fen*, blast-fried Rhizoma Zingiberis (*Pao Jiang*), 5 *fen*, sourthern Fructus Crataegi (*Nan Shan Zha*), 2 *qian*, Feces Trogopterori Seu Pteromi (*Wu Ling Zhi*), 2 *qian*, Pollen Typhae (*Pu Huang*), 2 *qian*

Course of treatment: On July 9, 1975, after taking four *ji* of medicinals, bleeding had already stopped. There was [still] lumbar pain. [Therefore,] Radix Dipsaci (*Chuan Duan*), 3 *qian*, was added to the above formula in order to secure [*i.e.*, consolidate] the therapeutic effect. One month later, her menses had come normally one time.

Case 3: Gen, female, 27 years old, a simple case in the out-patient department

Date of initial examination: June 19, 1975

[The patient] had had a spontaneous miscarriage on May 13. After seven days, the bleeding had stopped. On May 30, she began bleeding from her vaginal tract again. This had persisted for 30 days. The volume of the blood had gradually increased. Sometimes its amount was as profuse as a half a spittoon. This was accompanied by abdominal pain. [The patient] had previously had two miscarriages. The tongue body was purple and dark and the pulse was deep and choppy.

Western medical diagnosis: Vaginal tract bleeding after spontaneous miscarriage

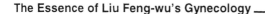

Chinese medical pattern discrimination: Blood vacuity and blood stasis, blood not returning to the channels

Treatment methods: Quicken the blood and transform stasis, nourish the blood and warmly free the flow

Formula & medicinals: Radix Angelicae Sinensis (*Dang Gui*), 3 *qian*, Radix Ligustici Wallichii (*Chuan Xiong*), 1 *qian*, Flos Carthami Tinctorii (*Hong Hua*), 1 *qian*, Herba Leonuri Heterophylli (*Yi Mu Cao*), 1 *qian*, Semen Pruni Persicae (*Tao Ren*), 1.5 *qian*, mix-fried Radix Glycyrrhizae (*Gan Cao*), 1 *qian*, Feces Trogopterori Seu Pteromi (*Wu Ling Zhi*), 2 *qian*, Pollen Typhae (*Pu Huang*), 2 *qian*, blast-fried Rhizoma Zingiberis (*Pao Jiang*), 5 *fen*

Course of treatment: On June 21, the blood volume was greatly reduced after having taken one *ji* of the formula. Bleeding was already stopped after administering three [more] *ji*.

Commentary: Both case #2 and case #3 [had to do with] vaginal bleeding after spontaneous miscarriage, and neither [patient] had had uterine curettage. The course of disease was 30-50 days, and both had a history of recurrent miscarriages. The volume of vaginal bleeding was sometimes scanty and sometimes profuse. Its color was purple and it contained clots. When the amount was profuse, it was as much as half a spittoon. Since the tongue was dull or dark purplish and the pulse was deep and choppy or fine and weak, there was blood vacuity and blood stasis. New blood was not being engendered and the blood was not returning to its channels. [Therefore,] *Chan Hou Sheng Hua Tang* was used in combination with *Shi Xiao San* (Loose a Smile Powder). This avoided the bitterness [*i.e.,* suffering] of a uterine curettage while achieving the effect of a "medicinal uterine curettage."

Case 4: Zhang, female, 44 years old, a simple case history in the out-patient department

Date of initial examination: April 6, 1974

Two days prior, [the patient] had had an electric uterine curettage due to incomplete miscarriage. Last night, she had suddenly felt pain in her lower abdomen. This was acute onset, severe pain [accompanied by] lumbar pain. She took pain-stopping tablets and tetramyacine, but the abdominal pain was not relieved. At present, she felt pain which wound around her low back and lower abdomen. When this pain occurred, her facial complexion was somber white and there was sweating. The amount of the lochia was profuse, her legs were flaccid and without strength, and there was dizziness, torpid intake, a dark yet pale tongue body, and a bowstring, relaxed pulse.

Western medical diagnosis: A) Incomplete postpartum abortion; B) abdominal pain to be examined

Chinese medical pattern discrimination: Blood stasis gathering internally, cold congelation abdominal pain

Treatment methods: Quicken the blood and transform stasis, nourish the blood and warm the channels

Formula & medicinals: Radix Angelicae Sinensis (*Dang Gui*), 3 *qian*, Radix Ligustici Wallichii (*Chuan Xiong*), 1 *qian*, Flos Carthami Tinctorii (*Hong Hua*), 3 *qian*, Herba Leonuri Heterophylli (*Yi Mu Cao*), 1 *qian*, Semen Pruni Persicae (*Tao Ren*), 5 *fen*, mix-fried Radix Glycyrrhizae (*Gan Cao*), 5 *qian*, blast-fried Rhizoma Zingiberis (*Pao Jiang*), 5 *fen*, Pollen Typhae (*Pu Huang*), 2 *qian*, Feces Trogopterori Seu Pteromi (*Wu Ling Zhi*), 3 *qian*

Course of treatment: On Apr. 7, 10 minutes after taking one *ji* of the above formula, her abdominal pain had decreased to the point where it was bearable. After taking two *ji*, the lochia had decreased and she discharged two black-colored clots. Now the patient felt sagging and distention in her lower abdomen and a frequent desire to defecate. Her

83

stools were loose, resolving two times each day. Her tongue was dark [or dull] and pale with slimy, yellow fur, while her pulse was bowstring and relaxed. Blast-fried Ginger (*Pao Jiang*) in the above formula was replaced by dry Ginger (*Gan Jiang*) and two *qian* of Rhizoma Atractylodis Macrocephalae (*Bai Zhu*) were added. [This formula] was continuously administered [until] Apr. 13, when the lochia had already ceased, the lower abdominal pain had already stopped, and her bowel movements were normal.

At present, [the patient] felt coolness in her lower legs, numbness, and lumbar soreness. Her intake of food was devitalized. Her tongue was dark red with slimy, yellow fur, and her pulse was deep, bowstring, and fine. Therefore, in order to supplement the qi and nourish the blood, harmonize the stomach and free the flow of the network vessels, and thus finish the treatment, the following formula and medicinals [were administered]: Radix Codonopsitis Pilosulae (*Dang Sheng*), 3 *qian*, Radix Angelicae Sinensis (*Dang Gui*), 3 *qian*, Radix Albus Paeoniae Lactiflorae (*Bai Shao*), 4 *qian*, Radix Ligustici Wallichii (*Chuan Xiong*), 1.5 *qian*, Rhizoma Atractylodis Macrocephalae (*Bai Zhu*), 3 *qian*, Radix Dioscoreae Oppositae (*Shan Yao*), 5 *qian*, Sclerotium Poriae Cocos (*Fu Ling*), 3 *qian*, Pericarpium Citri Reticulatae (*Chen Pi*), 2 *qian*, Herba Agastachis Seu Pogostemi (*Huo Xiang*), 3 *qian*, Caulis Milettiae Seu Spatholobi (*Ji Xue Teng*), 1 *liang*.

Case 5: Wang, female, 32 years old, a simple case history in the out-patient department

Date of initial examination: January 31, 1972

On Nov. 30, 1971, [the patient] had had an artificial abortion. After the operation, vaginal bleeding had continued unabated. On Dec. 10, the patient again had vacuuming of her uterus. Until then, there had been vaginal tract bleeding which had dribbled and dripped without cease for over two months. Her lower abdomen was slightly painful. The tongue was pale with white fur, and the pulse was choppy and bowstring.

Western medical diagnosis: Vaginal tract bleeding after artificial abortion, the cause of which is to be examined

Chinese medical pattern discrimination: Blood vacuity and blood stasis, blood not returning to the channels

Treatment methods: Quicken the blood and transform stasis, nourish the blood and warm the channels

Formula & medicinals: Radix Angelicae Sinensis (*Dang Gui*), 3 *qian*, Radix Ligustici Wallichii (*Chuan Xiong*), 1 *qian*, Semen Pruni Persicae (*Tao Ren*), 2 *qian*, Herba Leonuri Heterophylli (*Yi Mu Cao*), 2 *qian*, Flos Carthami Tincotrii (*Hong Hua*), 1 *qian*, blast-fried Rhizoma Zingberis (*Pao Jiang*), 1 *qian*, mix-fried Radix Glycyrrhizae (*Gan Cao*), 1 *qian*, sourthern Fructus Crataegi (*Nan Shan Zha*), 2 *qian*, Herba Lycopi Lucidi (*Ze Lan*), 2 *qian*, Feces Trogopterori Seu Pteromi (*Wu Ling Zhi*), 2 *qian*

Course of treatment: On Feb. 5, after taking three *ji* of the formula, bleeding was stopped and [all] the symptoms had been eliminated.

Case 6: Ning, female, 28 years old, a simple case history in the out-patient department

Date of initial examination: July 1, 1975

[The patient] had gotten married that Spring Festival. On June 3, after having been pregnant for over two months, she had had a spontaneous miscarriage and a uterine curettage. After the operation, there was vaginal tract bleeding which dribbled and dripped without cease. Till now, this had endured for one month. It was accompanied by lower abdominal pain, lumbar pain, no flavor in the stomach's intake, occasional nausea, a dark, red tongue with slimy, white fur, and a bowstring, slippery pulse.

Western medical diagnosis: Vaginal tract bleeding, the cause of which is to be examined

Chinese medical pattern discrimination: Blood vacuity and blood stasis, disharmony of the liver and stomach

Treatment methods: Quicken the blood and transform stasis, course the liver and regulate the stomach

Formula & medicinals: Radix Angelicae Sinensis (*Dang Gui*), 3 *qian*, Radix Ligustici Wallichii (*Chuan Xiong*), 1 *qian*, Flos Carthami Tincotrii (*Hong Hua*), 1 *qian*, Herba Leonuri Hetrophylli (*Yi Mu Cao*), 1 *qian*, Semen Pruni Persicae (*Tao Ren*), 5 *fen*, mix-fried Radix Glycyrrhizae (*Gan Cao*), 5 *fen*, blast-fried Rhizoma Zingiberis (*Pao Jiang*), 5 *fen*, Radix Bupleuri (*Chai Hu*), 2 *qian*, Radix Scutellariae Baicalensis (*Huang Qin*), 3 *qian*, Rhizoma Pinelliae Ternatae (*Ban Xia*), 3 *qian*, southern Fructus Crataegi (*Nan Shan Zha*), 2 *qian*

Course of treatment: On July 8, 1975, three days after taking these medicinals, the bleeding had already stopped. Intake of food was flavorful [again] and the abdominal and lumbar pains were diminished. She was administered another three *ji* continuously in order to secure the therapeutic effect.

Commentary: Cases #4, #5, and #6 were all vaginal tract bleeding due to incomplete abortion and uterine curettage. They were also able to be treated with *Chan Hou Sheng Hua Tang* with additions and subtractions. In case #4, abdominal pain was severe. [Therefore, this formula] was combined with *Shi Xiao San* (Loose a Smile Powder) and Carthamus, 3 *qian*, to increase and strengthen its action of quickening and breaking the blood. After taking these medicinals, two black clots flowed out, the bleeding immediately stopped, and the abdominal pain was relieved. However, because [the patient's] spleen and stomach were weak, as manifest by loose stool, increased frequency of defecation, and slimy, yellow tongue fur, blast-fried Ginger was changed to dry Ginger and

Atractylodes was added in order to fortify the spleen and warm the center and thus subsequently supplement the qi and fortify the blood.

In case #5, vaginal tract bleeding after uterine curettage had not stopped and the uterus was vacuumed a second time. But still the bleeding had not stopped. This had continued for approximately two months and was accompanied by slight lower abdominal pain, while the pulse was bowstring and choppy. This was categorized as static blood gathering internally with new blood not being calm. [Therefore,] *Chan Hou Sheng Hua Tang* with Flying Squirrel Droppings was used and got the effect.

Case #6 was accompanied by liver-stomach disharmony symptoms. Therefore, Bupleurum, Scutellaria, and Pinellia were added to this formula in order to soothe the liver and harmonze the stomach.

Case 7: Zhao, female, 29 years old, a case of consultant treatment for another hospital, hospitalization No. 162718

Date of initial examination: September 23, 1975

Due to toxemia during pregnancy with twin fetuses, [the patient's] uterus had begun contracting and her waters had broken prematurely 36 hours before. Because the delivery did not progress, she had had a Caesarean section on the morning of Sept. 20. The operation had gone smoothly and bleeding during the operation was 250ml. Her blood pressure was 160/100mmHg after returning to the ward. The postpartum lochia was not profuse but was accompanied by low-grade fever. Her temperature had been approximately 37.9°C for three days already. There was no pain in the abdominal region but there was occasional headache and dizziness. Vaginal tract bleeding was not profuse, the tongue fur was thin and white [*i.e.*, normal], and the pulse was bowstring and slippery.

Western medical diagnosis: Low-grade fever after Caesarean section that is to be examined

Chinese medical pattern discrimination: Blood vacuity and blood stasis, yin vacuity with liver effulgence

Treatment methods: Nourish the blood and transform stasis, enrich yin and level [or calm] the liver

Formula & medicinals: Radix Angelicae Sinensis (*Dang Gui*), 3 *qian*, Radix Ligustici Wallichii (*Chuan Xiong*), 1 *qian*, Herba Leonuri Heterophylli (*Yi Mu Cao*), 2 *qian*, Flos Carthami Tinctorii (*Hong Hua*), 1.5 *qian*, Radix Albus Paeoniae Lactiflorae (*Bai Shao*), 3 *qian*, uncooked Radix Rehmannia (*Sheng Di*), 3 *qian*, Radix Achyranthis Bidentatae (*Niu Xi*), 3 *qian*, Haematitum (*Dai Zhe Shi*), 5 *qian*, uncooked Os Draconis & Concha Ostreae (*Long Mu*), 1 *liang* each

Course of treatment: On September 24, after taking these medicinals, there was no discomfort, the blood pressure was 120/90mmHg, and her vaginal tract bleeding was not profuse. The highest body temperature was 37.5°C and the next day it was normal. By September 28, [the case] was cured and [the patient] was discharged from the hospital.

Commentary: This case can be used to explain the modification of *Chan Hou Sheng Hua Tang* with additions and subtractions. After Caesarean section, [the patient] suffered from low-grade fever and anemia. Before delivery, there was toxemia during pregnancy. After delivery, the blood pressure had only slightly gone down. Occasionally there was headache and dizziness. From the point of view of Chinese medicine, the pattern was categorized as blood vacuity and blood stasis with yin vacuity and liver effulgence. Therefore, *Chan Hou Sheng Hua Tang* was used without blast-fried Ginger, Lycopus, or mix-fried Licorice. [Instead,] White Peony was added to nourish the blood and astringe yin. Uncooked Rehmannia and Achyranthes [were added] to nourish yin and supplement the liver and kidneys and to simultaneously quicken the blood, level the liver, and lead yang to move downward. While Hematite and uncooked Dragon Bone and Oyster Shell [were added] to subdue and settle liver yang. After [taking] these medicinals, the low-grade fever abated and the blood pressure returned to normal.

Case 8: Wang, female, 44 years old, a simple case history in the out-patient department

Date of initial examination: July 8, 1975

[The patient] suffered from vaginal tract bleeding after external injury to the abdominal region in January. After emergency aid to stop bleeding, the volume of blood decreased. [However,] it had occurred intermittently for two months and hemostatic medicinals had to be constantly used. Since that June, her menses had dribbled and dripped without cease for over 40 days. Thus [this bleeding] had continued for four months in total. At this point, the hemostatic prescriptions were no longer effective. She had tried taking *Gui Pi Tang* (Restore the Spleen Decoction) type medicinals without effect. Her symptoms [consisted of] vaginal tract bleeding which was small in volume and dark brown in color with small black clots. There was insidious lower abdominal pain which was fixed in location. Sometimes this pain was related to [the patient's] emotions. Her eating and drinking and her two excretions were normal. Her sleep was not replete and there were profuse dreams. Sometimes she had fright palpitations, heart fluster, shortness of breath, and a tendency to sigh greatly. Her tongue body was dark red with red spots and static macules and scanty fur. Her pulse was deep, fine, and choppy.

Western medical diagnosis: Post-traumatic vaginal tract bleeding, the cause of which is to be examined

Chinese medical pattern discrimination: Static blood obstructing the network vessels, blood not returning to the channels

Treatment methods: Quicken the blood and transform stasis, lead the blood to return to the channels

Formula & medicinals: Radix Angelicae Sinensis (*Dang Gui*), 3 *qian*, Radix Ligustici Wallichii (*Chuan Xiong*), 1 *qian*, Flos Carthami Tinctorii (*Hong Hua*), 1 *qian*, Herba Leonuri Heterophylli (*Yi Mu Cao*), 1 *qian*, Herba Lycopi Lucidi (*Ze Lan*), 1 *qian*, Semen Pruni Persicae (*Xing Ren*), 5 *fen*, Radix Glycyrrhizae (*Gan Cao*), 5 *fen*

Course of treatment: After taking three *ji* of this formula, the vaginal tract bleeding had already stopped. Three more *ji* were administered continuously in order to secure the therapeutic effect and the condition was entirely eliminated. On follow-up on Jan. 5, 1976, there had been no recurrence and her menstruation was normal.

Commentary: This case was caused by external injury. [Thus] static blood was obstructing the uterus and this resulted in unstoppable vaginal tract bleeding which had gone on for a long period [of time]. This [case] did not relate to pregnancy and birth. However, it was due to blood stasis. Therefore, one can use *Chan Hou Sheng Hua Tang* with additions and subtractions [in any case] to treat it, quickening the blood and transforming stasis in order to stop bleeding.

Thus, based on a combination of the above views and the experience of these disease cases, it is clear that the *Chan Hou Sheng Hua Tang* used in the Beijing area suits clinical practice better than the *Sheng Hua Tang* in *Fu Qing Zhu Nu Ke (Fu Qing-zhu's Gynecology)*. Its therapeutic effect is comparatively ideal, its pattern discrimination is accurate, and its application is flexible.

8
Preliminary Observations on the Treatment of Uterine Myoma with *Qin Lian Si Wu Tang* (Scutellaria & Coptis Four Materials Decoction) with Additions & Subtractions

Uterine myomas [a.k.a., uterine fibroids] are one of the commonly-seen benign tumors in gynecology. The onset of this disease mostly occurs between 30-50 years of age. Western medicine mostly uses surgery and hormones to treat it. In Chinese medicine, this is typically categorized as "concretions and conglomerations, accumulations and gatherings." As it is said in "The Treatise on Bone Cavities" in the *Su Wen (Simple Questions)*, "When the *ren mai* is diseased... women [have] concretions and conglomerations below the belt." "The Chapter on Water Distention" in the *Ling Shu (Spiritual Axis)* says:

> If stone conglomerations arise in the uterus, cold qi has lodged in the fetal gate. [Thus] the fetal gate is blocked and obstructed. The qi cannot obtain free flow and malign blood which ought to be drained is not drained. This blood is retained and stopped. Over days it grows and enlarges and in form [the woman] becomes as if pregnant. The menses do not then periodically descend as they ought to.

In "Inquiry [Number] Two of Women's Miscellaneous Diseases" in the *Zhu Bing Yuan Hou Lun (Treatise on the Origins & Symptoms of Various Diseases)*, it says, "The eight conglomerations all are engendered in the uterus by the fetus's engenderment and birth, the coming and going of the menstrual water, and lack of regulation of the blood vessels and essence qi." It also says:

> Women's diseases are different from men's. They are due to postpartum visceral vacuity suffering cold, the comings and goings of the menstrual

water, and excessive choice of chilly [things] but not solely lack of discipline in eating and drinking. Their production is mostly mixed with the blood and qi.

In the *Fu Ren Liang Fang (Fine Formulas for Women)* it says:

> Women's concretions and conglomerations are caused by undisciplined eating and drinking, unregulated cold and warmth, and qi and blood damaged by [over]taxation. The viscera and bowels are vacuous and weak. Wind chill enters the abdomen and binds with the blood and thus they are engendered.

Based on the characteristic symptoms of this disease, it has preliminarily been thought that uterine myomas equal "stony conglomerations."

As to the onset of this disease, it is internally caused by postpartum visceral vacuity and externally by contraction of cold. "Cold qi may lodge in the fetal gate" or "choosing excessively chilly [things]" may result in the fetal gate becoming blocked and obstructed. The qi cannot obtain its free flow and the blood vessels and essence qi do not move. Malign blood is not drained but is retained and stops. Daily these grow and enlarge and result in conglomerations and gatherings. A few years ago, this [view] was reported [in the Chinese medical literature] based on both the ancient and modern literature. Thus the treatment methods and principles for "concretions and conglomerations" and formulas and medicinals for moving the qi, quickening the blood, and transforming stasis, dispersing the hard and scattering binding [*i.e.*, nodulation] were mechanically adhered to [in the treatment of this disease]. [However,] the outcomes were not fully satisfactory.[14]

---

[14] Although what the author says here is clearly and simply stated, it nevertheless should be pointed out that one of the main themes of Dr. Liu's work is that treatment should be based primarily on the patient's actual pattern discrimination and not on some generalized idea about their disease. It is debatable whether uterine myomas which cannot be palpated from outside should be categorized and, therefore, treated in all instances as concretions and conglomerations.

Therefore, in recent years, by further analyzing the main signs and symptoms, such as uterine bleeding, lumbar pain, abdominal pain, and abnormal vaginal discharge, and combining these with the above pathological materials [*i.e.*, theories], [I] have understood by experience what is meant by the saying in "The Treatise on Bone Cavities" in the *Su Wen (Simple Questions)*, "When the *ren mai* is diseased... in women [this results in] conglomerations and gatherings below the belt." [Alternative reading: "When the *ren mai* is diseased...(this results in) abnormal vaginal discharge and conglomerations and gatherings."] It can also be seen from practical cases that most of the patients [with this disease] manifest yin vacuity blood heat, liver-kidney yin deficiency, yin vacuity and liver effulgence, liver-spleen disharmony, and *chong* and *ren* irregularity patterns. It can also be seen that what is called visceral vacuity mainly manifests as depletion detriment and dysfunction of the three viscera of the liver, spleen, and kidneys. Although "cold qi lodged in the fetal gate" is due to blood's having obtained cold and thus congealed, static blood and malign blood congealing and binding and enduring for days contrarily [typically] brews and engenders heat. If due to cold qi damaging the spleen, the spleen's movement will lose its fortification. Dampness will then be engendered internally. If this brews and endures, it can [also] transform into heat.

If static blood and malign blood congeal and gather, are retained and stop, and grow and enlarge daily, one will see swollen lumps in the abdominal region and abdominal pain. If damp heat enters the blood division, it forces the blood to move frenetically. This then leads to the appearance of vaginal tract bleeding. Liver-kidney depletion detriment leads to the appearance of lumbar pain. Liver-spleen disharmony, yin and blood loss of regulation, and heat evils burning and consuming, consume and damage the qi and blood. This leads to *chong* and *ren* irregularity or yin vacuity and liver effulgence. Thus one should not base their treatment solely on the concept of "concretions and conglomerations." Based on the methods and principles of clearing heat and drying dampness, nourishing the blood and regulating the *chong* and *ren*, [I] now mainly use *Qin Lian Si Wu Tang* (Scutellaria & Coptis

Four Materials Decoction) to treat this [disease]. According to preliminary observations, the clinical treatment effect is higher when compared with the previous one. Using this formula and treatment, I have treated 22 cases as analyzed below.

In this group, there were 20 cases between 30-40 years of age. Of the [remaining] two cases, one was 50 years old and the other was 52 years old. Only one case was unmarried. The shortest disease course was one month, while the longest was two and a half years. In 21 cases, the tumor was located in the body of the uterus. In one case, it was located outside the uterine neck [*i.e.,* cervix].

I. Analysis of the clinical signs & symptoms

A. Abdominal region mass: All the patients were examined and a mass was found in the uterus [in all]. The smallest was the size of a walnut, and the largest made the uterus approximately the size of a three month pregnancy.

B. Uterine bleeding: All these patients had abnormal uterine bleeding. Nineteen cases had profuse menstruation. One case had continuous bleeding which had endured for three months. The menses dribbled and dripped without cease in one case. And the menses were scanty in amount in two cases. In those with profuse menstruation, the color [of the blood] was dark red or dark purple and was accompanied by clots.

C. Abnormal vaginal discharge: Six cases had yellow vaginal discharge which was large in volume. One case had a red vaginal discharge.

D. Lumbar & abdominal distention & pain: In 14 cases, there was a self-described [feeling] of lumbar and abdominal downward sagging or menstrual pain.

E. Other [symptoms]: In two cases, there was breast distention and pain. Six cases were complicated by pelvic inflammation. There were two cases of urinary tract infection. And 15 cases had the generalized symptoms of premenstrual tension and climacteric syndrome as well as heart fluster, heart palpitations, vexation and agitation, shortness of breath, lack of strength, and superficial edema.

II. Treatment

Based on the pattern discrimination of the above signs and symptoms, this condition was categorized as blood heat and dampness brewing with *chong* and *ren* irregularity. However, since the constitutional conditions and the accompanying symptoms were not the same, there was also simultaneous yin vacuity, liver-spleen disharmony, liver qi upward counterflow, yin vacuity with yang hyperactivity, and qi and blood dual vacuity patterns.

Treatment principles: Clear heat and disinhibit dampness, nourish the blood and harmonize the blood, regulate and rectify the *chong* and *ren*

Formula & medicinals: Radix Scutellariae Baicalensis (*Huang Qin*), 3 *qian*, Rhizoma Thalictri Foliosi (*Ma Wei Lian*), 3 *qian* (or powdered Rhizoma Coptidis Chinensis, *Huang Lian*, 1 *qian*), uncooked Radix Rehmanniae (*Sheng Di*), 3-5 *qian*, Radix Albus Paeoniae Lactiflorae (*Bai Shao*), 3-5 *qian*, Radix Angelicae Sinensis (*Dang Gui*), 3 *qian*, Radix Ligustici Wallichii (*Chuan Xiong*), 1.5 *qian*

Additions & subtractions following [different] patterns: If there was marked yin vacuity, Radix Scrophulariae Ningpoensis (*Xuan Shen*), Tuber Ophipogoni Japonici (*Mai Dong*), and Herba Ecliptae Prostratae (*Han Lian Cao*) were added. If there was marked cold and dampness, Radix Bupleuri (*Chai Hu*) and Herba Seu Flos Schizonepetae Tenuifoliae (*Jing Jie Sui*) were added. If there was marked kidney vacuity, Radix Dipsaci (*Chuan Duan*), Semen Cuscutae Chinensis (*Tu Si Zi*), cooked Radix Rehmanniae (*Shu Di*), and Semen Nelumbinis Nuciferae (*Shi Lian*) were added. If there was relatively [more] severe blood heat and profuse bleeding (or irregular bleeding), Dang Gui and Ligusticum Wallichium were removed and Cortex Radicis Lycii Chinensis (*Di Gu Pi*), Herba Artemisiae Apiaceae (*Qing Hao*), Cortex Cedrelae (*Chun Gen Pi*), Os Sepiae Seu Sepiellae (*Wu Zei Gu*), and uncooked Concha Ostreae (*Mu Li*) were added. If there was unstoppable bleeding, carbonized Cacumen Biotae Orientalis (*Ce Bai*), carbonized Fibra Stipulae Trachycarpi (*Zong Lu*), carbonized Rhizoma Guanchong (*Guan Zhong*), and Gelatinum Corii Asini (*E Jiao*) were added. If there was headache and dizziness [due to] marked liver effulgence, Folium Mori Albi (*Sang Ye*), Flos Chrysanthemi Morifolii (*Ju Hua*), Fructus Ligustri Lucidi (*Nu Zhen Zi*), Herba Ecliptae Prostratae (*Han Lian Cao*), uncooked Dens Draconis (*Long Chi*), and Concha Margaritiferae (*Zhen Zhu Mu*) were added. If there was marked spleen vacuity, Radix Pseudostellariae (*Tai Zi Shen*), Semen Nelumbinis Nuciferae (*Lian Zi*), and Rhizoma Atractylodis Macrocephalae (*Bai Zhu*) were added. If there was damp heat pouring downward, Herba Dianthi (*Qu Mai*), Semen Plantaginis (*Che Qian Zi*), and Caulis Akebiae Mutong (*Mu Tong*) were added. If there was marked aching and pain due to qi stagnation, Fructus Meliae Tosendan (*Chuan Lian Zi*), Rhizoma Corydalis Yanhusuo (*Yan Hu Suo*), Feces Trogopterori Seu Pteromi (*Wu Ling Zhi*), and Rhizoma Cyperi Rotundi (*Xiang Fu*) were added.

III. Treatment outcomes

Among these 22 cases, the shortest course of treatment was five days and the longest was five months. The smallest number of medicinals administered was five *ji* and the largest was 100 *ji*. In terms of the whole condition [*i.e.*, generalized symptoms], abdominal uterine bleeding was controlled and the clinical symptoms were improved in all [cases]. Through examination of the local condition, no myoma was found to have developed [further], while in one individual it had gotten somewhat smaller. In terms of improvement of the main symptoms, 13 out of the 19 cases of profuse menstruation returned to normal, while the volume of blood decreased in the [other] six cases. Thirteen cases of the 14 cases of menstrual movement enduring for days [*i.e.*, prolonged menstruation] returned to normal, while the duration of the menstrual movement in the [other] cases shortened. Two out of 14 cases of lumbar and abdominal pain [saw that pain] disappear, while in the [other] 12 cases, it markedly decreased. Five out of the six cases of profuse abdominal vaginal discharge returned to normal, and the amount of discharge in the [other] one case decreased. [Therefore,] in terms of the total outcomes, the improvement in clinical symptoms was relatively marked, while the disappearance or decrease in size of the uterine myomas was not marked. This may be due to the short time of observation or the formula and medicinals may need further adjustment.[15]

IV. Typical case

Ma, female, 51 years old, a simple case history in the out-patient department

Date of initial examination: May 26, 1973

In the last two years, [the patient] had suffered from irregular vaginal tract bleeding. In one month, profusely voluminous vaginal bleeding had occurred for half the month. Four times in the past she had hemorrhaged greatly. Based on gynecological examination, this was called [*i.e.*, diagnosed as] uterine myoma. The last menstruation had occurred on Apr. 19. This was accompanied by shortness of breath, lower leg flaccidity, a dry mouth, heat in the centers of the hands and feet [alternate reading: heat in the hands, feet, and heart], and oppression in the chest and venter [*i.e.*, epigastrium]. Compared to before, the vaginal tract bleeding was not excessive. An endometrial examination had occurred on Aug. 28, 1972 and there was said to be

---

[15] These outcomes are not as successful as some published on uterine myomas in the Chinese medical literature but are consistent with Bob Flaws's experience in treating Western patients over the last 17 years.

cystic hyperplasia of the endometrium. A gynecological examination had occurred on Sept. 22, 1972. [This revealed] a small amount of blood in the vaginal tract and two small polyps on the uterine mouth. The anterior of the uterus was as large as an eight week pregnancy and its body as hard. Its surface was level. [In terms of] both sides of the uterus, the right side was slightly purple while the left side was negative. This was diagnosed as early stage uterine myoma with uterine cervical polyps. [The patient] came to the out-patient department of our hospital on May 26, 1973. [At that time,] there was seen irregular vaginal tract bleeding which was profuse in amount and contained large blood clots. There was lumbar pain, generalized lack of strength, heart fluster, and shortness of breath. Examination of the uterus [showed it to be] approximately like a 10 week pregnancy. The tongue was pale red with dry, yellow fur, and the pulse was bowstring, slippery, and rapid.

Western medical diagnosis: A).Uterine myoma; B) cervical polyps

Chinese medical pattern discrimination: Blood heat and dampness brewing, *chong* and *ren* irregularity

Treatment methods: Clear heat and disinhibit damp, cool the blood and secure the *chong*

Formula & medicinals: Radix Scutellariae Baicalensis (*Huang Qin*), 3 *qian*, Rhizoma Thalictri Foliosi (*Ma Wei Lian*), 3 *qian*, Radix Angelicae Sinensis (*Dang Gui*), 3 *qian*, Radix Ligustici Wallichii (*Chuan Xiong*), 1.5 *qian*, cooked Radix Rehmanniae (*Shu Di*), 4 *qian*, Radix Albus Paeoniae Lactiflorae (*Bai Shao*), 3 *qian*, Herba Eecliptae Prostratae (*Han Lian Cao*), 4 *qian*, Gelatinum Corii Asini (*E Jiao*), 5 *qian*, carbonized Cacumen Biotae Orientalis (*Ce Bai*), 4 *qian*, carbonized Radix Sanguisorbae (*Di Yu*), 4 *qian*, Cortex Cedrelae (*Chun Gen Bai Pi*), 4 *qian*, Os Sepiae Seu Sepiellae (*Wu Zei Gu*), 4 *qian*, carbonized Rhizoma Guanchong (*Guan Zhong*), 4 *qian*

Course of treatment: On May 29, 1973, after taking three *ji* of the above formula, the vaginal tract bleeding was markedly decreased. However, the chest and venter oppression and devitalized intake of food were still seen. [Therefore,] carbonized Guanchong and carbonized Biota were removed from the above formula and Radix Auklandiae Lappae (*Mu Xiang*), 1 *qian*, and Fructus Amomi (*Sha Ren*), 5 *fen*, were added, [the latter ingredient taken] washed down [with the decoction]. On Jun. 1, 1973, there was self-described stomach venter [*i.e.,* epigastric] distention but desire for food had taken a turn for the better. [Thus] administration of the above formula was continued.

On July 6, 1973, on re-examination, it was said that the menses were still profuse and that menstruation had moved [*i.e.,* had lasted] for nine days. There were ulcers on the mouth and lips, the tongue was red with dry, yellow fur, and the pulse was bowstring and rapid. [Therefore,] the following formula and medicinals [were prescribed]: Radix Scutellariae Baicalensis (*Huang Qin*), 3 *qian*, Rhizoma Thalictri Foliosi (*Ma Wei Lian*), 3 *qian*, Radix Angelicae Sinensis (*Dang Gui*), 3 *qian*, Radix Ligustici Wallichii (*Chuan Xiong*), 1.5 *qian*, uncooked Radix Rehmanniae (*Sheng Di*), 4 *qian*, Radix Albus Paeoniae Lactiflorae (*Bai Shao*), 3 *qian*, Herba Ecliptae Prostratae (*Han Lian Cao*), 4 *qian*, Gelatinum Corii Asini (*E Jiao*), 3 *qian*, Os Sepiae Seu Sepiellae (*Wu Zei Gu*), 4 *qian*, Radix Glehniae Littoralis (*Sha Shen*), 5 *qian*, Radix Pseudostellariae (*Tai Zi Shen*), 3 *qian*

On re-examination on Jun. 15, 1973, [it was said that] the last menstruation had occurred on May 20 and had lasted 7-8 days with clots. On that day, the menstruation had come [again] and was small in volume with insidious pain in the lower abdomen. There was lack of strength, fatigue, a red tongue body with white fur, and a bowstring, slippery pulse. [Therefore,] Glehnia and Pseudostellaria were subtracted from the above formula and carbonized Cacumen Biotae Orientalis (*Ce Bai*), 3 *qian*, carbonized Rhizoma Guanchong (*Guan Zhong*), 3 *qian*, carbonized Radix Sanguisorbae (*Di Yu*), 3 *qian*, and Cortex Cedrelae (*Chun Gen Bai Pi*), 3 *qian*, were added along with powdered Radix Pseudoginseng (*San Qi*), 5 *fen*, taken washed down [with the decoction].

99

On Jun. 29, after taking three *ji* of the above formula, the abdominal pain had already stopped. The menses had moved for five days and their amount was normal. The tongue was slightly fat, but the fur was thin and white. The pulse was bowstring. The formulas and medicinals were as [follows] below: Radix Scutellariae Baicalensis (*Huang Qin*), 3 *qian*, Rhizoma Thalictri Foliosi (*Ma Wei Lian*), 3 *qian*, Radix Angelicae Sinensis (*Dang Gui*), 3 *qian*, Radix Ligustici Wallichii (*Chuan Xiong*), 1.5 *qian*, cooked Radix Rehmanniae (*Shu Di*), 4 *qian*, Radix Albus Paeoniae Lactiflorae (*Bai Shao*), 3 *qian*, Herba Ecliptae Prostratae (*Han Lian Cao*), 4 *qian*, Gelatinum Corii Asini (*E Jiao*), 5 *qian*, Cortex Cedrelae (*Chun Gen Bai Pi*), 4 *qian*.

On Oct. 25, [the patient] was re-examined and the above formula's administration was continued. In August and September, the menstruation came twice normally. On Oct. 22, the menstruation came, the amount of the menses was not profuse, but its color was black. It had already moved for four days and there was heart fluster and heart vexation. However, there was no other obvious discomfort. The tongue was red with yellow-white fur. The above formula was continued after removing Cedrela and adding Tuber Ophiopogonis Japonici (*Mai Dong*), 3 *qian*, Fructus Schisandrae Chinensis (*Wu Wei Zi*), 3 *qian*, and carbonized Fibra Stipulae Trachycarpi (*Zong Lu*), 3 *qian*. On re-examination on Dec. 25, it was said that the gynecological examination at the original hospital on Nov. 12 had found that the uterus had shrunk smaller to approximately the size of a six week pregnancy. Compared to how the volume of menses was profuse originally before, the present menstrual cycle was accurate [*i.e.*, on target], the volume of menses and the date for the beginning of the menstruation being normal. *Qin Lian Si Wu Tang* with added Cortex Cedrelae (*Chun Gen Bai Pi*), Os Sepiae Seu Sepiellae (*Wu Zei Gu*), Herba Ecliptae Prostratae (*Han Lian Cao*), and Gelatinum Corii Asini (*E Jiao*) was continuously administered to secure the therapeutic effect.

Knowledge gained based on this experience:[16]

The onset of this disease from the point of view of the condition was due to loss of regularity in the function of the three viscera of the liver, spleen, and kidneys plus, as an external cause, "cold qi" having lodged in the fetal gate. Static blood had congealed and bound. This had brewed and endured and transformed into heat. This had then combined with internal dampness. Malign blood had been retained and stopped and this had grown and increased daily [eventually resulting in] the onset of this disease. Therefore, in treating the above, the methods of quickening the blood, transforming stasis, and dispersing concretions that simply addresses local concretions and lumps had to be modified. Based on the whole condition and the principles of clearing heat and drying dampness, nourishing the blood and harmonizing the blood, and regulating and rectifying the *chong* and *ren*, *Qin Lian Si Wu Tang* was selected as the main [formula] with additions and subtractions following the condition. Regulation of viscera and bowel function resulted in promoting the improvement of the integrated functioning of the whole body. Thus the clinical symptoms improved, the local swelling of substance was controlled and somewhat reduced, and the treatment effect was high. This offers a new clue for further steps in the treatment of this disease.

---

[16] The term *ti hui* is a difficult one to translate in one or two words. *The Pinyin Chinese-English Dictionary*, The Commercial Press, Beijing & Hong Kong, 1991, defines it as knowledge from experience or what one has learned from experience.

9
Knowledge Based on Experience
in the Clinical Application of Bupleurum

Radix Bupleuri (*Chai Hu*) is bitter in flavor and level [*i.e.*, even] in nature [or temperature]. It enters the two channels of the liver and gallbladder. Its function is to harmonize, resolve, and abate fever. It soothes the liver and resolves depression, upbears and lifts yang qi. In clinic, its application is relatively wide. However, due to its disadvantage of "upbearing and scattering ", there are some people who will not use it at all or others who are too cautious to dare to use it in large amounts. I have also [in the past] experienced this negative psychological state in clinic. The main reason is that I had not grasped well Bupleurum's characteristic functions, its scope of application, its combination [with other medicinals], and its dosages. Most gynecological diseases are caused by [disorders of] the qi and blood, and, therefore, the opportunities for using Bupleurum are many. My initial knowledge based on experience is that what is called Bupleurum's disadvantage of "upbearing and scattering" is simply the effectiveness of its charac-teristic function of upbearing and emitting. The key [to its use] lies in grasping well the conditions for which it is suitable and the amount to use.

Because its flavor is acrid and its nature is level [*i.e.*, even or neutral], it is able to upbear and emit, course and scatter. This is the mechanism for the *shao yang's* pivotal conduction, dispelling evils and exiting [them] externally. Therefore, it is able to harmonize, resolve, and abate fever [or recede heat]. Because of its function of upbearing and emitting the yang qi, the qi mechanism orderly reaches. Therefore, it is able to soothe the liver and resolve depression, course the qi and regulate the channels [or menses]. In addition, this has the indirect action of boosting the qi, harmonizing the exterior and out-thrusting, coursing and freeing the flow of the channels and network vessels qi and blood, and harmonizing and regulating the fluids and humors. It is able to emit [the sweat] when there is no perspiration, while it is able to astringe [the sweat] when there is perspiration. Because it can upbear and emit, course and regulate, it cannot only upbear yang and boost the stomach, it assists the movement and lifting of the center in order to enable the middle burner to upbear and scatter damp obstruction, transforming dampness and making this into fluids and humors. Therefore, it is able to stop abnormal vaginal discharge.

Bupleurum is basically a qi division[17] medicinal. It enters the qi division and is able to course the qi and resolve depression, thus using the qi to treat the blood. In other words, it frees the flow and regulates the qi, thus treating blood division diseases. Since it also enters the foot *jue yin* liver channel and the liver is the blood viscus, therefore, it also enters the blood division, moving the qi within the blood. Depending on its different combinations, it is able to either dispel and scatter cold within the blood or push and stir depressive heat within the blood, out-thrusting this and resolving it externally. Thus it can be seen that the scope of [Bupleurum's] application is extraordinarily wide. Hence it is said in the *Ben Cao Chong Xin (Newly Revised Materia Medica)*, Bupleurum is able to:

> ...diffuse and smooth the flow of the qi and blood, scatter binding [or nodulation] and regulate the channels [or menses]... It treats cold damage and evil heat, phlegm heat binding and repletion, vexatious heat below the heart, all malaria-like cold and heat [*i.e.*, fevers and chills], dizziness and vomiting, red eyes, chest glomus, rib-side pain, a bitter [taste in the] mouth, and deafness.

---

[17] Wiseman suggests aspect for the Chinese *fen*. The Chinese character shows a knife dividing something in two. Therefore, we prefer the word division over aspect since it more clearly retains all the meanings of the Chinese no matter whether this word is used as a verb or a noun.

In terms of the dosage of Bupleurum, if it is being used to dispel evils and resolve heat, 3-4 *qian* are ok. If it is being used to resolve depression and upbear yang, 1-1.5 *qian* are sufficient. This refers to making use of this medicinal's nature in order to lead medicinals into the channels. If the amount is too large, it cannot be appropriate.

In regards to the clinical applications of the combinations of Bupleurum, my knowledge based on experience is described under the following headings.

1. [Bupleurum's] aspect of harmonizing, resolving & abating fever

The reason why Bupleurum is able to abate fever [or recede heat] is due to its acrid flavor. This has the function of acridly scattering, coursing, and resolving. Because its nature is level [or temperature is neutral] and depending on its different combinations, its ability to resolve heat mainly pertains to *shao yang* channel heat. The formulas and prescriptions which resolve heat in which Bupleurum is the main [ingredient] are as follows:

Xiao Chai Hu Tang (Minor Bupleurum Decoction) ([composed of] Radix Bupleuri, *Chai Hu,* Radix Scutellariae Baicalensis, *Huang Qin,* uncooked Rhizoma Zingiberis, *Sheng Jiang,* Rhizoma Pinelliae Ternatae, *Ban Xia,* Radix Panacis Ginseng, *Ren Shen,* Radix Glycyrrhizae, *Gan Cao,* and Fructus Zizyphi Jujubae, *Da Zao*) is the main formula in Zhang Zhongjing's *Shan Han Lun (Treatise on Damage [Due to] Cold)* for treating *shao yang* damage by cold. The *shao yang* is the initial engenderment of yang. "The *shao yang* is the pivot" means that it is the pivot for conduction [or transmission of evils]. The *shao yang* channel and network vessels lie neither in the exterior or interior. Rather, they are half-exterior and half-interior. Therefore, they are the pivot for the conduction of the channels and network vessels. They can channel and network with the internal and the external. The *shao yang* governs the gallbladder and the three burners. The three burners govern disease engendered by qi. If qi and blood are vacuous and weak, the interstices will be loose. If cold damage disease evils assail, they may depart from the *tai yang* to lodge in the *shao yang*. Therefore, the *shao yang* channels and network vessels' pivotal conduction become inhibited. [The evils] are not able to be out-thrust and it is difficult for them to enter internally. Thus disease evils are retained in the *shao yang*.

In clinic, the *shao yang* pattern which is seen is not as regular and typical as that described in the *Shang Han Lun (Treatise on Damage [Due to] Cold)* where it says, "In damage by cold, day one righteous yang [*i.e., tai yang*] suffers; day two, the *yang ming* suffers; day three, the *shao yang* suffers..." If external evils assail and enter, righteous and evils will struggle with each other, binding underneath the side of the ribs. The main type of heat [or fever] is alternating cold [*i.e.*, chills] and heat [*i.e.*, fever]. This is accompanied by the symptoms of chest and rib-side bitterness [*i.e.*, pain] and fullness, heart vexation, tendency to vomit, no desire to eat or drink, a bitter [taste in the] mouth, dry throat, veritgo, etc. In this case, Bupleurum is the main medicinal to harmonize and resolve the *shao yang*, upbear yang and out-thrust the exterior. It leads evils to be exited externally and restores the function of pivotal conduction.

When [Bupleurum] is combined with Ginseng, [these two] support the righteous in order to out-thrust evils and exit them externally. [When combined with] Scutellaria, [these two] clear heat and discharge half-interior heat from the *shao yang*. Therefore, it is said in "The Discrimination of *Yang Ming* Diseases, Pulses & Patterns and Their Treatment Methods" in the *Shang Han Lun (Treatise on Damage [Due to] Cold)*, "By using *Xiao Chai Hu Tang*, the upper burner obtains free flow, fluids and humors obtain descent, the stomach qi is harmonized, the body immediately exits sweat, and [the condition] is resolved." Therefore, it can be seen that, after administration of *Xiao Chai Hu Tang*, perspiration is obtained and the disease is resolved. However, this is not due to Bupleurum's function of emitting sweat. Rather, it is due to "the upper burner obtaining free flow, the fluids and humors obtaining descent, and the stomach qi being harmonized." This is why it is said that *Xiao Chai Hu Tang* is a harmonizing, resolving, abating fever prescription, and it is not able to be used as a diaphoretic prescription.

Da Chai Hu Tang (Major Bupleurum Decoction) ([composed of] Radix Bupleuri, *Chai Hu*, Radix Scutellariae Baicalensis, *Huang Qin*, Radix Albus Paeoniae Lactiflorae, *Shao Yao*, Rhizoma Pinelliae Ternatae, *Ban Xia*, uncooked Rhizoma Zingiberis, *Sheng Jiang*, Fructus Immaturus Citri Aurantii, *Zhi Shi*, Fructus Zizyphi Jujubae, *Da Zao*, and Radix Et Rhizoma Rhei, *Da Huang*) is made up from a combination of *Xiao Chai Hu Tang* and *Xiao Cheng Qi Tang* (Minor Order the Qi Decoction) with additions and subtractions. It is mainly for treating simultaneous *shao yang* and *yang ming* disease. Its action is to externally resolve the *shao yang* and internally discharge heat binding. In "The Discrimination *Tai Yang* Diseases, Pulse, & Patterns and Treatment Methods" in the *Shang Han Lun (Treatise on Damage [Due to] Cold)*, "If there is damage due to cold of more than 10 days [duration], heat has bound in the interior, and there is recurrent alternating cold and heat, use *Da Chai Hu Tang*." This explains that there are not only the symptoms of a *Xiao Chai Hu Tang* pattern but also heat bound in the interior. Therefore, there must be lack of free flow of the stools, the tongue fur is dry, and there is thirst and a desire for chilled drinks. This is categorized as a *shao yang-yang ming* simultaneous disease. From the clinical point of view presented above, there does not necessarily have to be stomach and intestinal dryness and binding if there is interior heat. However, only if there are symptoms of interior heat, is it ok to use *Da Chai Hu Tang*.

In terms of its composition, Ginseng and Licorice are removed from *Xiao Chai Hu Tang* (if there is interior heat, supplementing the qi will strengthen this heat) and Rhubarb, Immature Aurantium, and White Peony are added. Within [this formula], Rhubarb and Immature Aurantium discharge the interior and clear heat, thus ridding interior heat by resolving internally. Bupleurum still restores the *shao yang's* function of pivotal conduction, thus ridding heat via external resolution.

Xiao Cheng Qi Tang discharges the interior. Hence both exterior and interior are resolved.

Chai Hu Gui Zhi Tang (Bupleurum & Cinnamom Twig Decoction) ([is composed of] Radix Bupleuri, *Chai Hu*, Ramulus Cinnamomi Cassiae, *Gui Zhi*, Radix Albus Paeoniae Lactiflorae, *Shao Yao*, Radix Scutellariae Baicalensis, *Huang Qin*, Radix Panacis Ginseng, *Ren Shen*, Radix Glycyrrhizae, *Gan Cao*, Rhizoma Pinelliae Ternatae, *Ban Xia*, Fructus Zizyphi Jujubae, *Da Zao*, and uncooked Rhizoma Zingiberis, *Sheng Jiang*). It is used in "The Discrimination of *Tai Yang* Diseases, Pulses & Patterns and Their Treatment Methods" in the *Shang Han Lun (Treatise on Damage [Due to] Cold)* [where it says], "If there is damage due to cold for six or seven days with fever, slight aversion to cold, limb joint vexatious aching, slight vomiting, branch binding below the heart, this is an external pattern which has not been dispelled." This pattern is categorized as *tai yang-shao yang* simultaneous disease. Within this formula, Bupleurum emits and scatters the *shao yang*, while Cinnamon Twigs open the *tai yang*, thus regulating and harmonizing the constructive and defensive.

Chai Ge Jie Ji Tang (Bupleurum & Pueraria Resolve the Muscles Decoction) ([is composed of] Radix Bupleuri, *Chai Hu*, Radix Puerariae, *Ge Gen*, Radix Glycyrrhizae, *Gan Cao*, Radix Scutellariae Baicalensis, *Huang Qin*, Radix Et Rhizoma Notopterygii, *Qiang Huo*, Radix Angelicae Dahuricae, *Bai Zhi*, Radix Albus Paeoniae Lactiflorae, *Shao Yao*, Radix Platycodi Grandiflori, *Jie Geng*, uncooked Gypsum Fibrosum, *Shi Gao*, uncooked Rhizoma Zingiberis, *Sheng Jiang*, and Fructus Zizyphi Jujubae, *Da Zao*). It treats *shao yang* pattern and simultaneous *yang ming* pattern. Pueraria resolves the muscles and clears heat arising in the exterior of the *yang ming*. Based on this foundation, Bupleurum is able to give full play to its functions of coursing and resolving, thus out-thrusting evils and exiting them externally. The exterior of the *tai yang* is located in the skin and hair. The exterior of the *yang ming* is located in the interstices of the flesh. Uncooked Gypsum resolves heat in the interstices of the flesh by clearing heat and engendering fluids. Bupleurum and Pueraria combined upbear, scatter, and out-thrust. Bupleurum and uncooked Gyspum combined together course and resolve and clear heat.

The above two formulas are the ones to treat simultaneous disease of the *tai yang* and *shao yang* and the *shao yang* and *yang ming* [respectively]. In them, Bupleurum is able to perform the function of lightly diffusing, coursing, and resolving. However, if there were no Cinnamon Twig to regulate and harmonize the constructive and defensive, it would be hard to out-thrust external evils from the *tai yang*. While if there were no Pueraria to resolve the muscles, course and free the flow of external evils, Bupleurum could not play its role. And if there were no uncooked Gypsum to clear the qi and resolve the muscles, it would be difficult to disperse interior heat. Hence it is necessary to combine Bupleurum [with other medicinals] in order that its functions may be fully displayed.

Jing Fang Bai Du San (Schizonepeta & Ledebouriella Vanquish Toxins Powder) ([composed of] Radix Et Rhizoma Notopetrygii, *Qiang Huo*, Radix Angelicae Pubescentis, *Du Huo*, Radix Bupleuri, *Chai Hu*, Radix Peucedani, *Qian Hu*, Fructus Citri Aurantii, *Zhi Ke*, Sclerotium Poriae Cocos, *Fu Ling*, Herba Seu Flos Schizonepetae Tenuifoliae, *Jing Jie Sui*, Radix Ledebouriellae Divaricatae, *Fang Feng*, Radix Platycodi Grandiflori, *Jie Geng*, Radix Ligustici Wallichii, *Chuan Xiong*, and Radix Glycyrrhizae, *Gan Cao*) is made from *Ren Shen Bai Du San* (Ginseng Vanquish Toxins Powder) minus Ginseng and plus Schizonepeta and Ledebouriella. In clinic, this is mostly used for aversion to cold, fever, and cough of an external contraction exterior cold pattern. Schizonepeta and Ledebouriella are the root of this formula's acridly and warmly resolving the exterior. They can dispel evils and exit them externally. If Bupleurum's upbearing and scattering is placed therein, this can strengthen Schizonepeta and Ledebouriella's function of out-thrusting evils and exiting them externally. Schizonepeta scatters the exterior of the *tai yang*, while Ledebouriella dispels the exterior of the *yang ming*. Bupleurum harmonizes and resolves *shao yang* evils. Thus all three, *tai yang, yang ming*, and *shao yang*, are resolved. They acridly scatter but do not strengthen heat, and they scatter cold but do not damage the righteous.

Si Ni San (Four Counterflows Powder) ([composed of] Radix Bupleuri, *Chai Hu,* Fructus Citri Aurantii, *Zhi Ke,* Radix Glycyrrhizae, *Gan Cao,* and Radix Albus Paeoniae Lactiflorae, *Shao Yao*) contains within it Bupleurum. It mainly treats heat reversal. Due to channel conduction, heat evils fall into the interior and yang qi becomes depressed internally. It is thus not able to out-thrust externally to the four limbs. Therefore, the four limbs emit coolness [*i.e.,* are cool to the touch]. This is due to heat evils, but its clinical manifestations are reversal and counterflow of the four limbs. This is a false image. Within [this formua], Bupleurum's function is to harmonize and resolve the *shao yang,* thus restoring pivotal conduction and qi transformation. This results in the ability to out-thrust depressive heat. When combined together, Bupleurum and Aurantium can upbear the clear and downbear the turbid, course the liver and rectify the spleen. When the *shao yang* obtains pivotal conduction, the liver and spleen are automatically regulated. This leads to depressive heat being out-thrust and heat reversal is automatically cured. Although this formula comes from the chapter [of the *Shang Han Lun*] on *shao yang* disease, it actually uses medicinals for the *shao yang* and *yang ming.*

Sheng Yang San Huo Tang (Upbear Yang & Scatter Fire Decoction) (a Li Dong-yuan formula [composed of] Radix Bupleuri, *Chai Hu,* Radix Puerariae, *Ge Gen,* Radix Et Rhizoma Notopterygii, *Qiang Huo,* Radix Ledebouriellae Divaricatae, *Fang Feng,* Radix Angelicae Pubescentis, *Du Huo,* Radix Panacis Ginseng, *Ren Shen,* Radix Albus Paeoniae Lactiflorae, *Bai Shao,* mix-fried Radix Glycyrrhizae, *Gan Cao,* uncooked Rhizoma Zingiberis, *Sheng Jiang,* and Fructus Zizyphi Jujubae, *Da Zao*) is a formula which treats fire depression. In the *Nei Jing (Inner Classic)* it says, "Strong fire eats qi; qi eats lesser fire." In terms of strong fire, one can use bitter, cold, heat-clearing [medicinals] straightforwardly. In terms of lesser fire, because it is mostly engendered in the two channels of the liver and gallbladder, if liver qi has a surplus, it is able to engender fire. If lesser fire becomes depressed and accumulates internally and is not able to be scattered and emitted, it may manifest red eyes, headache, a bitter [taste in the] mouth, and other such symptoms of depressive heat. This type of heat cannot [be treated] straight-forwardly by bitter, cold [medicinals]. Therefore, Bupleurum is the main medicinal used to course the liver and scatter fire. Notopterygium and Ledebouriella scatter and emit *tai yang* fire. Cimicifuga [*sic*] and Pueraria upbear and emit *yang ming* fire. Angelica Pubescens scatters and emits *shao yang* fire. Ginseng and Licorice are added to supplement the center in order to discharge fire. White Peony discharges the liver and restrains the spleen. Thus there is supplementing in the midst of scattering and restraining in the midst of emitting. This results in depressive fire obtaining emission and scattering, while qi sufficiency obtains the erosion of fire. Hence, fire depression is automatically resolved. This is a typical formula of the method of using heat [*i.e.*, warm medicinals] to treat heat. [However,] it is prohibited to use this for replete heat patterns.

From the point of view of the above-mentioned formulas and prescriptions, Bupleurum mainly courses and resolves *shao yang* heat. However, when it is combined [with other medicinals], such as Bupleurum, Scutellaria and Ginseng, Bupleurum and Rhubarb, Bupleurum and Pueraria, Bupleurum and Cinnamon Twig, Bupleurum, Schizonepeta, and Ledebouriella, it can course and resolve the *shao yang* and the *yang ming*, the *shao yang* and the *tai yang*, or all three yang together when disease is due to external contraction with fever. Hence its scope of application is relatively wide. In addition, *Si Ni San* and *Sheng Yang San Huo Tang* contain Bupleurum within them in order to promote coursing, resolving, and out-thrusting heat evils which have fallen into the interior, yang qi depressed internally, or qi depression which has transformed into fire. By upbearing and scattering this, it is able to resolve this heat reversal or fire depression. This is another aspect of Bupleurum's resolving of heat. From a clinical point of view, in the pattern of fire reversal which *Si Ni San* mainly treats, the power of heat is relatively more exuberant than in the fire depression pattern.

Therefore, when using this [formula] it is important to grasp well its appropriate pattern if this formula is to be able to manifest its effect.

2. [Bupleurum's] aspect of soothing the qi & regulating menstruation

Menstrual diseases are mostly caused by loss of regularity in the function of the liver, spleen, and kidneys, the qi and blood, and the *chong* and *ren*, and this, [in turn,] is mostly due to emotional depression, fatigue and taxation beyond measure, and lack of discipline in bedroom affairs [*i.e.*, sex]. Bupleurum has the action of soothing the liver and regulating the qi. It is a qi division medicinal, but it is also able to enter the blood division and move the qi within the blood. Within the qi division, it is able to regulate the blood, while, within the blood division, it is also able to regulate the qi. Therefore, it can be used to course the qi and, [therefore,] treat blood diseases. When regulating and rectifying the menses, Bupleurum is usually combined with or goes to make up the formula. The commonly used formulas [for this purpose] are as follows below:

Xiao Chai Hu Tang (Minor Bupleurum Decoction): In "The Discrimination of *Tai Yang* Diseases, Pulses, Patterns & Their Treatment Methods" in the *Shang Han Lun (Treatise on Damage [Due to] Cold)*, it says:

> In women with wind stroke with cold and heat [*i.e.*, fever and chills] which have continued for seven or eight days with a [definite] peridocity for their occurrence, the menstrual water may be cut off. This is due to heat entering the blood chamber. The blood must necessarily have become bound. Therefore, there are malaria-like symptoms which occur at [definite] times. *Xiao Chai Hu Tang* rules this.

This explains that, for heat entering the blood chamber with blood binding internally, one must necessarily use *Xiao Chai Hu Tang* to harmonize the blood, scatter binding [or nodulation], and regulate the menses. From the clinical point of view, *Xiao Chai Hu Tang* is not only able to treat heat entering the blood chamber resulting in blood bindng, it can also treat heat entering the blood chamber resulting in flooding and leaking. [In other words,] it is important to use *Xiao Chai Hu Tang* whenever its pattern appears. Of course, it is essential that additions and subtractions be made following the [patient's] condition. Since Bupleurum is able to course and resolve heat in the *shao yang* gallbladder channel, and since the liver and gallbladder have an interior-exterior [relationship] and the *jue* yin vessel networks with the yin organs [*i.e.*, genitalia], Bupleurum is able to push outward heat in the blood chamber associated with the *jue yin* channnel via the *shao yang*. When heat is dispelled, flooding and leaking automatically stop.

Chai Hu Si Wu Tang (Bupleurum Four Materials Decoction): In this formula, Radix Angelicae Sinensis (*Dang Gui*), Radix Albus Paeoniae Lactiflorae (*Bai Shao*), Radix Ligustici Wallichii (*Chuan Xiong*), and uncooked Radix Rehmanniae (*Sheng Di*) nourish and harmonize the blood. Radix Scutellariae Baicalensis (*Huang Qin*) clears heat and quiets the *chong*. Radix Bupleuri (*Chai Hu*) soothes the liver, resolves depression, and regulates the menses. One can use this formula with additions and subtractions in order to treat uterine myomas categorized as blood heat.

Ding Jing Tang (Stabilize Menstruation Decoction)([composed of] Radix Bupleuri, *Chai Hu*, Herba Seu Flos Schizonepetae Tenuifoliae, *Jing Jie Sui*, Radix Angelicae Sinensis, *Dang Gui*, cooked Radix Rehmanniae, *Sheng Di*, Radix Albus Paeonies Lactiflorae, *Bai Shao*, Semen Cuscutae Chinensis, *Tu Si Zi*, Radix Dioscoreae Oppositae, *Shan Yao*, and Sclerotium Poriae Cocos, *Fu Ling*) is a commonly-used formula for treating menstruation which is [sometimes] early, [sometimes] late, [and comes at] no fixed schedule due to loss of regularity in the function of the three viscera of the liver, spleen, and kidneys. Within this formula, Bupleurum and Schizonepeta are the ruling [or main] medicinals which soothe the liver and regulate the qi, upbear yang and eliminate dampness, and scatter depression and binding in the liver channel.

113

Cooked Rehmannia, White Peony, and Dang Gui nourish the blood and emolliate the liver. Dioscorea and Poria fortify the spleen and eliminate dampness. When the spleen's movement function is normal, the engenderment and transformation of qi and blood has a source. Cuscuta, Dioscorea, and cooked Rehmannia supplement the kidneys. If the kidney qi is sufficient, the *chong* and *ren* are secure [or securing] and the menses are automatically regulated.

De Sheng Dan (Obtaining Life [*i.e.*, Birth] Elixir) ([composed of] Radix Angelicae Sinensis, *Dang Gui*, Radix Albus Paeoniae Lactiflorae, *Bai Shao*, Radix Ligustici Wallichii, *Chuan Xiong*, Fructus Citri Aurantii, *Zhi Ke*, Radix Bupleuri, *Chai Hu*, Radix Auklandiae Lappae, *Mu Xiang*, Radix Et Rhizoma Notopterygii, *Qiang Huo*, and Herba Leonuri Heterophylli, *Yi Mu Cao*) is a commonly used formula for nourishing the blood and rectifying the qi, soothing the liver and regulating the menses. Within this formula, Bupleurum is the main [medicinal] for soothing the liver, resolving depression, and orderly reaching the qi mechanism. Notopterygium is able to resolve depression and is also able to quicken the blood. Aurantium and Auklanida assist Bupleurum in opening the spleen qi and moving depression and binding. Dang Gui, White Peony, Ligusticum Wallichium, and Leonurus nourish and quicken the blood. Bupleurum's function of regulating and rectifying the qi mechanism thus results in the qi treating the blood.

3. [Bupleurum's] aspect of soothing the liver & resolving depression

[Bupleurum's] action of soothing the liver and resolving depression is similar to the previously described function, [since] depression and binding are mostly due to qi stagnation. The original causes of qi stagnation are many. Loss of regulation of cold and heat, emotional depression, worry and thinking beyond measure, phlegm rheum and damp turbidity may all result in the arising of qi stagnation depression and binding. In gynecology, liver qi depression and stagnation and spleen-stomach qi stagnation are commonly seen. Because Bupleurum is able to promote normal flow and its nature is to orderly reach, it effuses qi which is depressed and blocked. Thus it is able not only to soothe the liver but harmonize the spleen and resolve depression and binding. The commonly used formula [for this purpose] is as follows:

Xiao Yao San (Rambling Powder)([composed of] Radix Bupleuri, *Chai Hu*, Radix Angelicae Sinensis, *Dang Gui*, Radix Albus Paeoniae Lactiflorae, *Bai Shao*, Rhizoma Atractylodis Macrocephalae, *Bai Zhu*, Sclerotium Poriae Cocos, *Fu Ling*, Radix Glycyrrhizae, *Gan Cao*, uncooked Rhizoma Zingiberis, *Sheng Jiang*, and Herba Menthae Haplocalycis, *Bo He*) is the main formula for soothing the liver and resolving depression. Within [this formula], Bupleurum enters the two channels of the liver and gallbladder. It also enters the qi and the blood divisions. [Thus,] it is able to move the qi and quicken the blood. It not only treats the liver but also is able to harmonize the spleen. Therefore, it is frequently used to treat all conditions of liver-stomach depression and binding. This formula is derived from *Xiao Chai Hu Tang* with additions and subtractions. *Xiao Chai Hu Tang* is indicated for *shao yang* damage by cold with the simultaneous appearance of liver-stomach disharmony. The *Xiao Yao San* pattern also has symptoms of liver-stomach disharmony. These signs and symptoms are due to liver depression and discomfort [alternate reading: liver depression and lack of smooth flow] which affects spleen-stomach function. [In this case,] the aim of using *Xiao Yao San* is not to course the exterior but rather that Bupleurum should soothe the liver and resolve depression. Dang Gui and White Peony then nourish the blood and harmonize the liver. Atractylodes, Poria, and Licorice fortify the spleen and harmonize the stomach. And Mentha assists Bupleurum to upbear and scatter and to arouse the spleen and harmonize the stomach.

4. [Bupleurum's] aspect of upbearing yang & boosting the qi

The qi and blood and yin and yang of the human body are interdependent. [Therefore,] if yang is vacuous, in all [cases], qi vacuity must appear, while in most [cases] of qi vacuity, yang vacuity will appear. Qi vacuity and yang vacuity are mostly due to insufficiency of the organic qi transformation function. Hence, when supplementing the qi, one should also combine this with yang-upbearing medicinals in order to promote the qi transformation function. This then allows the action of supplementing the qi to display itself fully. Because Bupleurum has the function of upbearing yang and boosting the qi, it is typically used at the same time with qi-supplementing medicinals as the main [medicinals in the formula]. [In that case,] Bupleurum is the assistant which upbears yang. The commonly used formulas [for this aspect of Bupleurum's use] are as follows:

Bu Zhong Yi Qi Tang (Supplement the Center & Boost the Qi Decoction): ([This is composed of] Radix Astragali Membranacei, *Huang Qi*, Radix Glycyrrhizae, *Gan Cao*, Radix Panacis Ginseng, *Ren Shen*, Radix Angelicae Sinensis, *Dang Gui*, Pericarpium Citri Reticulatae, *Chen Pi*, Rhizoma Atractylodis Macrocephalae, *Bai Zhu*, Rhizoma Cimicifugae, *Sheng Ma,* and Radix Bupleuri, *Chai Hu*.) The spleen governs the central islet [*i.e.,* middle burner]. When the spleen is diseased, this leads to listlessness and an addiction to lying down, lack of strength in the four limbs, and loose stools. Because the spleen and stomach are the source of the engenderment and transformation of the constructive and defensive and qi and blood, if food and drink or taxation and fatigue damage the spleen, then the engenderment and transformation of the qi and blood will have no source. If spleen qi does not upbear, then the clear yang falls downward. Because Bupleurum has an action of upbearing and effusing the yang qi, when combined with Cimicifuga, it is able to upbear and boost yang qi. This can then assist Ginseng, Atractylodes, uncooked Astragalus, and Licorice's upbearing yang, supplementing the center, and boosting the qi. However, [for this] it should be used in a scanty [or lesser] amount.

Sheng Yang Yi Wei Tang (Upbear Yang & Boost the Stomach Decoction) ([composed of] Radix Astragali Membranacei, *Huang Qi*, Radix Panacis Ginseng, *Ren Shen*, Rhizoma Pinelliae Ternatae, *Ban Xia*, mix-fried Radix Glycyrrhizae, *Gan Cao*, Radix Et Rhizoma Notopterygii, *Qiang Huo*,

Radix Angelicae Pubescentis, *Du Huo,* Radix Ledebouriellae Divaricatae, *Fang Feng,* Radix Albus Paeoniae Lactiflorae, *Bai Shao,* Pericarpium Citri Reticulatae, *Chen Pi,* Rhizoma Atractylodis Macrocephalae, *Bai Zhu,* Sclerotium Poriae Cocos, *Fu Ling,* Rhizoma Alismatis, *Ze Xie,* Radix Bupleuri, *Chai Hu,* and Rhizoma Coptidis Chinensis, *Huang Lian*). This formula upbears and lifts the yang qi, [thus] increasing and strengthening the spleen and stomach function of moving and transforming. Therefore, it is called Upbear Yang & Boost the Stomach Decoction. If the spleen and stomach are vacuous and weak, movement and transformation lose their duty. Thus the finest essence of water and grains cannot be transported upward. Hence, uncooked Astragalus, Atractylodes, Ginseng, and Poria are used to boost the qi and fortify the spleen. Bupleurum upbears and lifts the yang qi, thus increasing and strengthening this action of boosting the qi. If the spleen and stomach are vacuous and weak, movement and transformation lose their duty. [Thus] dampness may easily lodge and gather. Hence Poria and Alisma are for fortifying the spleen and disinhibiting dampness. Ledebouriella and Notopterygium upbear and effuse stomach yang and eliminate dampness. Here, Bupleurum not only is able to upbear yang but is also able to scatter dampness, thus achieving the regulation and rectification of the spleen and stomach's function.

5. [Bupleurum's] aspect of upbearing, scattering, and eliminating dampness

Dampness is a yin evil. It is heavy, turbid, sticky, and slimy. External dampness usually invades the muscles and exterior and the channels and network vessels, resulting in disease. Internal dampness leads to the main symptoms of loss of regulation of the function of the viscera and bowels. If external dampness is heavy [*i.e.,* severe], it may affect the internal viscera. If internal dampness is heavy, it can spill over into the muscles and exterior. Disease due to damp evils may be located in the interior or exterior, above or below or may transform into heat or cold. Damp evils located above or externally should be diffused, resolved, and scattered. If [they] are located below or internally, one should fortify the spleen and move water in order to disinhibit [them]. As it is said in "The Great Treatise on Yin & Yang Correspondences & Images" in the *Su Wen (Simple Questions)*, "For those located in the skin, sweat and effuse"; "For those located below, lead and exhaust." Because spleen vacuity easily leads to the engenderment of dampness, kidney vacuity easily leads to the spilling over of water, lack of diffusion of the lungs leads to loss of command over free flow and regulation [of the water passageways], inhibition of the bladder leads to lack of free flow of the urination, or obstruction of the three burners' qi transformation leads to lack of authority to regulate the ditches [or drains], when treating dampness, one must necessarily address the essence of the patho-physiology. Because Bupleurum has the function of upbearing, scattering, and eliminating dampness, by upbearing and lifting spleen and stomach yang qi, movement and transformation are made normal, damp evils are transformed by yang qi and turned into fluids and humors, and damp evils are prevented from pouring downward. Therefore, in the treatment of gynecological abnormal vaginal discharge disease, Bupleurum is commonly combined with and makes up the following formula:

Wan Dai Tang (End Vaginal Discharge Decoction) ([composed of] Rhizoma Atractyodis Macrocephalae, *Bai Zhu*, Radix Dioscoreae Oppositae, *Shan Yao*, Sclerotium Poriae Cocos, *Fu Ling*, Radix Codonopsitis Pilosulae, *Dang Shen*, Radix Albus Paeoniae Lactiflorae, *Bai Shao*, Semen Plantaginis, *Che Qian Zi*, Rhizoma Atractylodis, *Cang Zhu*, Radix Glycyrrhizae, *Gan Cao*, Pericarpium Citri Reticulatae, *Chen Pi*, Radix Bupleuri, *Chai Hu*, Herba Seu Flos Schizonepetae Tenuifoliae, *Jing Jie Sui*) is a main formula for treating white vaginal discharge.[18] Within this formula, the two Atractylodes are the rulers which fortify

---

[18] Unfortunately, the authors use the single term *bai dai* both as a generic translation for leukorrhea and also to denominate specifically white-colored vaginal discharge. Sometimes it is clear which way they are using this term and sometimes it is not so clear. Therefore, in some cases we have translated this term as leukorrhea and in others as white vaginal discharge.

the spleen and dry dampness. Codonopsis boosts the qi and fortifies the spleen in order to increase and strengthen the movement and transformation of dampness. Poria and Dioscorea fortify the spleen and disinhibit dampness. Bupleurum and Schizonepeta are added in order to upbear yang and scatter dampness. This scattering of dampness strengthens the action of eliminating abnormal vaginal discharge.

From the above, it can be seen that Bupleurum is a medicinal which has a very wide scope of application in clinical practice. In particular, it is even more often used in gynecology. It is not difficult to obtain an effect [with Bupleurum] as long as one grasps well this medicinal's nature, combinations, dosage, and appropriate conditions. Bupleurum's harmful effect is that it upbears and scatters. If this harmful effect is turned into a benefit, then surely this will command an even better result when it is employed.

10

A Preliminary Exploration of the Treatment of Menstrual Irregularity Based on Chinese Medical Pattern Discrimination

Menstrual irregularities are commonly-seen, frequently encountered diseases in gynecology. [Therefore, we] must vigorously conduct preventive treatment [for them] in order to guarantee the greatest number of women good health. In our national medicine [*i.e.*, Chinese medicine], it is held that menstrual irregularities are mostly due to loss of regulation in the function of the three viscera of the liver, spleen, and kidneys, the qi and blood, and the two vessels of the *chong* and *ren* as well as external contraction of wind, cold, damp, and heat evils. Based on present clinical practice, [they] are treated not only on the basis of disease (such as functional uterine bleeding, amenorrhea, and dysmenorrhea) but also by analyzing the pathological changes in the menstrual cycle, the color of the menses, the consistency of the menses, and the amount of the menses. Menstrual irregularities include menstruation ahead of schedule, menstruation arriving [too] frequently, flooding and leaking, menstruation at no fixed schedule, menstruation behind schedule, sparse emission of menstruation [*i.e.*, infrequent menstruation], blocked menstruation, painful menstruation, etc. The color of the menstruate may be divided into pale-colored, red-colored, dark-colored, and purple-colored. The substance [or consistency] of the menstruate may be divided into thin [*i.e.*, dilute] or sticky and thick. The amount of the menstruate may be divided into scanty or profuse. Because these conditions may be complicated and the treatment methods and formulas are also many, it may seem difficult to grasp them. However, there are definite internal relationships between disease causes [of menstrual irregularities], their pathophysiology, and the tendencies and characteristics of their pathological manifestations. The difference [between them] lies only in the lightness or gravity of their degree and their replete or vacuous, cold or hot natures as well as their stage of mutual transformation.

Based on clinical practice, I have come to recognize that there are certain rules which can be explored in terms of menstrual irregularities. [Therefore,] I would like to say some things about my personal points of view based on knowledge gained through experience.

1. Menstrual physiology

Menstruation is a physiological phenomenon in women. Menstrual irregularities [on the other hand] are a manifestation of dysfunction of the integrated function of the body. Therefore, we must [first] deeply understand the state of the integrated functions of the body so that, via the manifestations of menstrual irregularities, we are able to grasp their pathological essence. [Thus] we can regulate and treat these at their root as well as grope our way in a step-by-step manner towards a rule [or protocol] for the treatment of menstrual diseases in Chinese medicine. Hence,we must have some understanding of menstrual physiology. In "The Treatise on the Former Ancient Heavenly Simplicity [*i.e.*, Age of Innocence]" in the *Su Wen (Simple Questions)*, it says:

> When females are seven, their kidney qi is exuberant. [Thus their adult or second] teeth are emitted and grow. At two [times] seven, the *tian gui* arrives, the *ren mai* is free-flowing, and the *tai chong mai* is exuberant. [Therefore,] the menses are precipitated periodically [alternate reading: descend periodically]... At seven [times] seven, the *ren mai* is vacuous, the *tai chong mai* is debilitated and scanty, and the *tian gui* is exhausted. [Thus] the earth passageways [*i.e.*, tunnels] are no longer free flowing.

This clearly explains that menstruation is directly related to the exuberance and decline of the kidney qi and the free flow and exuberance of the two vessels of the *chong* and *ren*. If we further consider this, we can see that the reason why the menstruation is able to descend periodically or the tunnels are not free-flowing is directly related to whether or not "the *tian gui* has arrived" or "the *tian gui* is exhausted." According to the *Nei Jing (The Inner Classic)*, both men and women have a *tian gui*. What is this *tian gui*? *Gui* is water.[19] Therefore, the *tian gui* is also called *gui* water. It is a type of yin fluid substance created by the human body's engenderment and transformation of qi and blood and fluids and humors. In women, it is the initial stage of the material basis which governs the function of reproduction and the production of menstrual blood. Because it is derived from the qi and blood and fluids and humors of the whole body, if the integrated function of the viscera and bowels (and especially of the three viscera of the liver, spleen, and kidneys) is harmonious and regulated and the qi and blood and fluids and humors are full and abundant, then the *tian gui* will be effulgent and exuberant. If [on the other hand] viscera and bowel function loses its regularity and the qi and blood and fluids and humors become depleted and lacking, then the *tian gui* will be insufficient. Since it is a yin fluid material substance derived from the qi and blood and fluids and humors, under normal circumstances, it has a definite constructing and nourishing action on the human body. [Therefore,] if the *tian gui* is insufficient or excessively exuberant, this will exert an influence on the whole body and particularly on the menstruation.

How does the *tian gui* transform itself into the menstrual blood? According to my experience, this is most closely related to the kidneys. If the integrated function of the viscera and bowels is harmonious and regulated and the qi and blood and fluids and humors are full and abundant, it will eventually come to pass that kidney yin (also called kidney water, the material substance of yin essence within the kidneys) will become full and replete and the *tian gui* is able to be produced. At this time, the *tian gui* is merely a yin fluid material substance and has no special function. Through the functional activity of kidney yang, the *tian*

_____

[19] *Gui* is one of the two heavenly stems which correspond to the water phase in five phase theory.

gui is able to be transformed red [yang corresponds to fire] and become the menstrual blood. This is then transported via the two vessels of the *chong* and *ren* to the *bao gong* [or uterus]. After the sea of blood is full and exuberant, at a certain time, it is expelled and discharged. This then is called the menstrual period.

Therefore, the menstrual blood and the origin of the blood are the same and yet not entirely the same. If the function of kidney yang qi transformation is insufficient, then the *tian gui* is not able to be completely transformed red and made into menstrual blood but is excreted in its original form, *e.g.*, a white, or pinkish colored secretion from the vagina during the premenstruum or postmenstruum. This is the *tian gui* substance which has not been completely transformed into the menstrual blood. If kidney yin is depleted and vacuous and there is no water to fill it, then the *tian gui* will not be produced in adequate amount. In that case, the secretion from the vaginal tract will be correspondingly scanty and poor. If yang heat is excessively exuberant, this can boil and scorch the menstrual blood after it has been transformed red. This then results in the menstrual blood's consistency becoming thick, congealed, and bound and produces blood clots. Therefore, if any link between the function of the three viscera of the liver, spleen, and kidneys, the qi and blood and fluids and humors, and the two vessels of the *chong* and *ren* becomes hindered or obstructed, this can result in the arising of menstrual irregularities.

2. Menstrual disease pathophysiology

The causes for the arising of menstrual diseases have many aspects but [all of these] are included under the two aspects [or headings] of internal causes and external causes. The internal causes are emotional dissatisfactions, [such as] worry, thinking, depression, and anger, bedroom taxation, excessive births, food and drink, and taxation and fatigue. The external causes are cold, heat, wind, and dampness of the six environmental excess evils which invade internally. As it is said in "The Heart Methods & Essential Secrets of Gynecology" in the *Yi Zong*

Jin Jian (Golden Mirror of Ancestral Medicine), "If heaven and earth are warm and harmonious, the menstrual water is quiet, while cold congeals, heat boils, and wind sweeps away." No matter which link in the physiological course of menstruation is affected by the above-mentioned factors, this may lead to the arising of menstrual irregularities. According to my clinical experience, abnormal changes in the menstrual cycle are related to dysfunction of the viscera and bowels. The profusion or scantiness of the menstrual volume is related to the vacuity and repletion of the qi and blood. And pathological changes in the consistency of the menstruate are related to the exuberance and decline of cold and heat. In addition, if the color of the menses is pale, this is mostly due to blood vacuity. If the color of the menses is black, this is mostly due to blood stasis.

Although menstrual irregularities may manifest an intermixing of vacuity and repletion, cold and heat, as a whole, (mainly in terms of pathological changes in the menstrual cycle) they can be greatly [*i.e.,* generally] divided into leaking menstruation types of menstrual irregularity and blocked menstruation types of menstrual irregularity. Menstruation which is [sometimes] early and [sometimes] late [and comes at] no fixed schedule can transform into either of these two extremes depending on its various causes. In terms of the influence of cold and heat, basically one may have either a tendency to cold or a tendency to heat. A tendency to heat mostly manifests as the leaking menstruation type of menstrual irregularity, while a tendency to cold mostly manifests as the blocked menstruation type of menstrual irregularity. However, even among these there may be abnormalities. For instance, a tendency towards vacuity cold can result in the arising of menstrual dribbling and dripping without cease, while a tendency to heat may desiccate the blood and lead to the arising of blocked menstruation. In addition, within loss of function of the viscera and bowels, there are differences in stress on the liver, spleen, or kidneys as well as the distinction between qi vacuity and blood vacuity or qi stagnation blood stasis and blood stasis qi obstruction.

Therefore, one should both observe the basic guidelines [as outlined above] at the same time as discriminating the pattern and analyzing the [individualized] bodily condition. Thus, when discriminating the pattern of menstrual irregularities, it is not only necessary to take into account abnormalities in the menstrual cycle, but one should also pay special attention to abnormal changes in the volume of the menses, the consistency of the menses, and the color of the menses.

3. The treatment of menstrual irregularities

In terms of the treatment of menstrual irregularities [in general], it should first be noted that the menstrual cycle, the color of the menses, the volume of the menses, and the time of any abnormal vaginal discharge in between are all only the epiphenomena, while loss of function of the viscera and bowels, the two vessels of the *chong* and *ren*, and the qi and blood and fluids and humors, and abnormalities in the engenderment and transformation of the *tian gui* are the root substance. According to the principle, "In treating disease, one must seek its root," the disease cause should be analyzed, thus grasping the basic rule [or principle] of [the disease's] pathophysiology. Based on such an analysis, treatment should [in turn] be based on the methods and principles that cold should be warmed, heat should be cleared, repletion and depression should be discharged (coursed), vacuity should be supplemented, descension should be ascended (upborne), ascension should be descended (downborne), flooding and leaking should be contracted, and blockage and stasis should be opened. That is to say, by warming, clearing, supplementing, discharging (coursing), upbearing, downbearing, contracting, and opening, the integrated function of the body is balanced, the qi and blood are regulated and harmonized, and thus the menstruation is able to return to normal. Therefore, the regulation and treatment of menstruation is the treatment of the blood, while the treatment of the blood is the treatment of the *tian gui* and the harmonization and regulation of the function of the integrated viscera and bowels.

In terms of the leaking type of menstrual irregularity, this includes menstruation ahead of schedule, menstruation which arrives [too] frequently, and flooding and leaking. The difference in these diseases is only one of degree, and mostly they are due to a tendency to heat. Their main symptoms are heart vexation, tension and agitation, feverish skin, dry mouth with lack of fluids, black or purplish colored menses containing clots, and a slippery, fine, somewhat rapid pulse. During treatment, *Qing Jing Tang* (Clear the Menses Decoction) can be used as the main [or ruling] formula. If qi depression is marked, add Radix Bupleuri (*Chai Hu*) and stir-fried Herba Seu Flos Schizonepetae Tenuifoliae (*Jing Jie Sui*) to course the qi, or use *Dan Zhi Xiao Yao San* (Moutan & Gardenia Rambling Powder) with additions and subtractions. If mixed with stasis, one can use *Sheng Hua Tang* (Engendering & Transforming Decoction), omitting the blast-fried Rhizoma Zingiberis (*Pao Jiang*) and adding *Shi Xiao San* (Loose a Smile Powder) to open.

If qi vacuity leads to its arising, mostly the manifestations are heart palpitations, shortness of breath, fatigue and listlessness, torpid intake, a pale red colored menstruate, a greenish-bluish, white, or yellow, and dark [or dull] facial complexion, and a relaxed, weak pulse. During treatment, *Si Wu Tang* (Four Materials Decoction) is the ruler. In order to boost the qi in case of qi vacuity flooding and leaking, use *Gui Pi Tang* (Restore the Spleen Decoction). If there is great flooding which will not stop, add carbonized Cacumen Biotae Orientalis (*Ce Bai*), carbonized Radix Sanguisorbae (*Di Yu*), and carbonized Fibra Stipulae Trachycarpi (*Zong Lu*) or Os Draconis (*Long Gu*), Concha Ostreae (*Mu Li*), and Cortex Cedrelae (*Chun Gen Bai Pi*) to stop bleeding and treat the branch by contracting. If there is simultaneous qi fall and no lifting, one can add Rhizoma Cimicifugae (*Sheng Ma*) and Radix Bupleuri (*Chai Hu*) to upbear. If due to kidney vacuity (opening but not closing) with unstoppable leaking of blood, it is ok to use *San Jiao Si Wu Tang* (Three Gelatins & Four Materials Decoction) plus Radix Dipscai (*Chuan Duan*), Semen Cuscutae Chinensis (*Tu Si Zi*), and Radix Dioscoreae Oppositae (*Shan Yao*) to contract and supplement.

In terms of the blocked menstruation type of menstrual irregularity, including menstruation behind schedule, sparse onset of menstruation [*i.e.*, infrequent menstruation], and blocked menstruation, these diseases differ only in degree and mostly tend towards cold. If the blood vessels congeal, the menstrual blood will become stagnant and will not move. Hence [the menses] are not able to come on time. Therefore, one [also] sees lower abdominal emission of coolness, lack of warmth in the four limbs, or menstrual movement abdominal pain. During treatment, *Wen Jing Tang* (Warm the Channels [or Menses] Decoction) is the ruling formula in order to warm. If mixed with depression, it is ok to use *De Sheng Dan* (Obtaining Birth Elixir) or *Xiao Yao San* (Rambling Powder) in order to course. If menstrual block endures for [many] days, it is ok to add Semen Pruni Persicae (*Tao Ren*), Flos Carthami Tinctorii (*Hong Hua*), and Radix Achyranthis Bidentatae (*Niu Xi*) in order to lead the blood to move downward so as to open blockage.

If due to liver heat leading to upward counterflow of the *chong* qi, it is ok to use the experiential formula, *Gua Shi Tang* (Trichosanthes & Dendrobium Decoction). If heat tends to be heavy, this may lead to erroneous [*i.e.*, vicarious] menstruation, spitting of blood, spontaneous external ejection of blood [*i.e.*, nosebleed], headache, agitation and sweating, and blocked menstruation which has lasted for [many] days. In that case it is ok to use *Dang Gui Long Hui Wan* (Dang Gui & Aloe Pills) plus Radix Achyranthis Bidentatae (*Niu Xi*) in order to downbear.

If due to spleen vacuity, [in which case] the source of engenderment and transformation of the qi and blood and fluids and humors is insufficient, it is ok to use *Ba Zhen Yi Mu Wan* (Eight Pearls Leonurus Pills) or *Gui Pi Tang* (Restore the Spleen Decoction) in order to supplement. If blood vacuity-kidney deficiency menstrual block arises due to postpartum great bleeding (Sheehan's syndrome), it is ok to use the experiential formula, *Si Er Wu He Fang* (Four, Two, Five Combined Formula) in order to warm and supplement.

In terms of the menstrual irregularity of menstruation [sometimes] early, [sometimes] late, [coming at] no fixed schedule, this mostly results due to loss of function of the viscera of the liver, spleen, and kidneys and is closely associated with emotional factors. At the same time, it is an earlier manifestation of either leaking menstruation type or blocked menstruation type menstrual irregularity which can transform into either of these. During treatment, it is ruled by *Ding Jing Tang* (Stabilize the Menses Decoction). This [formula] stresses the return [to normalcy] and the harmonization and regulation of the function of the three viscera of the liver, spleen, and kidneys.

In addition, cases in which the menstrual cycle is normal but the volume of the menstruate is relatively profuse can be divided into the two types of that tending towards vacuity and that tending towards heat. The vacuity one is mostly due to spleen-kidney insufficiency and lack of security of the *chong* and *ren*. Treatment should fortify the spleen and supplement the kidneys. The formula to use is *Si Jun Zi Tang* (Four Gentlemen Decoction) plus Radix Dipsaci (*Chuan Duan*) and cooked Radix Rehmanniae (*Shu Di*) to supplement. Or one can add Os Draconis (*Long Gu*), Concha Ostreae (*Mu Li*), and Cortex Cedrelae (*Chun Ge Bai Pi*) in order secure the *chong* and *ren* and thus contract. If tending towards heat, this is mostly due to heat forcing the blood to move [frenetically]. One should use *Qing Jing Tang* (Clear the Menses Decoction) plus Herba Ecliptae Prostratae (*Han Lian Cao*) and Os Sepiae Seu Sepiellae (*Wu Zei Gu*). One [of these medicinals] clears and the other contracts.

If the menstrual cycle is normal but the volume of the menses is scanty, one mostly sees the two types of blood vacuity and blood stasis. In terms of blood vacuity, one can use *Ba Zhen Tang* (Eight Pearls Decoction) to supplement. Blood stasis may also be distinguished into simultaneous cold or simultaneous heat [types]. If there is simultaneous cold, one should use *Shao Fu Zhu Yu Tang* (Lower Abdomen Dispel Stasis Decoction) in order to warm and course. If there is simultaneous heat, one should use *Qin Lian Si Wu Tang* (Scutellaria & Coptis Four Materials Decoction) plus Semen Pruni Persicae (*Tao Ren*), Flos Carthami Tinctorii (*Hong Hua*), Herba Lycopi Lucidi (*Ze Lan*), and Herba Leonuri Heterophyllii (*Yi Mu Cao*) in order to clear and course.

If the menstrual cycle is normal but the menses dribble and drip and move for many days, this is mostly categorized as kidney vacuity with *chong* and *ren* insecurity. One should use *San Jiao Si Wu Tang* (Three Gelatins & Four Materials Decoction) plus Radix Dipsaci (*Chuan Duan*) and Semen Cuscutae Chinensis (*Tu Si Zi*) or Os Draconis (*Long Gu*) and Concha Ostreae (*Mu Li*) in order to supplement and contract. If there is simultaneous heat, one should use *Liang Di Tang* (Two *Di* Decoction) plus Os Sepiae Seu Sepiellae (*Wu Zei Gu*), Herba Ecliptae Prostratae (*Han Lian Cao*), and Gelatinum Corii Asini (*E Jiao*) in order to clear, supplement, and contract.

In a word, although the symptoms of menstrual irregularity are complex, certain rules [or protocols] can still be discerned. There are eight therapeutic methods, [namely] warming, clearing, supplementing, discharging, coursing, upbearing, downbearing, contracting, and opening. If one is able to grasp the basic rule [or general principles and patterns] of menstrual irregularities and the above methods are flexibly used based on pattern discrimination, then one can also gradually find a rule [or protocol] for treating this disease. This then will supply the valuable source material for treating menstrual diseases and regulating the hormones with integrated Chinese-Western medicine.

BOOK TWO
CASE HISTORIES

Premenstrual Tension: Five Cases

Premenstrual tension refers to symptoms such as vexation and agitation, easy stimulation, headache, insomnia, dizziness, breast distention and pain, devitalized stomach intake, chest oppression, rib-side distention, lower abdominal discomfort, edema, diarrhea, etc. which appear 7-10 days before the onset of menstruation and which disappear automatically after the menstruation comes like a tide.[20] The cause of this disease [in Western medicine] is not yet completely clear. It seems to be related to dysfunction of the nervous system and reproductive hormones. Ancient [Chinese] medical books do not contain any description of this. It is usually distributed over [chapters in the premodern Chinese medical literature on] premenstrual spitting of blood and spontaneous external ejection of blood [i.e., nosebleed], premenstrual bloody stools, premenstrual fever, premenstrual bodily pain, premenstrual diarrhea, etc. These are categorized as miscellaneous diseases in gynecology.

According to his experience, Old Doctor[21] Liu preliminarily held that the occurrence of such conditions relates to loss of function of the viscera and bowels during the premenstruum and is essentially due to liver

---

[20] In Chinese medicine, the coming of menstruation is likened to a tide. This is due to both its periodicity and the fact that the menstrual blood ebbs and flows as the sea of blood becomes empty and full respectively. Therefore, the phrase, "comes like a tide," simply refers to the onset of menstruation.

[21] *Lao yi sheng* or Old Doctor is a term of respect for older Chinese doctors with many years of clinical experience. This reflects the fact that it takes deep learning, many years of experience, and mature judgement in order to become an especially good Chinese doctor. The fact that Old Doctor Liu is referred to in the third person shows that these cases were compiled and written up by Dr. Liu's students. This is a common practice in the People's Republic of China where most professional doctors still think of themselves as students or disciples of senior physician mentors.

depression qi stagnation. If liver depression obstructs and causes stagnation in the breast network vessels, then there is breast distention. If liver qi counterflows horizontally and assails the spleen, the spleen and stomach function will be affected and one may see spleen vacuity with liver effulgence resulting in diarrhea which must be [accompanied] by pain. One may also see spleen vacuity water dampness not transforming resulting in edema. If liver qi remains depressed for some time, it can transform into fire. Then one may see liver yang ascendant hyperactivity resulting in headache, or heat may enter the blood network vessels leading to bloody stools, spontaneous external ejection of blood [*i.e.*, nosebleed], or shifted menstruation [*i.e.*, vicarious menstruation]. If spleen vacuity losing its movement endures for [many] days, the engenderment and transformation of qi and blood will have no source. This may manifest as qi and blood dual vacuity symptoms.

Typically, these [symptoms] occur [in women] before menstruation. This is because, premenstrually, the *chong* and *ren* vessels are exuberant. The qi is full and the blood is flowing urgently. In many [cases], this easily leads to the channels and vessels becoming congested, stagnant, and not freely flowing. This [in turn] easily results in the occurrence of the above conditions. Once the menstrual blood comes and the *chong* and *ren* qi and blood flow freely and are regulated, these symptoms are automatically eliminated.

Case 1: Chan, female, 32 years old, a simple case in the out-patient department

Date of initial examination: July 5, 1973

Major complaints: Premenstrual dizziness, breast distention, and lower abdominal distention for two years

Present case history: There was premenstrual dizziness, breast distention, lower abdominal distention, numbness in her hands and feet, easy contraction of colds, and fear of chill 7-10 days before each menstruation for the last two years. Her sleep was still good, and she gradually recovered after menstruation. Each time premenstrually she experienced all these same [symptoms]. Previous gynecological examination had not shown any abnormalities. The last menstruation was on Jun. 13.

Tongue image: Slightly yellow fur

Pulse image: Bowstring and fine

Western medical diagnosis: Premenstrual tension

Chinese medical pattern discrimination: Liver depression qi stagnation, blood vacuity and network vessel obstruction

Treatment methods: Nourish the blood and course the liver, rectify the qi and free the flow of the network vessels

Formula & medicinals: Radix Angelicae Sinensis (*Dang Gui*), 3 *qian*, Radix Albus Paeoniae Lactiflorae (*Bai Shao*), 4 *qian*, Radix Ligustici Wallichii (*Chuan Xiong*), 2 *qian*, Radix Bupleuri (*Chai Hu*), 1.5 *qian*, Radix Scutellariae Baicalensis (*Huang Qin*), 3 *qian*, Radix Glycyrrhizae (*Gan Cao*) 2 *qian*, Radix Disocoreae Oppositae (*Shan Yao*), 5 *qian*, Rhizoma Atractylodis Macrocephalae (*Bai Zhu*), 3 *qian*, Sclerotium Poriae Cocos (*Fu Ling*), 3 *qian*, Sclerotium Polypori Umbellati (*Zhu Ling*), 4 *qian*, Rhizoma Alismatis (*Ze Xie*), 4 *qian*, Fructus Liquidambaris Taiwaniae (*Lu Lu Tong*), 3 *qian*, Caulis Trachelospermi Jasminoidis (*Luo Shi Teng*), 4 *qian*, Rhizoma Thalictri Foliosi (*Ma Wei Lian*), 3 *qian*

Course of treatment: On July 13, nine *ji* of the above formula had been administered and the menstruation had come like a tide that day. Since the medicinals were taken before menstruation, the above-mentioned symptoms did not manifest and any symptoms of the approach of her period were improved.

Commentary: This case was blood vacuity and liver depression, qi stagnation and obstruction of the network vessels. Because of liver depression qi stagnation, the qi and blood were not flowing smoothly and the channels and network vessels were congested and stagnant. Therefore, breast and lower abdominal distention were seen. Because of qi depression, the vessels and network vessels were not flowing smoothly and the sinew vessels lost their nourishment. Therefore, numbness of the hands and feet was seen. Because liver depression transformed into fire and attacked the head and eyes above, headache was seen. Due to habitual blood vacuity, the constructive and defensive had lost their harmony and the defensive external was insecure [or was not securing]. Therefore, there was easy contraction of external evils with the appearance of fear of chill.

Treatment was in order to nourish the blood and course the liver, rectify the qi and free the flow of the network vessels. The formula used was *Xiao Yao San* (Rambling Powder) with additions and subtractions. Within this formula, Dang Gui, Ligusticum Wallichium, and White Peony nourish the blood and emolliate the liver. Bupleurum soothes the liver and resolves depression. Scutellaria and Thalictrum clear heat and discharge the liver. Dioscorea, Atractylodes, Poria, and Licorice fortify the spleen and harmonize the stomach. Polyporus and Alisma fortify the spleen and disinhibit dampness. Trachelospermum and Liquidambar quicken the blood, course and free the flow of the channels and network vessels, and thus assist the regulation and harmonization of the qi and blood.

Case 2: Qu, female, 27 years old, a simple case in the out-patient department

Date of initial examination: June 18, 1972

Major complaints: Premenstrual diarrhea for 3-4 years

Present case history: In the past, [the patient's] menstrual cycle had been normal. The color [of the menses] was pale, its consistency was thin [*i.e.*, dilute], there was severe lower abdominal pain, and there were blood clots [in the menstruate]. In the last 3-4 years, diarrhea occurred three times each day during the 5-7 days before each menstruation. Abdominal pain must cause diarrhea. After the diarrhea, the pain is relieved. [The patient's] eating and drinking were [also] devitalized. Her facial complexion was somber white. She had been married for two years but had not yet conceived.

Tongue image: A pale tongue body

Pulse image: Deep and relaxed

Western medical diagnosis: Premenstrual tension

Chinese medical pattern discrimination: Spleen vacuity with liver effulgence, damp heat brewing internally

Treatment methods: Fortify the spleen and repress the liver, clear heat and eliminate dampness

Formula & medicinals: Stir-fried Rhizoma Atractylodis Macrocephalae (*Bai Zhu*), 3 *qian*, Sclerotium Poriae Cocos (*Fu Ling*), 5 *qian*, Radix Ledebouriellae Divaricatae (*Fang Feng*), 2 *qian*, Pericarpium Citri Reticulatae (*Chen Pi*), 2 *qian*, Radix Albus Paeoniae Lactiflorae (*Bai Shao*), 4 *qian*, Radix Scutellariae Baicalensis (*Huang Qin*), 3 *qian*, Radix Glycyrrhizae (*Gan Cao*), 2 *qian*, Radix Dipsaci (*Chuan Duan*), 3 *qian*, Semen Cuscutae Chinensis (*Tu Si Zi*), 3 *qian*

Course of treatment: On August 29, [the patient] was examined once again. Ten *ji* of the above-mentioned formula had been taken orally. On Aug. 18, the menstruation came like a tide but premenstrual diarrhea had not occurred. The stools were formed and were resolved [*i.e.*, excreted] once per day. In December 1972, during follow-up, [the

137

patient] reported that there had not been any premenstrual diarrhea since the last treatment and that her menstruation had been normal.

Commentary: This case was categorized as liver depression repressing the spleen resulting in spleen vacuity. [This, in turn] had led to stomach and intestinal damp heat brewing internally which had then resulted in painful diarrhea and torpid stomach intake. Since spleen vacuity was not able to fill and nourish the skin, the facial complexion was a somber white. Since spleen vacuity led to damp exuberance, therefore the menses were pale in color and thin [or watery] in consistency.

Treatment was in order to repress the liver, fortify the spleen, and eliminate dampness using *Tong Xie Yao Fang* (Painful Diarrhea Essential Formula) plus *Huang Qin Shao Yao Gan Cao Tang* (Scutellaria, Peony & Licorice Decoction) with additions and subtractions. Within this formula, Atractylodes and Poria fortify the spleen and eliminate dampness. Orange Peel rectifies the qi and arouses the spleen. All of these together supplement the spleen. White Peony nourishes the blood and represses the liver. Ledebouriella upbears yang and eliminates dampness. Both of these together harmonize the spleen. Dipsacus and Cuscutae supplement the kidneys and harmonize the liver. Scutellaria, White Peony, and Licorice clear and rectify stomach and intestinal damp heat.

Case 3: Shu, female, 25 years old, a simple case in the out-patient department

Date of initial examination: July 9, 1973

Major complaints: Premenstrual breast distention for four years

Present case history: Premenstrual breast distention had endured for four years already. Her menstrual cycle was normal. Its amount was not profuse [or excessive]. Its color was red. Breast distention and pain and headache began one week before menstruation. The onset [of this] had occurred four years ago after contracting wind during the premenstruum. The menses were accompanied by lumbar and abdominal distention and pain. Previous gynecological examination had not revealed any abnormalities.

Tongue image: Thin, white fur

Pulse image: Deep, bowstring, and relaxed

Western medical diagnosis: Premenstrual tension

Chinese medical pattern discrimination: Qi and blood dual vacuity, enduring retention of wind evils

Treatment methods: Boost the qi and nourish the blood, scatter wind and free the flow of the network vessels

Formula & medicinals: Radix Et Rhizoma Ligustici Chinensis (*Gao Ben*), 2 *qian*, Radix Angelicae Dahuricae (*Bai Zhi*), 2 *qian*, Radix Ledebouriellae Divaricatae (*Fang Feng*), 2 *qian*, Fructus Viticis (*Man Jing Zi*), 4 *qian*, Radix Astragali Membranacei (*Huang Qi*), 5 *qian*, Radix Angelicae Sinensis (*Dang Gui*), 3 *qian*, Radix Ligustici Wallichii (*Chuan Xiong*), 1.5 *qian*, Fructus Tribuli Terrestris (*Bai Ji Li*), 4 *qian*, Herba Equiseti Hiemalis (*Mu Zei Cao*), 3 *qian*

Course of treatment: [The patient] was re-examined on July 26. Twelve *ji* of this formula had been taken orally. On July 16, menstruation had come once. No symptoms of premenstrual headache, etc. had occurred.

Commentary: The case was categorized as qi and blood dual vacuity with enduring retention of wind evils. The main manifestation of this was premenstrual headache. Because she was habitually [or constitutionally] blood vacuous, when the menses came like a tide,

139

blood had already moved downward and blood vacuity in the region of the head became even more severe. This is actually the internal cause of the onset of this disease. Another cause was the contraction of wind affection in the region of the head during the premenstruum four years before. These wind evils had endured and been retained and had not been resolved. Each premenstruum, therefore, there was the onset of this disease. The premenstrual breast distention with scanty menstrual blood volume were both images of liver depression and blood vacuity.

Hence the above treatment was based on simultaneously supporting the righteous and dispelling evils. Within this formula, Dang Gui, Ligusticum Wallichium, Equisetum, and Tribulus nourish the blood, quicken the blood, and dispel wind. Astragalus supplements the qi so that the qi carries the blood. Ligusticum Chinensis, Angelica Dahurica, Ledebouriella, and Vitex scatter wind and quicken the network vessels. Thus branch and root were addressed simultaneously.

Case 4: Du, female, 30 years old, a simple case in the out-patient department

Date of initial examination: January 31, 1974

Major complaints: Heart fluster [*i.e.*, heart palpitations], shortness of breath, premenstrual dizziness, headache for over half a year

Present case history: In the last half year, [the patient] had felt dizziness, headache, heart fluster, shortness of breath, nausea, chest oppression and pain, a dry mouth, preferance for chilled drinks, vexation and agitation, easy anger, fatigue and listlessness of the four limbs, and lack of strength before each menstruation. Her blood pressure was sometimes high and sometimes low (the systolic pressure [fluctuated between] 120-189mmHg, while the diastolic pressure was 80-120mmHg) whenever she was premenstrual. Due to high blood pressure, the patient had previously fallen down two times. After her menses came, all these symptoms decreased. Her menstrual period was 3-7 days early, its color was blackish red, and its volume was medium. At the time of menstruation, there was lumbar aching and pain. During the premenstruum, she was not able to work.

Examination: [The patient's] general condition was good. Urine examination [showed] 4.5mg of phosphorus benzene diphenoamine. Her basic metabolism was +10%. ECG was normal with sinus tachycardia. Liver function was normal and the eye ground was normal. Abdominal x-ray imaging was normal.

Western medical diagnosis: A) Premenstrual tension; B) pheo-chromocytoma not excluded[22]

Chinese medical pattern discrimination: Liver depression transforming into fire, yin vacuity with yang hyperactivity

Treatment methods: Nourish yin and clear heat, cool the blood and level [or calm] the liver

Formula & medicinals: Folium Mori Albi (*Sang Ye*), 3 *qian*, Flos Chrysanthemi Morifolii (*Ju Hua*), 3 *qian*, Radix Scutellariae Baicalensis (*Huang Qin*), 3 *qian*, Rhizoma Thalictri Foliosi (*Ma Wei Lian*), 3 *qian*, uncooked Radix Albus Paeoniae Lactiflorae (*Bai Shao*), 3 *qian*, uncookd Radix Rehmanniae (*Sheng Di*), 4 *qian*, Fructus Trichosanthis Kirlowii (*Gua Lou*), 5 *qian*, Cortex Radicis Moutan (*Dan Pi*), 3 *qian*, Fructus Gardeniae Jasminoidis (*Zhi Zi*), 3 *qian*, Radix Achyranthis Bidentatae (*Niu Xi*), 3 *qian*, Fructus Ligustri Lucidi (*Nu Zhen Zi*), 3 *qian*, Herba Ecliptae Prostatae (*Han Lian Cao*,) 3 *qian*

---

[22] This is a tumor of the chromaffin cells that secrete catecholamines, thus causing hypertension. Although they may appear at any age, their maximum incidence is between 30-60 years of age. They are usually benign.

Course of treatment: On Mar. 10, after taking three *ji* of the above formula, the dizziness, headache, heart fluster, vexation and agitation, insomnia, and chest oppression were all reduced. Trichosanthes was removed from the above formula and Gelatinum Corii Asini (*E Jiao*), 5 *qian*, was added. On Apr. 13, [the patient] was re-examined and she was advised to take 3-6 doses of the above formula a few days before each menstruation. [At that time,] the dizziness, headache, heart fluster, shortness of breath, etc. were all decreased. The chest oppression and pain were decreased, and her blood pressure was 110-130/70-90mmHg. Her essence spirit had become good again and she was able to work the entire day. Her menstrual cycle was normal.

Commentary: This case was categorized as liver depression transforming into fire with ascendant hyperactivity of liver yang. The liver is the indomitable viscus. It depends on its enrichment and nourishment from kidney yin. If kidney yin is insufficient, blood does not nourish the liver. This leads to liver yin insufficiency. If liver yang becomes hyperactive and ascends, it harasses the clear portals above. Therefore, dizziness and headache are seen. If liver fire upbears and leaps, one may see vexation and agitation and easy anger. There is oral thirst and a preference for chilled drinks. If liver heat leads to stirring of blood heat, the menses may be early. If liver yin is insufficient and kidney yin is deficient and vacuous, they may not be able to aid the heart above. Thus the heart and kidneys do not interact and heart fluster, shortness of breath, and insomnia may be seen.

Treatment was in order to nourish yin and clear heat, cool the blood and level the liver. Within this formula, Mulberry Leaves, Chrysanthemum Flowers, Scutellaria, Thalictrum, Moutan, and Gardenia clear heat, cool the blood, and level the liver. Uncooked Rehmannia, White Peony, Ligustrum Lucidum, and Eclipta enrich yin and nourish the blood. Achyranthes enriches and supplements the liver and kidneys and leads heat to move downward. Donkey Skin Glue nourishes the blood and quiets the spirit. Trichosanthes rectifies the qi, broadens the middle, and clears heat. Thus, not only were all the symptoms improved, but the blood pressure was also stabilized.

Case 5: Luo, female, 42 years old, a simple case in the out-patient department

Date of initial examination: August 22, 1975

Major complaints: Severe premenstrual abdominal pain for more than one year

Present case history: [The patient] had a history of pelvic inflammation [*i.e.,* pelvic inflammatory disease or PID] for more than 10 years which treatment had not cured. In 1969, she had become pregnant and had had an artificial abortion. After surgery, she had hemorrhaged and this had caused her symptoms to get heavier [*i.e.,* worse]. There was wringing pain constantly in her lower abdomen which emitted coolness. After heat was applied, the aching and pain decreased. One year previously, her menses had become sparse [*i.e.,* infrequent], coming like a tide only once every 3-4 months. There volume had [also] become scanty. A half month before menstruation, her lower abdominal pain would become even more severe. This pain was sometimes so heavy she would faint and she was not able to work. After the menstrual movement, the abdominal pain disappeared. In general, [the patient] reported that she had bodily heat (although her temperature was normal), dizziness, nausea, a dry mouth with bitter [taste], heart vexation and tension, agitation and sweating, scanty intake [of food], and loose stools.

Tongue image: A dark red tongue

Pulse image: Deep, bowstring, and slippery

Chinese medical pattern discrimination: Liver depression qi stagnation, cold lodged in the *chong* and *ren*

143

Treatment methods: Course the liver and resolve depression, warm the channels [or menses] and scatter cold

Formula & medicinals: Radix Bupleuri (*Chai Hu*), 1.5 *qian*, Rhizoma Pinelliae Ternatae (*Ban Xia,*) 3 *qian*, Pericarpium Citri Reticulatae (*Chen Pi*), 2 *qian*, Radix Rubrus Paeoniae Lactiflorae (*Chi Shao*), 2 *qian*, Radix Angelicae Sinensis (*Dang Gui*), 3 *qian*, Radix Scutellariae Baicalensis (*Huang Qin*), 3 *qian*, processed Rhizoma Cyperi Rotundi (*Xiang Fu*), 3 *qian*, Rhizoma Corydalis Yanhusuo (*Yan Hu Suo*), 3 *qian*, Fructus Meliae Toosendan (*Chuan Lian Zi*), 3 *qian*, Resina Myrrhae (*Mo Yao*), 1 *qian*, Fructus Citri Aurantii (*Zhi Ke*), 2 *qian*, Radix Auklandiae Lappae (*Mu Xiang*), 1.5 *qian*, Feces Trogopterori Seu Pteromi (*Wu Ling Zhi*), 3 *qian*

Course of treatment: On August 28, after taking five *ji* of the above formula, the symptoms had not improved. [The patient] felt bodily heat and lower leg flaccidity. The pulse and [tongue] fur were the same as before. Groping towards a [new] pattern discrimination, [the case] was categorized as liver depression qi stagnation, stomach and intestines brewing heat. Therefore, the treatment methods used were to soothe the liver and resolve depression, clear heat and harmonize the stomach. The formula and medicinal were as follows: Radix Bupleuri (*Chai Hu*), 2 *qian*, Radix Scutellariae Baicalensis (*Huang Qin*), 3 *qian*, Rhizoma Pinelliae Ternatae (*Ban Xia*), 3 *qian*, Radix Glycyrrhizae (*Gan Cao*), 1.5 *qian*, Radix Et Rhizoma Rhei (*Da Huang*), 1 *qian*, Radix Albus Paeoniae Lactiflorae (*Bai Shao*), 4 *qian*, Folium Mori Albi (*Sang Ye*), 3 *qian*, Flos Chrysanthemi Morifolii (*Ju Hua*), 3 *qian*, Caulis Bambusae In Taeniis (*Zhu Ru*), 3 *qian*, Pericarpium Citri Reticulatae (*Ju Pi*), 2 *qian*, uncooked Rhizoma Zingiberis (*Sheng Jiang*), 3 slices, and Fructus Zizyphi Jujubae (*Da Zao*), 3 pieces.

On September 6, after taking five *ji* of the above formula, the dizziness, nausea, and bodily heat were all less. However, since the day before yesterday, they had become heavier again along with scanty intake and loose stools. Caulis Bambusae was removed from the above formula and

Fructus Gardeniae Jasminoidis (*Zhi Zi*), 3 *qian*, Fructus Forsythiae Suspensae (*Lian Qiao*), 3 *qian*, and Radix Gentianae Scabrae (*Long Dan Cao*), 1 *qian*, were added.

On September 20, after taking 15 *ji* of the above formula, the symptoms were greatly decreased. The dizziness, nausea, and bodily heat were all light. However, the stools were still loose. Uncooked Ginger and Red Dates were removed from the above formula and Herba Leonuri Heterophylli (*Yi Mu Cao*), 5 *qian*, was added.

On September 27, after taking five *ji* of the above formula orally, [the patient reported that] her menstruation had come like a tide on Sept 21. Their volume was less, their color was blackish red, their consistency was thick, and they moved for four days. The premenstrual abdominal pain had completely disappeared and there was only a very slight amount of abdominal pain with the menses. She had been able to go to work. Since all the symptoms had become lighter, administration of the original formula was continued in order to secure the treatment effect.

Commentary: This case's disease condition was more complicated than that of the previous four cases. In the beginning, Old Doctor Liu, based on the symptoms of lower abdominal wringing pain with emission of coolness, sparse menstruation, worsening of the pain during the premenstruum with dizziness and fainting, and inability to work *and not on the pulse*, discriminated the pattern as liver depression qi stagnation with cold lodged in the *chong* and *ren*. Therefore, the methods used were to soothe the liver and resolve depression, warm the channels and scatter cold. However, after administering five *ji* of medicinals, the symptoms had not improved. Through true [*i.e.*, serious or deep] analysis, it was found that [although] the pain was alleviated after menstruation, [the patient still] reported bodily heat, dizziness, nausea, a dry mouth with bitter [taste], vexation and tension, and agitation exiting sweat [*i.e.*, nervous perspiration]. A bowstring, slippery pulse was also seen.[23]

By synthesizing the pulse [image] and the symptoms, it was found these [symptoms] were caused by qi stagnation transforming fire. Depressive heat existed in the interior which was not able to be effused or emitted. Dry heat was bound internally and the channels and network vessels were blocked and obstructed. Therefore, severe pain in the abdominal region was seen. After the menses moved and the *chong* and *ren* were free-flowing, the abdominal pain decreased and depressive heat was somewhat able to obtain effusion and scattering. The self-reported bodily heat, dizziness, nausea, dry mouth with bitter [taste], vexation and tension, agitation, and perspiration were all symptoms of liver heat internally depressed.

[Therefore,] after this, the methods of coursing the liver and clearing heat, downbearing counterflow and discharging fire were used. *Da Chai Hu Tang* (Major Bupleurum Decoction) with additions and subtractions was used. On the one hand, Bupleurum and Scutellaria were used to course the liver and resolve depression. On the other hand, Mulberry Leaves, Chrysanthemum Flowers, and Rhubarb were used to clear the exterior and free the flow of the interior. Thus clearing and coursing and freeing the flow and discharging were combined together, and afterwards, Gardenia, Gentiana, and Forsythia were added to clear the liver and downbear fire. Then the symptoms were improved. This was continued and Leonurus was [added] in order to quicken the blood and regulate the menses. The severe premenstrual abdominal pain completely disappeared and all the other symptoms were seen to be lighter. Thus the pathological essence of premenstrual tension was gradually rectified and resolved.

---

[23] A slippery pulse may indicate any of a number of things. It may mean there is healthy stomach qi. It may mean there is evil dampness and phlegm. And, as in this case, it may mean the presence of evil heat.

Ovulatory Bleeding: Two Cases

Case 1: Zhang, female, 27 years old, a simple case in the out-patient department

Date of initial examination: July 13, 1974

Major complaints: Vaginal bleeding in the middle of the menstrual cycle for more than a half year; in the last two days, a scanty amount of vaginal tract bleeding

Present case history: For the last half year, a small amount of vaginal tract bleeding had appeared in the middle between two menstruations. Each time this lasted for 2-3 days. The amount was scanty and its color was blackish purple. Usually the lower abdomen emitted coolness and was painful. Before the menses and during the menses this abdominal pain got heavier. There was [also] a white vaginal discharge which was profuse in amount. There was a past history of pelvitis [*i.e.*, PID]. [The patient] had been married for more than one year but had not conceived. Previously, she had been administered more than 10 *ji* of warming the uterus and scattering cold method medicinals, but the signs of ovulatory bleeding had not taken a turn for the better.

Tongue image: White, slimy fur with slightly red tongue body

Pulse image: Bowstring and slippery

Western medical diagnosis: Ovulatory bleeding

Chinese medical pattern discrimination: Damp heat pouring downward, heat damaging the blood network vessels

147

Treatment methods: Clear heat and disinhibit dampness, move the qi and quicken the blood

Formula & medicinals: Herba Dianthi (*Qu Mai*), 4 *qian*, Herba Polygoni Avicularis (*Bian Xu,*) 3 *qian*, Caulis Akebiae Mutong (*Mu Tong*), 1 *qian*, Semen Plantaginis (*Che Qian Zi*), 3 *qian*, Fructus Meliae Toosendan (*Chuan Lian Zi*), 4 *qian*, Rhizoma Corydalis Yanhusuo (*Yan Hu Suo*), 3 *qian*, Herba Taraxaci Mongolici Cum Radice (*Pu Gong Ying*), 5 *qian*, Herba Patriniae Heterophyllae Cum Radice (*Bai Jiang Cao*), 4 *qian*, Radix Rubrus & Albus Paeoniae Lactiflorae (*Chi Bai Shao*), 3 *qian* each

Course of treatment: On Aug. 26, Radix Bupleuri (*Chai Hu*), Herba Seu Flos Schizonepetae Tenuifoliae (*Jing Jie Sui*), Rhizoma Cyperi Rotundi (*Xiang Fu*), Semen Plantaginis (*Che Qian Zi*), Cortex Cedrelae (*Chun Gen Bai Pi*), or Rhizoma Atractylodis (*Cang Shu*) had been either added or subtracted from the above formula and more than 30 *ji* had been administered. The coolness emitted from the lower abdomen was already decreased but there was still occasional very slight abdominal pain. At that time, it was just the middle of the menstrual cycle. There was lower abdominal pain and white vaginal discharge in which were seen threads [*i.e.,* streaks] of blood. Dandelion and Patrinia were removed from the above formula and Rhizoma Dioscoreae Hypoglaucae (*Bi Xie*) and Herba Leonuri Heterophylli (*Yi Mu Cao*), 4 *qian* each, and Radix Achryanthis Bidentatae (*Niu Xi*) and Feces Trogopterori Seu Pteromi (*Wu Ling Zhi*), 3 *qian* each, were added.

On Sept. 26, after taking 10 *ji* of the above formula, vaginal bleeding was not seen at the middle of the menstrual cycle. On Oct. 13, a pregnancy antibody test was positive. Later, birth occurred at full term. On follow-up, [the patient's] postpartum condition was typically good and no sign of ovulatory bleeding was seen.

Case 2: Li, female, 24 years old, a simple case in the out-patient department

Date of initial examination: December 25, 1974

Major complaints: A small amount of vaginal tract bleeding for three days

Present case history: In the last three days, during the middle of the menstrual cycle, there had been a small amount of vaginal tract bleeding. This had been diagnosed as ovulatory bleeding by a hospital. Half a month before menstruation, [the patient] felt marked itching of her external genitalia and a dry mouth and thirst. [Sometimes] menses were early, [sometimes] they were late, [and they came at] no fixed schedule. During the premenstruum there was abdominal pain which became relatively severe on day one of the menstrual movement. There was [also] distention of her perineal and anal region.

Tongue image: A red tongue tip with thin, yellow fur

Pulse image: Bowstring and slippery

Western medical diagnosis: Ovulatory bleeding

Chinese medical pattern discrimination: Damp heat pouring downward, heat damaging the blood network vessels

Treatment methods: Clear heat and disinhibit dampness, move the qi and quicken the blood

Formula & medicinals: Herba Dianthi (*Qu Mai*), 4 *qian*, Herba Polygoni Avicularis (*Bian Xu*), 3 *qian*, Caulis Akebiae Mutong (*Mu Tong*), 1 *qian*, Semen Plantiginis (*Che Qian Zi*), wrapped, 3 *qian*, Radix Rubrus & Albus Paeoniae Lactiflorae (*Chi Bai Shao*), 1 *qian* each, Rhizoma Dioscoreae Hypoglaucae (*Bi Xie*), 4 *qian*, Rhizoma Corydalis Yanhusuo (*Yan Hu Suo*), 2 *qian*, Fructus Meliae Toosendan (*Chuan Lian Zi*), 3 *qian*, Radix

Scutellariae Baicalensis (*Huang Qin*), 2 *qian*, Radix Bupleuri (*Chai Hu*), 1 *qian*, Herba Seu Flos Schizonepetae Tenuifoliae (*Jing Jie Sui*), 1.5 *qian*

Course of treatment: After administering four *ji* of this formula, the vaginal tract bleeding had already stopped. On follow-up, there had been no sign of midcycle bleeding.

Commentary: Ovulatory bleeding mostly occurs in the middle between two menstruations or, in other words, on days 12-16 after the menses [come]. There are not many discussions of this disease in Chinese medical books. Patients who have midcycle vaginal tract bleeding typically also have lower abdominal chilly pain or menstrual pain. Therefore, [Dr. Liu] initially used the methods and principles of warming the uterus and scattering cold to treat this. However, the effects were not ideal. Gradually, through further analysis, he observed that the main symptoms of patients with midcyle vaginal tract bleeding are lower abdominal pain and chill with a white vaginal discharge which is profuse in amount. Their tongue fur is usually white and slimy or thin and yellow, and their pulse image is mostly bowstring and slippery. Although symptoms of lower abdominal chilly pain are seen, [the doctor] should clearly differentiate the preponderance of heat or cold and whether these are true or false in nature. One cannot discriminate every case which is seen as a cold condition. This is because, in the true cold pattern of lower abdominal chilly pain, there is mostly a somber white facial complexion, a bowstring, fine pulse, and thin, white [tongue] fur. [However,] in this type of patient, the facial complexion is either normal or slightly red, the pulse image is mostly bowstring and slippery, and the tongue fur is white and slimy or thin and yellow.

The reason for this kind of lower abdominal chilly pain is damp heat obstructing and stagnating in the channels and network vessels. The qi and blood of the two vessels of the *chong* and *ren* are thus not freely flowing and hence [lower abdominal chilly pain] results. At each midcycle (*i.e.*, at ovulation), if there is vaginal tract bleeding, this is because dampness and heat are hidden or deeply lying inside the *chong* and *ren*. After midcycle, the *chong* and *ren* vessels and passageways gradually become full and exuberant and their function gradually [also] becomes effulgent and exuberant. Function is yang. Yang exuberance leads to heat. This then leads to internal stirring of deep-lying dampness and heat. Dampness and heat pour downwards and thus a profuse, white vaginal discharge can be seen. If this damp heat enters the blood network vessels, it may damage and stir the blood which then frenetically spills over outside the vessels and passageways of the *chong* and *ren*. Hence, vaginal tract bleeding is seen.

Therefore, on the basis of his past failures and based on a dialectical analysis of the integrated whole body and all the manifestations of the disease, Old Doctor Liu came to recognize that midcycle bleeding should mostly be categorized as damp heat pouring downward with heat damaging the blood network vessels. Therefore, it is the methods of clearing heat and disinhibiting dampness, moving the qi and quickening the blood that affect its treatment. Thus, when Old Doctor Liu treated [this disease], he used an experiential formula [called] *Qing Gan Li Shi Tang* (Clear the Liver & Disinhibit Dampness Decoction) with additions and subtractions and this has obtained a definite treatment effect. As a whole, this accords with the rule of treating free flow [*i.e.*, diarrhea, vaginal discharge, bleeding, etc.] by freeing the flow. Thus damp heat obtains clearing, qi and blood obtain free flow, the blood vessels are coursed and reach, and the *chong* and *ren* are regulated and harmonized. This leads to the stoppage of bleeding and the elimination of the disease.

In case #1, besides ovulatory bleeding, there was a history of pelvic inflammation and infertility. At the very beginning, [the patient's] main complaint and diagnosis was infertility, and Old Doctor Liu only paid attention to this disease diagnosis (*i.e.*, infertility). Therefore, at the beginning, he used medicinals for warming the uterus and scattering

151

cold, such as Semen Citri Reticulatae (*Ju He*), Fructus Foeniculi Vulgaris (*Xiao Hui Xiang*), Semen Trigonellae Foeni-graeci (*Hu Lu Ba*), etc. The result was that, not only was the infertility not effectively treated, but the ovulatory bleeding also became aggravated. Through further pattern discrimination, the treatment method was changed to the application of *Qing Gan Li Shi Tang* with additions and subtractions. Then, not only was ovulatory bleeding cured, but [the patient] also got pregnant and had [a normal] birth.

Although bleeding was seen [in this case], medicinals for stopping bleeding were not used. Rather, medicinals for quickening the blood, such as Achyranthes, Leonurus, Red Peony, and Flying Squirrel's Droppings, were used to quicken blood, course, free the flow, and dispel stasis, and transform stagnation. This is what is meant by the saying, "When bleeding is seen, it is not ok to stop bleeding." Thus damp heat deep-lying internally is dispelled and eliminated in the midst of coursing and freeing the flow. However, it is not advisable to use [such medicinals] in excessively large amounts in order to prevent damp heat from spreading or profuse bleeding.

In case #2, the disease course was relatively short and, [therefore,] the effect was achieved quickly. In both the above two cases, Schizonepeta was used. This is because Schizonepeta has the function of clearing deep-lying heat within the blood.

Shifted [*i.e.*, Vicarious] Menstruation: One Case

Case: Zhong, female, 20 years old, a simple case in the out-patient department

Date of initial examination: September 16, 1974

Major complaints: Nosebleeding during menstruation for six years

Present case history: Menarche had occurred at 12 years of age. [The patient's] menstruation was 10 days early. Its volume was scanty and its color was black. The menses moved for two days. During the menstrual period, there was nosebleeding. Whenever [the patient] was affected by her emotions, her nosebleeding was relatively more profuse. It [also] contained clots. Premenstrually, there was vexation and agitation, easy anger, and dizziness. She habitually had profuse leukorrhea, lumbar pain, and abdominal pain. Her last menstruation had come on Sept. 8 and had moved for [only] one day.

Tongue image: A pale tongue with red edges

Pulse image: Bowstring and slippery

Chinese medical pattern discrimination: Liver effulgence and blood heat, counterflow menstruation moving erroneously

Treatment methods: Level [or calm] the liver and clear the menses

Formula & medicinals: Rhizoma Imperatae Cylindricae (*Bai Mao Gen*), 1 *liang*, Nodus Rhizomatis Nelumbinis Nuciferae (*Ou Jie*), 1 *liang*, uncooked Radix Rehmanniae (*Sheng Di*), 5 *qian*, Cortex Radicis Moutan (*Dan Pi*), 2 *qian*, Radix Gentianae Scabrae (*Long Dan Cao*), 3 *qian*, Radix Achyranthis Bidentatae (*Niu Xi*), 4 *qian*, Radix Scutellariae Baicalensis (*Huang Qin*), 3 *qian*, Fructus Citri Aurantii (*Zhi Ke*), 2 *qian*, Tuber Ophiopogonis Japonici (*Mai Dong*), 3 *qian*, Fructus Gardeniae Jaminoidis (*Zhi Zi*), 3 *qian*

Course of treatment: On November 7, [the patient reported that] after taking the above formula, on October 15 her menses had come like a tide. There had been no appearance of shifted menstruation and her menses were normal. There was [also] no appearance of abdominal pain. On follow-up after more than half a year, there had been no sign of the occurrence of shifted menstruation.

Commentary: Shifted menstruation [*i.e.*, vicarious menstruation] refers to symptoms of spontaneous ejection of blood [*i.e.*, nosebleed] or spitting of blood [*i.e.*, hematemesis] 1-2 days before the menstruation or during menstruation.[24] This is also called "counterflow menstruation" and "premenstrual spitting and spontaneous ejection of blood." Shifted menstruation is mostly related to liver channel depressive heat forcing the blood to move frenetically. [It may also be due to] dryness damaging the lung network vessels with blood spilling outside the channels or to yin vacuity blood heat damaging the blood network vessels. These result in blood heat with qi counterflow. Since the blood follows the movement of the qi, if qi counterflows, this leads to blood counterflow ascending and spilling over [alternate reading: spilling over above].

---

[24] Vicarious menstruation refers to cyclic perimenstrual bleeding from an orifice other than the vagina. This is actually one of the less frequently encountered symptoms of endometriosis. In this case, endometrial tissue is located in the nose, throat, bronchi, large intestine, or bladder. At the end of the luteal phase, when the ovaries' production plummets, this endometrial tissue necroses and sheds along with the endometrial tissue lining the uterus and hence there is bleeding. Thus the ancient Chinese were quite right in calling such non-vaginal bleeding shifted or counterflow menstruation.

When the menses come like a tide or before the menstrual movement, because the *chong* qi is relatively exuberant and the sea of blood is full and exuberant, blood may be heated and [its movement thus] forced. It then follows the *chong* qi counterflowing upward. Hence there is counterflow of the menstrual movement.

In this case, there was liver effulgence and blood heat, counterflow menstruation and erroneously shifted movement. Therefore the menstruation was 10 days ahead of schedule. Because the yin and blood had been boiled and cooked, the amount of the menses was scanty, their color was black, and their movement was short. Premenstrual dizziness, vexation and agitation, and easy anger were due to liver channel depressive fire upbearing and soaring. Each time the qi became more depressed, the amount of shifted menstruation was heavier. This is because anger leads the qi to penetrate and counterflow upward.

Old Doctor Liu used the experiential formula, *Liang Xue Zhi Nu Tang* (Cool the Blood & Stop Spontaneous Ejection of Blood) with additions and subtractions to treat [this case]. Because the signs of heat in this case were not heavy and the duration of its course was long, and also because there was the simultaneous appearance of leukorrhea and lumbar pain, signs of internal vacuity, [Dr. Liu] removed Radix Et Rhizoma Rhei (*Da Huang*) from the basic *Liang Xue Zhi Nu* [*Tang*] above and added Ophiopogon in order to nourish yin. In addition, because the qi depression symptoms were heavy, he added Aurantium to move the qi and open depression. [Thus,] not only was the shifted menstruation treated and cured, but the menstrual cycle also returned to normal.

Frequent Arrival of Menstruation: Three Cases

Case 1: Wang, female, 26 years old, a simple case in the out-patient department

Date of initial examination: June 21, 1975

Major complaints: Frequent and excessive menstruation for four years already

Present case history: Menarche had occurred at 13 years of age and [the menses had come sometimes] early, [sometimes] late, and at no fixed schedule. Four years previously, the menses had become [too] frequent and profuse in amount, moving every 12-23 days. The menstrual movement last 5-7 days, their color was blackish, and they contained clots. Sometimes they dribbled and dripped without cease and there was lumbar and lower leg aching and pain. Occasionally, she had lower abdominal sagging pain, heart and chest opression and vexation, shortness of breath, tension and agitation, and profuse leukorrhea which was sometimes yellow in color. For the last three months [*i.e.*, periods], her menses had come on April 20, May 3, and May 15. Gynecological examination had not shown any abnormality.

Tongue image: A dark tongue body with white fur

Pulse image: Bowstring, fine, and slippery

Western medical diagnosis: Irregular menstruation

Chinese medical pattern discrimination: Yin vacuity and blood heat, *chong* and *ren* loss of regulation

Treatment methods: Enrich yin and clear heat, quiet the *chong* and secure menstruation

Formula & medicinals: Uncooked Radix Rehmanniae (*Sheng Di*), 4 *qian*, Radix Scutellariae Baicalensis (*Huang Qin*), 3 *qian*, Rhizoma Thalictri Foliosi (*Ma Wei Lian*), 3 *qian*, Pericarpium Trichosanthis Kirlowii (*Gua Lou Pi*), 5 *qian*, Herba Dendrobii (*Shi Hu*), 3 *qian*, Tuber Ophiopogonis Japonici (*Mai Dong*), 3 *qian*, Radix Scrophulariae Ningpoensis (*Xuan Shen*), 3 *qian*, Fructus Ligustri Lucidi (*Nu Zhen Zi*), 3 *qian*, Herba Ecliptae Prostratae (*Han Lian Cao*), 3 *qian*, Cortex Radicis Moutan (*Dan Pi*), 3 *qian*, Gelatinum Corii Asini (*E Jiao*), 5 *qian*

Course of treatment: On re-examination on July 13 it was said that, after taking 20 *ji* of the above formula, her menses had come on time on June 11 and July 11. [Thus,] her menstrual cycle was normal, the amount of blood was moderate, and the menses had moved for three days.

Case 2: Cui, female, 12 years old, a simple case in the out-patient department

Date of initial examination: July 22, 1973

Major complaints: Frequent arrival of menstruation with the menses moving for 10 days or more without stopping

Present case history: Menarche had occurred at 11 years of age. Right from the beginning it had come [too] frequently and its volume was profuse. The menses moved for more than 20 days each time. This was accompanied by no flavor for the food taken in, bodily lassitude, and lack of strength. During the premenstruum and the menstrual period there was lumbar and abdominal pain and vexation and agitation. [The patient also] had leukorrhea. The last menses had occurred on July 11 and had not stopped for already now 11 days.

Tongue image: Thin, white fur and a dark tongue body

Pulse image: Bowstring, slippery, and rapid

Western medical diagnosis: Irregular menstruation

Chinese medical pattern discrimination: Yin vacuity and blood heat, *chong* and *ren* not securing [or insecure]

Formula & medicinals: Uncooked Radix Rehmanniae (*Sheng Di*), 5 *qian*, Tuber Ophiopogonis Japonici (*Mai Dong*), 3 *qian*, Radix Scrophulariae Ningpoensis (*Xuan Shen*), 3 *qian*, Herba Artemisiae Apiaceae (*Qing Hao*), 3 *qian*, Cortex Radicis Moutan (*Dan Pi*), 3 *qian*, Gelatinum Corii Asini (*E Jiao*), 5 *qian*, Herba Ecliptae Prostratae (*Han Lian Cao*), 3 *qian*, Cortex Cedrelae (*Chu Gen Bai Pi*), carbonized Rhizoma Cimicifugae (*Sheng Ma*), 3 *qian*, carbonized Rhizoma Guanchong (*Guan Zhong*), 3 *qian*, Radix Dioscoreae Oppositae (*Shan Yao*), 3 *qian*, Semen Nelumbinis Nuciferae (*Shi Lian*), 3 *qian*

Course of treatment: After taking a total of 16 *ji* of the above formula, the menstrual cycle became normal and the amount of the menstruate became normal. On follow-up after more than one year, no abnormality was seen.

Case 3: Zhang, female, 41 years old, a simple case in the out-patient department

Date of initial examination: June 23, 1972

Major complaints: Menstruation arriving [too] frequently with profuse volume

Present case history: Nine years previously, after great bleeding during birthing, [the patient's] menses moved one time every 22 days.

159

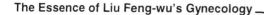

The menses moved for 4-5 days, their color was fresh red, and their amount was profuse. There was menstrual period lumbar and lower leg aching. Habitually, there was shortness of breath and lack of strength. Her last menstruation had occurred on Jun. 5.

Tongue image: A pale tongue body with thin, white fur

Pulse image: Bowstring and relaxed

Western medical diagnosis: Irregular menstruation

Chinese medical pattern discrimination: Spleen-kidney insufficiency, *chong* and *ren* loss of regulation

Treatment methods: Fortify the spleen and boost the kidneys, secure, contain, and quiet the *chong*

Formula & medicinals: Radix Dioscoreae Oppositae (*Shan Yao*), 5 *qian*, scorched Rhizoma Atractylodis Macrocephalae (*Bai Zhu*), 4 *qian*, Herba Ecliptae Prostratae (*Han Lian Cao*), 3 *qian*, Radix Dipsaci (*Chuan Duan*), 4 *qian*, Semen Cuscutae Chinensis (*Tu Si Zi*), 3 *qian*, cooked Radix Rehmanniae (*Shu Di*), 3 *qian*, Gelatinum Corii Asini (*E Jiao*), 5 *qian*, Fructus Ligustri Lucidi (*Nu Zhen Zi*), 3 *qian*, Radix Pseudostellariae (*Tai Zi Shen*), 3 *qian*, Radix Scutellariae Baicalensis (*Huang Qin*), 3 *qian*, Cortex Cedrelae (*Chun Gen Bai Pi*), 3 *qian*, Os Sepiae Seu Sepiellae (*Wu Zei Gu*), 3 *qian*

Course of treatment: On July 4, after taking 11 *ji* of this formula, cycles were 28 days apart. The menses had come like a tide on July 2 and their amount was normal. They moved for five days.

Commentary: All three of the above-mentioned cases were categorized as menstruation arriving [too] frequently with profuse volume. In terms of its development, this may be a manifestation of cycles which are relatively [too] short apart after menarche due to the menstrual movement enduring for [too many] days each time. Thus the time between them is too short. It is also possible that, due to excessive postpartum bleeding and other such factors, spleen and kidney function is affected. This results in the *chong* and *ren* losing their regulation and not being able to contain the blood. Hence the menses arrive too frequently. It is relatively common to see this condition begin from [sometimes] early, [sometimes] late, no fixed schedule [menstruation]. Due to being mixed with heat, this gradually develops into menstruation arriving [too] frequently and in profuse amount. If this develops further, it may eventually turn into flooding and leaking, [in other words,] either menstruation which dribbles and drips without ceasing or flooding strike of downward bleeding.

In case #1, after menarche there had been [sometimes] early, [sometimes] late, no fixed schedule [menstruation]. After four years, her menses had become too frequent and profuse in volume. For the last three months, the time between cycles was so short that her menses moved two times each month. Lumbar and lower leg aching and pain, lower abdominal sagging pain, a dark tongue, and a bowstring, fine, slippery pulse were also seen. The color of the menstrual blood was black and it was thick [in consistency]. There was heart and chest vexation and oppression and easy agitation. Leukorrhea was habitually profuse and yellow in color. [These symptoms] were categorized as the pattern of yin vacuity blood heat, *chong* and *ren* loss of regulation. [Dr. Liu] used the methods of clearing heat and enriching yin, quieting the *chong* and regulating the menses to treat this. The formula [Dr. Liu] used was *Gua Shi Tang* (Trichosanthes & Dendrobium Decoction) plus Ligustrum Lucidum and Eclipta to nourish yin and supplement the liver and kidneys and Moutan and Donkey Skin Glue to nourish the blood, cool the blood, and stop bleeding. Because [this case] was one of menstruation arriving [too] frequently, [Dr. Liu] therefore removed Achyranthes, Dianthus, Leonurus, and Plantago, [*i.e.,*] freeing the flow

161

and disinhibiting ingredients, from within this formula. In addition, he added Scutellaria to strengthen the effect of clearing heat.

In case #2, compared to the previous case, blood heat was marked. This resulted in the *chong* and *ren* not securing and the menses moved each time for more than 20 days. Therefore, [Dr. Liu] mainly used *Liang Di Tang* (Two *Di* Decoction) plus carbonized Cimicifuga and carbonized Guanchong to cool the blood and stop bleeding. Cedrela and Semen Nelumbinis [were also used] to fortify the spleen, supplement the kidneys, and secure the *chong* and *ren*.

Case #3 was categorized as spleen-kidney insufficiency, *chong* and *ren* loss of regulation. The formula used Pseudostellaria, scorched Atractylodes, and Dioscorea to fortify the spleen; Dipsacus, cooked Rehmannia, Cuscuta, Ligustrum Lucidum, and Eclipta to supplement the liver and kidneys; and Cuttlefish Bone, Cedrela, Donkey Skin Glue, and Semen Nelumbinis to nourish the blood and secure the *chong* and *ren*. Taken as a whole, this formula heavily [*i.e.*, strongly] regulates and supplements the function of the three viscera of the liver, spleen, and kidneys, and [thus] the menstruation was automatically regulated.

Flooding & Leaking (Functional Uterine Bleeding): Four Cases

Case 1: Shi, female, 41 years old, a simple case in the out-patient department

Date of initial examination: June 6, 1975

Major complaints: Menstruation [sometimes] early, [sometimes] late, [coming] at no fixed schedule; the menstrual movement was enduring [*i.e.*, continuing for too many] days for more than one year

Present case history: In the past [this patient's] menstruation had been normal. In the last year, [however,] the menstruation had become profuse in amount and its color was purple. It [also] contained blood clots. In eight months out of the [last] year, there had been great bleeding for more than 10 days, because of which the menstruation was arriving too frequently. When this was severe, it would arrive two times in one month, its amount was profuse, and its movement endured for [many] days (more than 10 days). During one month in the last year, vaginal bleeding had been so great, she had had uterine curettage surgery. The pathology report was "endometrial hyperplasia." After this, her menstruation had become blocked and stopped for two months. Then there was continuous vaginal tract dribbling and dripping for more than 10 days. She was treated with progesterone and, when her menses came like a tide, it [again] dribbled and dripped without stop. Its color was black and its amount tended to be profuse. It [also] contained small blood clots. For the past two years her emotions had been vexed and tense and she was easily angry. This was accompanied by chest and rib-side distention and fullness, torpid intake, abdominal distention, lumbar aching and pain, and dry stools which came one time every 2-3 days. The date of her last menstruation was April 22. Since then, she had had blocked menstruation [*i.e.*, amenorrhea] for 54 days.

Tongue image: A pale red tongue body

Pulse image: Bowstring and slippery

Western medical diagnosis: Functional uterine bleeding

Chinese medical pattern discrimination: Spleen-kidney insufficiency, blood heat and liver effulgence

Treatment methods: Fortify the spleen and supplement the kidneys, cool the blood and course the liver

Formula & medicinals: Radix Dioscoreae Oppositae (*Shan Yao*), 5 *qian*, Semen Nelumbinis Nuciferae (*Shi Lian*), 3 *qian*, Semen Cuscutae Chinensis (*Tu Si Zi*), 3 *qian*, Radix Dipsaci (*Chuan Duan*), 3 *qian*, uncooked and cooked Radix Rehmanniae (*Sheng Shu Di*), 3 *qian* each, Radix Albus Paeoniae Lactiflorae (*Bai Shao*), 4 *qian*, stir-fried Herba Seu Flos Schizonepetae Tenuifoliae (*Jing Jie Sui*), 1.5 *qian*, Radix Bupleuri (*Chai Hu*), 1.5 *qian*, Radix Scutellariae Baicalensis (*Huang Qin*), 3 *qian*, Cortex Radicis Moutan (*Dan Pi*), 3 *qian*, Herba Leonuri Heterophylli (*Yi Mu Cao*), 2 *qian*

Course of treatment: On June 26, 1975, after taking three *ji* of the above formula, the menses came like a tide and moved for four days. Their color was red and their amount was moderate. Because chest and rib-side distention and aching were marked, [Dr. Liu] added Fructus Meliae Toosendan (*Chuan Lian Zi*), 3 *qian*, to the previous formula and continued its administration for seven *ji*. On July 1, 1975, after these medicinals, the menses had come two times (June 18-22 and July 16-19). The volume of the blood was less and the menses moved for [only] four days. [Dr. Liu] continued administering the above formula [another] five *ji*. On September 27, 1975, [the patient] was re-examined. From June 19-August 1, she had taken a total of 23 *ji* of Chinese medicinals and all her symptoms had disappeared. Her menstruation moved on time and its amount was decreased. It moved for 3-5 days and had moved normally three times. The medicinals were stopped for observation. The menstruation came like a tide two more times. The menstrual cycle was a little early (23-25 days). The last menstruation had occurred on September 24.

Case 2: Zou, female, 46 years old, a simple case in the out-patient department

Date of initial examination: May 28, 1975

Major complaints: Profuse menstruation with menstrual movement enduring for [many] days for a half year already

Present case history: In the past, [this patient's] menstruation had been normal. A half year before, after having gotten angry and anxious, her menstruation had become [somtimes] early, [sometimes] late, [and came] at no fixed schedule. Its amount was profuse and the menstrual movement had been dribbling and dripping already for half a year. [The patient's] last menstruation had come like a tide on May 26. Its amount was exceptionally profuse, its color was fresh red, and there were no blood clots. This was accompanied by heart fluster [*i.e.*, palpitations], shortness of breath, bodily lassitude and lack of strength, lumbar aching and lower leg flaccidity, vacuity sweating, and comparatively poor sleep. Her food intake was typical [*i.e.*, normal], and her two excretions were normal. Her hematochrome was 8g.

Tongue image: A pale tongue body

Pulse image: Bowstring and relaxed

165

Western medical diagnosis: Functional uterine bleeding

Chinese medical pattern discrimination: Spleen-kidney insufficiency, *chong* and *ren* not securing [or insecure]

Treatment methods: Fortify the spleen and supplement the kidneys, boost the qi and secure the *chong*

Formula & medicinals: Radix Astragali Membranacei (*Huang Qi*), 8 *qian*, Radix Codonopsitis Pilosulae (*Dang Shen*), 4 *qian*, scorched Rhizoma Atractylodis Macroceephalae (*Bai Zhu*), 4 *qian*, mix-fried Radix Glycyrrhizae (*Gan Cao*), 3 *qian*, Radix Polygalae Tenuifoliae (*Yuan Zhi*), 3 *qian*, Arillus Euphoriae Longanae (*Gui Yuan Rou*), 3 *qian*, stir-fried Semen Zizyphi Spinosae (*Zao Ren*), 3 *qian*, Radix Dipsaci (*Chuan Duan*), 4 *qian*, cooked Radix Rehmanniae (*Shu Di*), 4 *qian*, calcined Concha Ostreae (*Mu Li*), 1 *liang*, Os Sepiae Seu Sepiellae (*Wu Zei Gu*), 4 *qian*, Gelatinum Corii Asini (*E Jiao*), 5 *qian*, carbonized Fibra Stipulae Trachycarpi (*Zong Lu*), 4 *qian*, carbonized Cacumen Biotae Orientalis (*Ce Bai*), 3 *qian*, carbonized Radix Sanguisorbae (*Di Yu*), 3 *qian*, Pulvis Radicis Pseudoginseng (*San Qi Mian*), 5 *fen* (taken separately washed down [by the decoction])

Course of treatment: On May 31, after taking three *ji* of the above formula, the amount of blood was markedly decreased. She only had a few drops which had not cleared [at this moment. Therefore, Dr. Liu] continued administering the above formula for three [more] *ji*. On re-examination on June 5, it was said that, after these medicinals, her menstruation had cleared on June 2. [However,] she still had shortness of breath, lack of strength, poor sleep, a pale tongue body, and a deep, weak pulse. Therefore, based on the methods of fortifying the spleen and supplementing the kidneys, nourishing the heart and quieting the spirit, the formula and medicinals were as follows: Radix Astragali Membranacei (*Huang Qi*), 1 *liang*, Radix Codonopsitis Pilosulae (*Dang Shen*), 5 *qian*, Rhizoma Atractylodis Macrocephalae (*Bai Zhu*), 3 *qian*,

Radix Dioscoreae Oppositae (*Shan Yao*), 4 *qian*, Radix Dipsaci (*Chuan Duan*), 4 *qian*, cooked Radix Rehmanniae (*Shu Di*), 3 *qian*, Semen Cuscutae Chinensis (*Tu Si Zi*), 3 *qian*, Radix Polygalae Tenuifoliae (*Yuan Zhi*), 3 *qian*, stir-fried Semen Zizyphi Spinosae (*Gui Yuan Rou*), 3 *qian*, Fructus Schisandrae Chinensis (*Wu Wei Zi*), 3 *qian*, and Radix Polygoni Multiflori (*He Shou Wu*), 1 *liang*.

On June 14, after taking the above formula, the heart fluster and shortness of breath had taken a turn for the better. However, she had a slight degree of facial edema and her four limbs were distended. Her tongue and pulse were the same as before. Therefore, based on the methods of fortifying the spleen and nourishing the heart, upbearing yang and eliminating dampness, the formula and medicinals were as follows: Radix Astragali Membranacei (*Huang Qi*), 5 *qian*, Radix Codonopsitis Pilosulae (*Dang Shen*), 3 *qian*, Rhizoma Atractylodis Macrocephalae (*Bai Zhu*), 5 *qian*, mix-fried Radix Glycyrrhizae (*Gan Cao*), 2 *qian*, Sclerotium Poriae Cocos (*Fu Ling*), 5 *qian*, Radix Polygalae Tenuifoliae (*Yuan Zhi*), 3 *qian*, Arillus Euphoriae Longanae (*Gui Yuan Rou*), 4 *qian*, Radix Et Rhizoma Ligustici Chinensis (*Gao Ben*), 2 *qian*, Herba Seu Flos Schizonepetae Tenuifoliae (*Jing Jie Sui*), 1.5 *qian*, and Radix Ldebouriellae Divaricatae (*Fang Feng*), 1.5 *qian*.

On June 23, she reported lumbar aching for the last day or so. [Thinking perhaps the menstruation was about to come, Dr. Liu] prescribed the following formula in order to prevent the menstrual blood from being excessive: Radix Astragali Membranacei (*Huang Qi*), 8 *qian*, Radix Codonopsitis Pilosulae (*Dang Shen*), 4 *qian*, scorched Rhizoma Atractylodis Macrocephalae (*Bai Zhu*), 4 *qian*, mix-fried Radix Glycyrrhizae (*Gan Cao*), 3 *qian*, Radix Polygalae Tenuifoliae (*Yuan Zhi*), 3 *qian*, Arillus Euphoriae Longanae (*Gui Yuan Rou*), 3 *qian*, stir-fried Semen Zizyphi Spinosae (*Zao Ren*), 3 *qian*, Radix Dipsaci (*Chuan Duan*), 4 *qian*, cooked Radix Rehmanniae (*Shu Di*), 4 *qian*, Os Sepiae Seu Sepiellae (*Wu Zei Gu*), 4 *qian*, carbonized Radix Sanguisorbae (*Di Yu*), 3 *qian*, carbonized Fibra Stipulae Trachycarpi (*Zong Lu*), 3 *qian*, carbonized

167

Cacumen Biotae Orientalis (*Ce Bai*), 3 *qian*, calcined Concha Ostreae (*Mu Li*), 1 *liang*, Gelatinum Corii Asini (*E Jiao*), 5 *qian*, and Pulvis Radicis Pseudoginseng (*San Qi Miao*), 5 *fen* (taken separately washed down [by the decoction]).

On July 9, after these medicinals, menstruation had come like a tide from June 26 to July 2. The menses had moved for six days. Compared to previously, the volume of the blood was only one third as much. [The patient's] essence spirit and bodily strength had become good [again], and lumbar aching and lower leg flaccidity had improved. Therefore, in order to secure the treatment effect, the following formula was prescribed: Radix Astragali Membranacei (*Huang Qi*), 8 *qian*, Radix Codonopsitis Pilosulae (*Dang Shen*), 4 *qian*, scorched Rhizoma Atractylodis Macrocephalae (*Bai Zhu*), 4 *qian*, mix-fried Radix Glycyrrhizae (*Gan Cao*), 2 *qian*, Radix Polygalae Tenuifoliae (*Yuan Zhi*), 3 *qian*, Arillus Euphoriae Longanae (*Gui Yuan Rou*), 3 *qian*, stir-fried Semen Zizyphi Spinosae (*Zao Ren*), 3 *qian*, Radix Dipsaci (*Chuan Duan*), 3 *qian*, cooked Radix Rehmanniae (*Shu Di*), 4 *qian*, Os Sepiae Seu Sepiellae (*Wu Zei Gu*), 4 *qian*, calcined Concha Ostreae (*Mu Li*), 1 *liang*, Gelatinum Corii Asini (*E Jiao*), 5 *qian*, and carbonized Radix Sanguisorbae (*Di Yu*), 4 *qian*.

Case 3: Yang, female, 28 years old, a simple case in the out-patient department

Date of initial examination: August 23, 1975

Major complaints: Uterine tract bleeding for more than 50 days

Present case history: In the past, [the patient's] menstruation had been normal. Her last menstruation had occurred on June 2 and the menses had moved for seven days. Their amount tended to be scanty. On July 1, her menses had come and [then] had dribbled and dripped without stop. She already had a diagnostic uterine curettage [which had shown] "hyperplasia of the endometrium." After this surgery, blood still dribbled and dripped without stop from her vaginal tract. This had been going on for more than 50 days and [prior] treatment had not cured it. Urine pregnancy test was negative.

Tongue image: A dark yet pale tongue body with white fur

Pulse image: Fine and relaxed

Western medical diagnosis: Functional uterine bleeding

Chinese medical pattern discrimination: Blood vacuity and blood stasis, *chong* and *ren* loss of regulation

Treatment methods: Nourish the blood and quicken the blood, transform stasis and regulate menstruation

Formula & medicinals: Radix Angelicae Sinensis (*Dang Gui*), 3 *qian*, Radix Ligustici Wallichii (*Chuan Xiong*), 1.5 *qian*, Semen Pruni Persicae (*Tao Ren*), 1 *qian*, Flos Carthami Tinctorii (*Hong Hua*), 1 *qian*, Herba Leonuri Heterophylli (*Yi Mu Cao*), 2 *qian*, Herba Lycopi Lucidi (*Ze Lan*), 2 *qian*, Radix Salviae Miltiorrhizae (*Dan Shen*), 2 *qian*, Radix Rubrus Paeoniae Lactiflorae (*Chi Shao*), 2 *qian*, Resina Myrrhae (*Mo Yao*), 1.5 *qian*, Radix Bupleuri (*Chai Hu*), 1 *qian*, stir-fried Herba Seu Flos Schizonepetae Tenuifoliae (*Jing Jie Sui*), 2 *qian*, carbonized Pollen Typhae (*Pu Huang*), 2 *qian*

Course of treatment: After taking five *ji* of these medicinals the bleeding stopped. [Dr. Liu prescribed another] three *ji* of the above formula in order to secure the treatment effect. On follow-up after [taking] these medicinals it was determined that menstruation had moved at regular intervals three times and no abnormal bleeding had appeared.

169

Case 4: Sun, female, 29 years old, a simple case in the out-patient department

Date of initial examination: March 2, 1974

Major complaints: The menstrual movement had endured for [many] days for the last 10 years

Present case history: For the last 10 years, [this patient's] menstrual movement had endured for [too many] days. Each time it continued for 15-70 days, and there was no regular intervals to her cycle. [Sometimes] it was early, [sometimes] it was late. It had no fixed schedule ([coming anywhere] between 20-70 days). The previous menstruation had occurred from January 13 to January 28, while the most recent menstruation had come on February 21 and had not yet cleared. Its amount was profuse, its color was red, and it contained blood clots. This was accompanied by dizziness, profuse dreams, vexation and tension, chest oppression, heat in the hands, feet, and heart [alternate reading: heat in the center of the hands and feet], and a dry mouth. For the last five months, her basal body temperature had been monophasic. She had been diagnosed at another hospital as [suffering from] functional uterine bleeding.

Tongue image: A dark tongue body with red tip

Pulse image: Bowstring and slippery

Western medical diagnosis: Functional uterine bleeding

Chinese medical pattern discrimination: Yin vacuity and blood heat, *chong* and *ren* not securing [or insecure]

Treatment methods: Nourish yin and clear heat, quiet the *chong* and regulate menstruation

170

Formula & medicinals: Herba Artemisiae Apiaceae (*Qing Hao*), 3 *qian*, Cortex Radicis Lycii Chinensis (*Di Gu Pi*), 3 *qian*, Radix Scutellariae Baicalensis (*Huang Qin*), 3 *qian*, Cortex Radicis Moutan (*Dan Pi*), 3 *qian*, Radix Albus Paeoniae Lactiflorae (*Bai Shao*), 3 *qian*, Herba Ecliptae Prostratae (*Han Lian Cao*), 3 *qian*, Cortex Cedrelae (*Chun Gen Bai Pi*), 3 *qian*, calcined Concha Ostreae (*Mu Li*), 8 *qian*, Gelatinum Corii Asini (*E Jiao*), 5 *qian*, carbonized Cacumen Biotae Orientalis (*Ce Bai*), 3 *qian*

Course of treatment: On March 13, after taking three *ji* of these medicinals, the vaginal tract bleeding had already stopped. Administration of [another] three *ji* was continued. On March 23, her menses again came like a tide. The menses moved for six days. Thus both the menstrual cycle and the amount of blood had returned to normal. The basal body temperature was now biphasic (indicating that she had ovulated). Whether the treatment effect was enduring had yet to be observed.

Commentary: All four of the above-mentioned cases had been diagnosed in Western medicine as [suffering from] functional uterine bleeding. The diagnostic criteria of this disease are [divided into] the following three varieties [or categories]:

1. Any reproductive pathological change or generalized disease leading to the arising of abnormal uterine bleeding which has continued for three months or more

2. An endometrial pathology examination [which shows] a hyperplastic condition of the uterine endometrium

3. A monophasic or atypical biphasic basal body temperature with body temperature gradually lowering after the start of menstruation, thus showing dysfunction of the corpus luteum

In Chinese medicine, functional uterine bleeding is categorized as "flooding and leaking."

In case #1, besides the clinical symptoms, endometrial pathology examination had diagnosed endometrial hyperplasia. This confirmed the diagnosis of functional uterine bleeding. [The patient's] menstrual cycles were not regularly spaced, their volume was profuse, and the menstrual movement endured for [many] days. The color was purple and [the menstruate] contained clots. This was the result of spleen-kidney insufficiency with liver effulgence and blood heat. The bowstring, slippery pulse and dark red tongue were categorized as blood heat signs. The chest and rib-side distention and pain were the result of liver depression qi stagnation. The vexation and tension and easy anger and the dry stools were the result of liver depression having endured for [many] days transfoming fire. While the torpid intake and abdominal distention were signs of spleen vacuity. Therefore, this case's pattern was categorized as spleen-kidney insufficiency with liver effulgence and blood heat. Treatment, [therefore,] should fortify the spleen and supplement the kidneys, cool the blood and clear the liver.

Within the formula, cooked Rehmannia, Cuscuta, and Dipsacus supplement the kidneys and quiet the *chong*. Dioscorea supplements the spleen and stomach. Semen Nelumbinis fortifies the spleen and supplements the kidneys. Uncooked Rehmannia, White Peony, Bupleurum, and Schizonepeta nourish the blood and soothe the liver. Moutan clears heat and cools the blood. Scutellaria clears blood heat. Leonurus quickens the blood and regulates menstruation. When used in small [amounts], it simultaneously has the action of nourishing the blood. After administering a total of 23 *ji* of these medicinals, the menstrual movement came three times regularly spaced with moderate volume. The menses moved for 3-5 days. The medicinals were stopped in order to observe if the menses were able to move at normal intervals [which they were].

In case #2, its onset was the same as the previous case's in that menstruation was [sometimes] early, [sometimes] late, and [came at] no fixed schedule, its amount was profuse, and the menstrual movement endured for [many] days. This then had gradually developed into functional uterine bleeding. The last menstruation had been exceptionally profuse and [the patient] had manifest symptoms of anemia (her hematochrome was 8g). These were signs of spleen-kidney dual vacuity with *chong* and *ren* not securing [or insecure]. Therefore, the formula [Dr. Liu] used was *Gui Pi Tang* (Restore the Spleen Decoction) with Dipsacus, cooked Rehmannia, and Donkey Skin Glue to supplement the kidneys and nourish the blood. Calcined Oyster Shell and Cuttlefish Bone were to nourish yin and secure the *chong*. Thus the root was treated. Carbonized Cacumen Biotae, carbonized Trachycarpus, carbonized Sanguisorba, and powdered Pseudoginseng cooled the blood and stopped bleeding, thus treating the branch. After three *ji* of these medicinals, the amount of blood was markedly decreased. After the bleeding stopped, [Dr. Liu] removed the blood-cooling, stop-bleeding prescriptions [*i.e.,* medicinals]. [Then] he heavily used fortifying the spleen and supplementing the kidneys, nourishing the heart and quieting the spirit. After that, in order to prevent excessive bleeding with the next menstrual movement, he again used the first formula, and, when the menstruation arrived, its amount was markedly less. Because, from start to finish, the essence of the pathology was spleen-kidney dual vacuity, he made heavy use of fortifying the spleen and supplementing the kidneys combined with modifications with additions and subtractions based on [the stage in] the menstrual cycle.

In case #3, the course of disease was relatively short. There had been vaginal tract bleeding for only 50 days. Thus it had not yet exceeded three months. However, a diagnostic uterine curettage [had shown] "hyperplasia of the endometrium." This had, therefore, confirmed the diagnosis of functional uterine bleeding. The next time her menses had moved, they still dribbled and dripped without stop. Their color was purple and they contained clots. The tongue was dark red with white fur, and the pulse was bowstring and relaxed. The pattern was categorized as blood vacuity and blood stasis with loss of regulation of the *chong* and *ren*. Static blood had not transformed and new blood [thus] did not abide [in its channels. Rather,] it left its channels and moved. Therefore, Dr. Liu used *Chan Hou Sheng Hua Tang* (Postpartum Engendering & Transforming Decoction) with additions and subtractions in order to nourish the blood and transform stasis.

Within this formula, Dang Gui, Ligusticum Wallichium, Leonurus, Myrrh, Lycopus, and Persica nourish the blood and quicken the blood, dispel stasis and engender the new. Carthamus transforms stasis. When used in small [amounts], it nourishes the blood. Red Peony and Moutan cool the blood, quicken the blood, and transform stasis. Carbonized Pollen Typhae quickens the blood, transforms stasis, and stops bleeding. Bupleurum and Schizonepeta are able to upbear yang and eliminate dampness. They are also able to course and resolve blood heat. [Taken as] a whole, this formula nourishes the blood and cools the blood, quickens the blood and dispels stasis, and [this] engenders the new. After five *ji* of these medicinals, the bleeding was stopped and the symptoms were eliminated. On follow-up the menstruation had moved at proper intervals three times. This clearly shows that, when the disease course is relatively short, the treatment effect and prognosis are relatively fully satisfactory.

In case #4, the disease course was comparatively long. There was [sometimes] early, [sometimes] late, no fixed schedule menstruation, the amount was profuse, and the menstrual movement endured for [many] days. The color [of the menstruate] was red and it contained clots. This was accompanied by profuse dreams, vexation and tension, chest oppression, heat in the hands, feet, and heart, and other such symptoms of liver yin vacuity heat brewing in the blood division pattern. Therefore, [Dr. Liu] mainly used *Qing Jing Tang* (Clear the Menses Decoction) with cooked Rehmannia and Poria removed and Cortex Phellodendri (*Huang Bai*) changed to Scutellaria. [In addition,] he added

Eclipta to supplement the yin of the liver and kidneys; Donkey Skin Glue to supplement the blood and secure menstruation, and Cedrela, calcined Oyster Shell, and carbonized Cacumen Biotae to nourish yin and secure the *chong* and *ren*. After administering six *ji* of these medicinals, the result of stopping bleeding was achieved and the basal body temperature became biphasic.

Threatened Miscarriage: Three Cases

Case 1: Li, female, 30 years old, a simple case in the out-patient department

Date of initial examination: January 22, 1972

Major complaints: Having been pregnant for 48 days, in the last three days, lumbar and abdominal aching and pain, blood flowing from the vaginal tract

Present case history: [The patient] had been pregnant for 48 days. In the last three days, there had been lumbar and abdominal pain and a bloody secretion from her vaginal tract. Pregnancy antibody test was positive.

Tongue image: A red tongue body

Pulse image: Fine and slippery

Western medical diagnosis: Threatened abortion

Chinese medical pattern discrimination: Spleen vacuity and blood heat

Treatment methods: Fortify the spleen and clear heat, cool the blood and quiet the fetus

Formula & medicinals: Uncooked Radix Disocoreae Oppositae (*Shan Yao*), 8 qian, Semen Nelumbinis Nuciferae (*Shi Lian*), 3 qian, Radix Scutellariae Baicalensis (*Huang Qin*), 3 qian, Rhizoma Thalictri Foliosi (*Ma Wei Lian*), 3 qian, Cortex Cedrelae (*Chun Gen Bai Pi*), 3 qian, carbonized Cacumen Biotae Orientalis (*Ce Bai*), 3 *qian*, Gelatinum Corii Asini (*E Jiao*), 5 *qian* (dissolved)

Course of treatment: On January 26, after oral intake of three *ji* of the above formula, the bloody secretion from the vaginal tract had stopped and the lumbar and abdominal aching and pain had been relaxed and resolved. Three more *ji* of the above formula were continued to be administered in order to secure the treatment effect.

Case 2: Qi, female, 32 years old, a case from another hospital, hospitalization No: 166629

Date of consultant examination: August 29, 1975

Major complaints: Amenorrhea for 28 days, a small amount of blood flowing from the vaginal tract for the last three days

Present case history: [The patient] was married in 1970. After the marriage, she had had four miscarriages. Each time, these were caused by overtaxation. All had occurred within the first three months [of pregnancy]. The last miscarriage had occurred on Jun. 9, 1975. After having blocked menstruation [*i.e.*, no menstruation] for 40 days, nausea, vomiting and a positive pregnancy antibody test were seen. On July 26, a small amount of blood flowed from her vaginal tract. Immediately progesterone was injected intramuscularly and had been every day from then till now. On Aug. 26, she was admitted to the hospital to preserve the fetus since she had been pregnant two months earlier and had a history of habitual miscarriage. After entering the hospital, besides the original treatment, 500 units of chorionic gonadotropin were injected intramuscularly and oral administration of vitamins and sedatives were added. Nevertheless, [the patient] still suffered from lumbar ache, abdominal region downward sagging, dizziness, sweating, and a small amount of vaginal tract bleeding. Her intake [of food] was scanty, but her two excretions were self-regulated [*i.e.*, normal].

Tongue image: A pale red tongue body

Pulse image: Deep, fine, and slightly rapid

Western medical diagnosis: A) Threatened miscarriage; B) habitual miscarriage

Chinese medical pattern discrimination: Qi and blood dual depletion, spleen-kidney insufficiency

Treatment methods: Supplement the qi and nourish the blood, fortify the spleen and boost the kidneys

Formula & medicinals: Stir-fried Radix Dioscoreae Oppositae (*Shan Yao*), 5 *qian*, Semen Nelumbinis Nuciferae (*Lian Rou*), 3 *qian*, Semen Cuscutae Chinensis (*Tu Si Zi*), 3 *qian*, Radix Dipsaci (*Chuan Duan*), 3 *qian*, Ramulus Loranthi Seu Visci (*Sang Ji Sheng*), 5 *qian*, Radix Angelicae Sinensis (*Dang Gui*), 2 *qian*, Rhizoma Atractylodis Macrocephalae (*Bai Zhu*), 3 *qian*, Gelatinum Corii Asini (*E Jiao*), 5 *qian* (dissolved)

Course of treatment: On September 5, after orally taking five *ji* of the above formula, the lumbar ache and downward sagging sensation in her lower abdomen were reduced but her urination was frequent. [Therefore,] Atractylodes and Dang Gui were removed from the above formula and Cortex Eucommiae Ulmoidis (*Du Zhong*), 3 *qian*, and Ramulus Loranthi Seu Visci (*Sang Ji Sheng*), 4 *qian*, were added. Administration was continued.

On September 9, after taking 3 *ji* of the above formula, the frequency of urination had decreased and the lumbar ache had diminished, but there was still a downward sagging sensation in her lower abdomen. Radix Astragali Membranacei (*Huang Qi*), 8 *qian*, was added to the above formula.

On September 16, after taking three *ji* of the above formula, the symptoms had almost disappeared, but there was still a slight sensation of downward sagging in the abdomen after activity.

On September 19, after taking three *ji* of the above formula, the downward sagging sensation in the abdomen had disappeared. In the last two days, [the patient had caught] a common cold [accompanied by] bodily [*i.e.*, generalized] lassitude, runny nose, and lumbar ache. The formula and medicinals were as follows: Herba Seu Flos Schizonepetae Tenuifoliae (*Jing Jie Sui*), 2 *qian*, Herba Menthae Haplocalycis (*Bo He*), 1 *qian*, Radix Disocoreae Oppositae (*Shan Yao*), 5 *qian*, Semen Nelumbinis Nuciferae (*Lian Rou*), 3 *qian*, Ramulus Loranthi Seu Visci (*Sang Ji Sheng*), 5 *qian*, Gelatinum Corii Asini (*E Jiao*), 5 *qian* (dissolved)

On September 26, after taking three *ji* of the above formula, the common cold was already cured. Schizonepeta and Mentha were subtracted from the above formula and Rhizoma Atractylodis Macrocephalae (*Bai Zhu*), 3 *qian*, and Semen Cuscutae Chinensis (*Tu Si Zi*), 3 *qian*, were added. Administration was continued.

On October 3, [the patient] was prepared for being discharged from the hospital. Due to being bathed, rushing upstairs and downstairs, and the increased activity, on Oct. 4 she again felt abdominal pain, lumbar ache, and occasional uterine contractions. Her tongue was pale red. Her right pulse was bowstring and slippery, while her left pulse was deep and slippery. The formula and medicinals were as follows: Radix Disocoreae Oppositae (*Shan Yao*), 8 *qian*, Radix Albus Paeoniae Lactiflorae (*Bai Shao*), 3 *qian*, Radix Scutellariae Baicalensis (*Huang Qin*), 3 *qian*, Cortex Cedrelae (*Chun Gen Bai Pi*), 3 *qian*, and Gelatinum Corii Asini (*E Jiao*), 5 *qian*.

On October 7, after taking two *ji* of the above formula, the abdominal pain had disappeared and the lumbar pain was decreased. [However,] there was still a sensation of downward sagging in the abdomen and scanty intake. [Therefore,] administration of the above formula was continued.

On October 9, after taking two *ji* of the above formula, the uterine contractions had disappeared but there was still lumbar pain and scanty intake. The formula and medicinals were as follows: Radix Disocoreae Oppositae (*Shan Yao*), 5 *qian*, Semen Nelumbinis Nuciferae (*Shi Lian*), 8 *qian*, Semen Cuscutae Chinensis (*Tu Si Zi*), 3 *qian*, Cortex Eucommiae Ulmoidis (*Du Zhong*), 3 *qian*, Gelatinum Corii Asini (*E Jiao*), 5 *qian* (dissolved), Ramulus Loranthi Seu Visci (*Sang Ji Sheng*), 4 *qian*, and Radix Dipsaci (*Chuan Duan*), 3 *qian*.

At present, the bottom of the uterus is parallel to the umbilicus. The heart of the fetus can be heard from the right lower abdomen (144 beats per minute). The pregnancy is at five months. On follow-up, the baby was delivered automatically [*i.e.*, without C-section or other such surgical intervention].

Case 3: Ma, female, 30 years old, a simple case in the out-patient department

Date of initial examination: November 1, 1973

Major complaints: Pregnant for 70 days, abdominal pain and vaginal tract bleeding for seven days

Present case history: The last menstruation had been normal. [The patient] had been pregnant for 70 days. Seven days ago, there appeared lower abdominal pain, lumbar ache, blood flowing from the vaginal tract which was fresh red in color, yellow urination, and dry stools. Re-examination for pregnancy was positive.

Tongue image: A red tongue body with scanty fur

Pulse image: Deep, slippery, and forceless

Western medical diagnosis: Threatened miscarriage

Chinese medical pattern discrimination: Blood heat damaging the fetus

Formula & medicinals: Radix Disocoreae Oppositae (*Shan Yao*), 5 *qian*, Semen Nelumbinis Nuciferae (*Shi Lian*), 3 *qian*, Radix Scutellariae Baicalensis (*Huang Qin*), 3 *qian*, carbonized Cacumen Biotae Orientalis (*Ce Bai*), 3 *qian*, Rhizoma Thalictri Foliosi (*Ma Wei Lian*), 3 *qian*, carbonized Cortex Cedrelae (*Chun Gen Bai Pi*), 3 *qian*, Gelatinum Corii Asini (*E Jiao*), 5 *qian* (dissolved), Radix Albus Paeoniae Lactiflorae (*Bai Shao*), 4 *qian*

Course of treatment: On November 4, after taking four *ji* of the above formula, the lumbar and abdominal pain had decreased and the vaginal tract bleeding had diminished. After continuing to administer three [more] *ji*, the vaginal tract bleeding had already stopped.

Commentary: Threatened abortion is called "fetal leakage" or "fetal stirring restlessness" in Chinese medicine. Old Doctor Liu held that fetal leakage is mostly caused by kidney qi insufficiency or spleen-stomach vacuity weakness. This then results in the fetal source not securing. It may also be caused by habitual bodily yang exuberance and heat forcing the blood to move.

If there is spleen qi vacuity weakness with blood heat damaging the fetus, mostly one will see bodily heat, a preference for chilled drinks, scanty eating, yellow urine and dry stools, lower abdominal sagging, distention, and pain, low back aching and pain, fresh red blood exiting from the vaginal tract, a red tongue body, and a bowstring, slippery, slightly rapid pulse. Treatment is in order to fortify the spleen and clear heat, cool the blood and quiet the fetus. To treat [this, Dr. Liu] commonly used the experiential formula, *Qing Re An Tai Yin* (Clear Heat & Quiet the Fetus Drink). If bleeding was profuse, he added carbonized Rhizoma Guanchong (*Guan Zhong*), carbonized Fibra Stipulae Trachycarpi (*Zong Lu*), uncooked Radix Rehmanniae (*Sheng Di*), and Herba Ecliptae Prostratae (*Han Lian Cao*).

If there is spleen-kidney dual vacuity and the fetal ligature is insecure, one will see scanty intake of food, lumbar aching and pain, lower abdominal sagging and distention, and continuous vaginal tract bleeding which is pale red in color. The tongue body is pale with white fur, and the pulse is slippery and forceless or deep and weak. Treatment is in order to fortify the spleen and boost the kidneys, nourish the blood and quiet the fetus. The formula [Dr. Liu] used was *Shou Tai Wan* (Long-life Fetus Pills) ([composed of] Semen Cuscutae Chinensis, *Tu Si Zi*, Radix Dipsaci, *Chuan Duan*, Ramulus Loranthi Seu Visci, *Sang Ji Sheng*, and Gelatinum Corii Asini, *E Jiao*) plus Radix Dioscoreae Oppositae (*Shan Yao*) and Semen Nelumbinis Nuciferae (*Shi Lian*). If the volume of bleeding was profuse, he added Cortex Cedrelae (*Chun Gen Bai Pi*) and carbonized Fibra Stipulae Trachycarpi (*Zong Lu*). If qi vacuity was marked, he added Radix Codonopsitis Pilosulae (*Dang Sheng*) and Radix Astragali Membranacei (*Huang Qi*). If there was lower abdominal downward sagging, [he] added carbonized Rhizoma Cimicifugae (*Sheng Ma*).

If there is yin vacuity blood heat, this mostly appears as fetal stirring restlessness or lower abdominal aching and pain with occasional dizziness, a tongue body tending towards red, and a fine, slippery pulse. Treatment is in order to nourish yin and emolliate the liver, clear heat and quiet the fetus. The formula [Dr. Liu] used was *Qin Lian Shao Yao Gan Cao Tang* (Scutellaria, Coptis, Peony & Licorice Decoction) with additions and subtractions.

Case #1 was categorized as spleen vacuity and blood heat. [Therefore,] the formula used was *Qing Re An Tai Yin*.

Case #2 was categorized as spleen-kidney insufficiency with insecurity of the fetal ligation. Treatment was in order to fortify the spleen and boost the kidneys, nourish the blood and quiet the fetus. Within its formula, Loranthus, Cuscuta, Dipsacus, and Eucommia enrich and supplement the liver and kidneys and quiet the fetus. Dioscorea, Lotus Seed, and scorched Atractylodes fortify the spleen, boost the kidneys, and quiet the fetus. Astragalus supplements the qi. Cedrela secures and astringes and stops bleeding. Donkey Skin Glue nourishes the blood and stops bleeding. Besides supplementing the qi and fortifying the spleen based on the rationale of the ancient formula, *Tai Shan Pan Shi San* (Mt. Tai Bedrock Powder), this formula also has a heavy power of securing the kidneys. [Therefore,] after [administering] these medicinals, the lumbar and abdominal pain resolved, while the vaginal tract bleeding had already stopped.

During the course of treatment, [the patient caught] a common cold with runny nose. However, there was no fever. This was categorized as a vacuity person with external contraction. Therefore, the original formula was used as a basis for supporting the righteous, while Schizonepeta and Mentha were added to course and resolve external evils. {Hence,] the righteous was supported and evils were dispelled.

In case #3, there was the simultaneous appearance of yin vacuity. Therefore, *Qing Re An Tai Yin* [was used] to which White Peony was added in order to nourish liver yin.

Infertility: Five Cases

Old Doctor Liu held that the main reasons why women are not able to get pregnant are kidney qi insufficiency, essence depletion and blood scantiness, uterus vacuity cold, yin vacuity and blood heat, liver depression qi stagnation, and loss of regulation of the *chong* and *ren*.

If the kidneys are vacuous and blood is scanty, mostly one will see an extremely scanty menstrual volume. The menstrual cycle will be normal and the menses will move for [only] 1-2 days. The color of the blood is pale and the bodily form is thin and weak. There is lumbar aching and lower leg pain. [The woman] has been infertile for many years, while her pulse is vacuous and fine. The tongue body is pale. To treat the above, [Dr. Liu] mostly used *Ba Zhen Tang* (Eight Pearls Decoction) without Rhizoma Atractylodis Macrocephalae (*Bai Zhu*) and Sclerotium Poriae Cocos (*Fu Ling*) but with the addition of Rhizoma Cyperi Rotundi (*Xiang Fu*), Flos Carthami Tinctorii (*Hong Hua*), Fructus Rubi Chingii (*Fu Pen Zi*), and Herba Epimedii (*Yin Yang Huo*), administering this for 6-7 *ji* after each menstruation.

If there is yin vacuity with blood scantiness, mostly one will see a normal menstrual cycle. The volume of the menses will [also] be extremely scanty but its color will be dark and brown. The bodily form is thin and weak, the mouth is dry, and there is vexatious heat or low-grade fever. The pulse is fine and vacuous or fine and rapid. The tongue body is red. To treat the above, [Dr. Liu] commonly used the following formula and medicinals: uncooked Radix Rehmanniae (*Sheng Di*), 4 *qian*, Radix Albus Paeoniae Lactiflorae (*Bai Shao*), 4 *qian*, Cortex Radicis Lycii Chinensis (*Di Gu Pi*), 3 *qian*, Radx Scrophulariae Ningpoensis (*Xuan Sheng*), 3 *qian*, Tuber Ophiopogoni Japonici (*Mai Dong*), 4 *qian*, Herba Artemisiae Apiaceae (*Qing Hao*), 3 *qian*, Fructus Lycii Chinensis (*Gou Qi Zi*), 5 *qian*, and Herba Leonuri Heterophylli (*Yi Mu Cao*), 4 *qian*. [These were used] in order to enrich yin and boost the kidneys, nourish the blood and clear heat.

If the uterus is cold and chilled, mostly one will see lower abdominal icy chill or chilly pain, a white facial complexion, a pale tongue with white fur, and a fine, relaxed pulse. To treat the above, [Dr. Liu] mostly used *Ai Fu Nuan Gong Wan* (Artemisia & Aconite Warm the Uterus Pills) or [he] used Radix Astragali Membranacei (*Huang Qi*), Fructus Evodiae Rutecarpae (*Wu Zhu Yu*), Radix Dipsaci (*Chuan Duan*), Semen Litchi Chinensis (*Li Zhi*), Herba Leonuri Heterophylli (*Yi Mu Cao*), and Fructus Foeniculi Vulgaris (*Xiao Hui Xiang*).

If there is yin vacuity and blood heat, one will mostly see menstruation ahead of schedule. If severe, [it may come] two times in one month. The color [of the menstruate] will be black and purple and it will contain large clots. During menstruation, there is vexatious heat or there may be menstrual pain. [Typically,] there are many years of infertility, and the pulse is slippery and rapid. To treat the above, [Dr. Liu] mostly used *Qing Jing Tang* (Clear the Menses Decoction) plus Semen Plantaginis (*Che Qian Zi*) and Herba Dianthi (*Qu Mai*).

If there is liver depression qi stagnation, one mostly will see menstruation behind schedule with chest and rib-side distention and pain, heart vexation and tension, and pale colored menstrual blood. There is abdominal pain with the menstrual movement, low back and lower leg aching and pain, many years infertility, and a deep, bowstring pulse. For treatment of the above, [Dr. Liu] mostly used *De Sheng Dan* (Obtaining Birth Elixir) plus Cortex Cinnamomi Cassiae (*Rou Gui*) and Rhizoma Cyperi Rotundi (*Xiang Fu*).

Case 1: Ren, female, 35 years old, married, a simple case in the out-patient department

Date of initial examination: April 5, 1973

Major complaints: Infertility for the last five years

Present case history: [The patient's] menarche occurred when she was 17 years old. Her menstrual cycle had been normal, but with her menses came lumbar and abdominal pain. Before her menses there appeared dizziness, nausea, and vomiting. After having been treated with Chinese and Western medicines, these symptoms had improved. After she was married, she gave birth to a baby boy in 1968. After that birth, her menses were [sometimes] early, [sometimes] late, and [came at] no fixed schedule. Their amount was scanty and their color was pale red. During the menstrual period, there was lumbar and abdominal pain with a preference for warmth and a preferance for pressure. [There was also] heart fluster [*i.e.,* heart palpitations], shortness of breath, lack of strength, and profuse dreams during sleep at night. After giving birth to this first child, she had not conceived for five years. Gynecological examinaton showed her uterus was retroverted and tended to be small.

Tongue image: A dark yet pale tongue body with thin, white fur

Pulse image: Fine and relaxed

Western medical diagnosis: Secondary infertility

Chinese medical pattern discrimination: Qi and blood dual vacuity, heart-spleen insufficiency

Treatment methods: Boost the qi and nourish the blood, supplement and boost the heart and spleen

Formula & medicinals: Radix Angelicae Sinensis (*Dang Gui*), 3 *qian*, Radix Astragali Membranacei (*Huang Qi*), 5 *qian*, Sclerotium Poriae Cocos (*Fu Ling*), 4 *qian*, Radix Glycyrrhizae (*Gan Cao*), 2 *qian*, Radix Codonopsitis (*Dang Sheng*), 4 *qian*, Rhizoma Atractylodis Macrocephalae

(*Bai Zhu*), 4 *qian*, Radix Disocoreae Oppositae (*Shan Yao*), 3 *qian*, Semen Zizyphi Spinosae (*Suan Zao*), 4 *qian*

Course of treatment: After taking eight *ji* of the above formula orally, *Kun Shun Dan* (*Kun* [*i.e.*, Female] Normalizing Elixir), 20 pills, was added.[25] The menstrual cycle was normal, its color was normal, and it did not contain blood clots. The lumbar and abdominal pain had already stopped. On July 12, 1973, due to blocked menstruation [*i.e.*, no menstruation] for more than one month, a pregnancy antibody test was given which was positive. On Mar. 5, 1974, after sufficient months, [she] gave birth to a baby girl.

Commentary: This case was categorized as qi and blood dual vacuity, heart-spleen insufficiency. After [the patient] had given birth the first time, her menses had come [sometimes] early, [sometimes] late, and at no fixed schedule. Their amount was scanty and their color was pale. This was due to postpartum qi and blood dual vacuity. The sea of blood was empty and vacuous and the uterine vessels had lost their nourishment. This had led to abdominal pain coming with menstruation which preferred pressure and preferred warmth. Due to heart-spleen insufficiency, there was heart fluster, shortness of breath, lack of strength, profuse dreams during sleep at night, a dark yet pale tongue with thin, white fur, and a fine, relaxed pulse. Because the sea of blood was empty and vacuous, essence had lost its place of nourishment and thus there was inability to conceive a second time. Treatment was in order to boost the qi and nourish the blood, supplement and boost the heart and spleen.

The formula used to treat this was *Gui Pi Tang* (Restore the Spleen Decoction) with additions and subtractions. Within this formula, Dang

---

[25] *Kun* is the name of one of the eight trigrams (*ba gua*) of the *Yi Jing* (*Classic of Change*). It is the most yin of all the trigrams and, therefore, is sometimes used to imply femininity or females in the Chinese medical literature.

Gui, White Peony, and Ligusticum Wallichium nourish the blood. Astragalus supplements the qi. Codonopsis, Atractyloodes, Poria, Licorice, and Dioscorea fortify the spleen and supplement the qi. Longans and Zizyphus Spinosa nourish the heart and quiet the spirit, while Leonurus quickens the blood and regulates menstruation. [Therefore, taken as] a whole, this formula boosts the qi and supplements the heart and spleen, quickens the blood and regulates the menses. Afterwards, *Kun Shun Dan* was used in addition and this treatment was continued for two whole months. Since the qi and blood and *chong* and *ren* had obtained fullness and nourishment, the menstruation was normal, lumbar and abdominal pain stopped, and, therefore, [she] conceived.

Case 2: Sun, female, 32 years old, married, a simple case in the out-patient department

Date of initial examination: November 23, 1971

Major complaints: No pregnancy after eight years of marriage

Present case history: The menses had been coming habitually late by more than 10 days. Their amount was moderate, their color was black, and there was premenstrual breast distention. Sometimes there was lumbar and abdominal chilliness. After having been married for eight years, she had never conceived. Previous gynecological examination showed that the uterus tended to be small.

Tongue image: Thin, white fur

Pulse image: Bowstring and slippery

Western medical diagnosis: Primary infertility

Chinese medical pattern discrimination: Liver depression qi stagnation, loss of regulation of the qi and blood

189

Treatment methods: Soothe the liver and resolve depression, nourish the blood, and regulate menstruation

Formula & medicinals: Radix Angelicae Sinensis (*Dang Gui*), 3 *qian*, Radix Albus Paeoniae Lactiflorae (*Bai Shao*), 3 *qian*, Radix Ligustici Wallichii (*Chuan Xiong*), 2 *qian*, Fructus Citri Aurantii (*Zhi Ke*), 2 *qian*, Radix Et Rhizoma Notopterygii (*Qiang Huo*), 1 *qian*, Radix Auklandiae Lappae (*Mu Xiang*), 1 *qian*, Herba Leeonuri Heterophylli (*Yi Mu Cao*), 6 *qian*, Radix Bupleuri (*Chai Hu*), 2 *qian*, Fructus Evodiae Rutecarpae (*Wu Zhu Yu*), 2 *qian*, Cortex Cinnamomi Cassiae (*Rou Gui*), 1 *qian*

Course of treatment: [The patient] conceived after taking 15 *ji* of this formula and delivered a boy normally after sufficient months. On follow-up in December 1974, she was pregnant [again]. This second time, she gave birth to twins in September 1973.

Commentary: This case was categorized as liver depression qi stagnation, loss of regulation of the qi and blood. The liver's storing of the blood, its preference for orderly reaching, and the menses are all closely related. If the emotions are not soothed, the liver may lose its orderly reaching and the qi and blood may lose their regulation. The *chong* and *ren* are not able to supply one another and, therefore, one is not able to conceive. Treatment was in order to soothe the liver and resolve depression, nourish the blood and regulate the menses. To treat [this, Dr. Liu] mostly used *De Sheng Dan* with added flavors. Within this formula, Dang Gui and White Peony nourish the blood. Ligusticum Wallichium courses and frees the flow of the qi within the blood. Aurantium and Auklandia regulate the qi and soothe depression. Bupleurum soothes the liver and resolves depression. Notopterygium courses and frees the flow of the qi and blood of the channels and vessels. Leonurus was used in place of cooked Radix Rehmanniae (*Shu Di*) in order to nourish the blood and regulate the menses without [causing] stagnation. Because there was simultaneously seen yang vacuity lumbar and abdominal chill, Evodia and Cortex Cinnamomi were added to warm the channels, scatter cold, and warm the uterus. After [taking] these medicinals, conception was obtained.

Case 3: Gong, female, 28 years old, married

Date of initial examination: March 1, 1973

Major complaints: No pregnancy after five years of marriage

Present case history: Menarche had occurred at age 15. The menstrual cycle was 30 days and the menses moved for 5-6 days. Their amount was profuse and their color was deep purple. They contained clots. With the menses came lumbar and abdominal distention, sagging, and aching and pain. There was whole body fear of chill, lower abdominal emission of coolness, icy chilling of the hands and feet, torpid intake, nausea, and loose stools. After five years of marriage, there had been no pregnancy.

Tongue image: A dark tongue body

Pulse image: Deep and relaxed

Western medical diagnosis: Primary infertility

Chinese medical pattern discrimination: Liver depression and blood vacuity, cold lodged in the uterus

Treatment methods: Resolve depression and nourish the blood, warm the channels and scatter cold

Formula & medicinals: Radix Angelicae Sinensis (*Dang Gui*), 3 *qian*, Radix Ligustici Wallichii (*Chuan Xiong*), 1.5 *qian*, stir-fried Radix Albus Paeoniae Lactiflorae (*Bai Shao*), 3 *qian*, Herba Leonuri Heterophylli (*Yi Mu Cao*), 4 *qian*, Fructus Citri Aurantii (*Zhi Ke*), 1.5 *qian*, Radix Auklandiae Lappae (*Mu Xiang*), 1.5 *qian*, processed Rhizoma Cyperi

191

Rotundi (*Xiang Fu*), 3 *qian*, Semen Cuscutae Chinensis (*Tu Si* Zi), 3 *qian*, Rhizoma Atractylodis Macrocephalae (*Bai Zhu*), 3 *qian*, dry Rhizoma Zingiberis (*Gan Jiang*), 2 *qian*, Semen Trigonellae Foeni-graeci (*Hu Lu Ba*), 3 *qian*

Course of treatment: On August 4, after taking 30 *ji* of these medicinals, the intake of food had increased. There was no nausea with the menses or loose stools, and the [patient's] essence spirit was already improved. However, there was still lower abdominal sagging pain, lumbar pain, and emission of a cool sensation in the lower abdomen. In order to increase the power of warming the uterus and scattering cold, the following formula and medicinals [were given]: Fructus Foeniculi Vulgaris (*Xiao Hui Xiang*), 3 *qian*, Semen Citri Reticulatae (*Ju He*), 3 *qian*, Semen Litchi Chinensis (*Li Zhi He*), 3 *qian*, Semen Trigonellae Foeni-graeci (*Hu Lu Ba*), 3 *qian*, Radix Linderae Strychnifoliae (*Wu Yao*), 3 *qian*, Rhizoma Corydalis Yanhusuo (*Yan Hu Suo*), 3 *qian*, Feces Trogopterori Seu Pteromi (*Wu Ling Zhi*), 3 *qian*, Herba Leonuri Heterophylli (*Yi Mu Cao*), 3 *qian*, and Semen Cuscutae Chinensis (*Tu Su Zi*), 3 *qian*.

On June 1, after taking 13 *ji* of the above formula, blocked menstruation [*i.e.*, no menstruation] had occurred for more than one month and pregnancy antibody test was positive. On follow-up in December 1974, [the patient] had given birth normally after sufficient months to a child. Her menstrual cycle was normal, its amount was slightly profuse, and its color was red. It did contain clots.

Commentary: In this case, there was originally a history of painful menstruation. When the menses came, there was lower abdominal sagging, distention, aching, and pain, nausea, and loose stools due to liver depression not being soothed affecting the spleen and stomach. The kidney qi was insufficient and the uterus was cold and chilled. Therefore, there was lower abdominal emission of coolness, fear of chill, and lack of warmth in the four limbs. In treating the above, besides soothing the liver, one needs to use warming the channels and scattering cold prescriptions.

[Dr. Liu] again used *De Sheng Dan* with added flavors to treat this. Within this formula, Dang Gui, Ligusticum Wallichium, White Peony, and Leonurus nourish the blood and regulate the menses. Aurantium, Auklandia, and Cyperus rectify the qi. Cuscuta and Fenugreek supplement the kidney qi. Atractylodes and dry Ginger warm and move spleen yang. After [taking] these medicinals, all the symptoms decreased. The intake of food increased and there was no nausea or loose stools with the coming of the menses. However, lower abdominal emission of coolness did not seem to be lessened and with the coming of the menses there was a sensation of sagging pain in the abdomen. This clearly evidenced that this formula's warming of the uterus was insufficient. [Therefore, Dr. Liu] used a prescription for warming the uterus and scattering cold, assisted by rectifying the qi and regulating the menses with the addition of Orange Seeds, Litchi, and Fennel to warm the lower source. Once the uterus obtained warmth and the *chong* and *ren* obtained regulation, afterwards there was conception.

Case 4: Wang, female, 29 years old, married

Date of initial examination: March 18, 1972

Major complaints: No pregnancy after 10 years of marriage

Present case history: Typically, [the patient's] menstrual cycle was normal, the color [of her menses] was normal, and their amount was moderate. [However,] there was profuse leukorrhea which was yellow in color and had a foul flavor [*i.e.*, odor]. There was [also] bilateral lower abdominal pain and lumbar pain accompanied by heat in the hands, feet, and heart [alternate reading: the centers of the hands and feet], headache, nausea, no desire to open the eyes, and frequent, numerous urination. Already having been married for 10 years, there had been no

193

pregnancy. Previous gynecological examination showed lack of free flow bilaterally in the fallopian tubes.

Tongue image: A dark red tongue body

Pulse image: Slippery

Western medical diagnosis: Primary infertility

Chinese medical pattern discrimination: Damp heat pouring downward, qi stagnation and blood stasis

Treatment methods: Clear heat and disinhibit dampness, course and free the flow of the qi and blood

Formula & medicinals: Herba Dianthi (*Qu Mai*), 4 *qian*, Herba Polygoni Avicularis (*Bian Xu*), 4 *qian*, Caulis Akebiae Mutong (*Mu Tong*), 1 *qian*, Semen Plantaginis (*Che Qian Zi*), 3 *qian*, Fructus Meliae Toosendan (*Chuan Lian Zi*), 3 *qian*, Radix Linderae Strychnifoliae (*Wu Yao*), 3 *qian*, Rhizoma Corydalis Yanhusuo (*Yan Hu Suo*), 3 *qian*, Rhizoma Dioscoreae Hypoglaucae (*Bi Xie*), 4 *qian*, Radix Rubrus & Albus Paeoniae Lactiflorae (*Chi Bai Shao*), 3 *qian* each, Flos Lonicerae Japonicae (*Yin Hua*), 5 *qian*

Course of treatment: On March 22, after taking three *ji* of the above formula, the pain on both sides of the lower abdomen was reduced, and the number of times of urination had decreased. The pulse was [now] relaxed. Red and White Peony were removed from the above formula, Herba Violae Yedoensis Cum Radice (*Di Ding*), 5 *qian*, and Herba Patriniae Heterophyllae Cum Radice (*Bai Jiang Cao*), 5 *qian*, were added, and administration was continued.

On March 27, the abdominal pain and frequent urination had basically disappeared. The yellow vaginal discharge had already stopped. [However,] there was still lumbar pain. In order to strengthen the above formula's power of moving the qi and quickening the blood, the following formula and medicinals [were given]: processed Rhizoma Cyperi Rotundi (*Xiang Fu*), 3 *qian*, Fructus Meliae Toosendan (*Chuan Lian Zi*), 3 *qian*, Radix Linderae Strychnifoliae (*Wu Yao*), 3 *qian*, Rhizoma Corydalis Yanhusuo (*Yan Hu Suo*), 3 *qian*, Feces Trogopterori Seu Pteromi (*Wu Ling Zhi*), 3 *qian*, Resina Myrrhae (*Mo Yao*), 1 *qian*, Semen Pruni Persicae (*Tao Ren*), 2 *qian*, Radix Auklandiae Lappae (*Mu Xiang*), 1.5 *qian*, and Pericarpium Citri Reticulatae (*Ju Pi*), 2 *qian*.

After taking 12 *ji* of the above formula continuously, blocked menstruation [*i.e.*, no menstruation] occurred for over one month until May 12, [at which time] pregnancy antibody test was positive. Afterwards, she gave birth to a child after sufficient months.

Commentary: This case was categorized as damp heat pouring downward with qi stagnation and blood stasis. Due to damp heat pouring downward, a profuse, yellow vaginal discharge was seen which had a foul odor. There was [also] frequent urination. Dampness and heat had bound together with qi stagnation and blood stasis, and, therefore, lumbar and abdominal aching and pain were seen. Damp heat assailed above but clear yang was not upborne. Therefore, there was headache, nausea, and no desire to open the eyes. Treatment was in order to clear and disinhibit dampness and heat, course and free the flow of the qi and blood.

The formula used was *Ba Zheng San* (Eight [Ingredients] Correcting Powder) with additions and subtractions. Within this formula, Dianthus, Polygonum Avicularis, Akebia, Plantago, and Dioscorea Hypoglauca clear heat and disinhibit dampness. Melia, Lindera, and Corydalis rectify the qi and quicken the blood. Red and White Peony nourish the blood and quicken the blood. Lonicera, Viola, and Patrinia clear heat and resolve toxins. After [taking] these medicinals, the yellow vaginal discharge, frequent urination, and abdominal pain all were decreased. This clearly evidenced that damp heat was gradually being

195

cleared. After further regulating and rectifying the qi and blood by using a qi-rectifying, blood-quickening prescription, the result was acheived.

Case 5: Wang, female, 28 years old, married

Date of initial examination: December 15, 1959

Major complaints: Infertility after three years of marriage

Present case history: [The patient's] menarche had occurred at age 16. The menstrual cycle was 40-50 days. Menstruation lasted 5-6 days, and the menses were scanty in volume and purplish red in color with clots. There was lower abdominal aching and pain before and during menstruation. [There was also] lumbar aching and, typically, there was a profuse, white vaginal discharge which was sticky and thick and had an odor. After having been married for three years, there had been no pregnancy. Her husband was healthy.

Examination: The external genitalia and vaginal tract were normal. The cervix was slightly eroded and its mouth was small. The body of the uterus was anteriorly flexed and uterine development was somewhat small. There was bilateral adnexal thickening. There was a loop-like thing on the left side, and the distal part was enlarged. In terms of endometrial examination, during menstruation there was late secretory stage endometrium. In terms of fallopian tube free flow examination [*i.e.*, histosalpingogram], the tubes on both sides were not free flowing.

Tongue image: A pale red tongue body with thin, white fur

Pulse image: Deep and relaxed

Western medical diagnosis: A) Primary infertility; B) chronic pelvic inflammation and bilateral fallopian tube blockage

Chinese medical pattern discrimination: Kidney depletion and blood vacuity, qi stagnation and blood stasis

Treatment methods: First nourish the blood and regulate the liver, soothe qi and transform stasis

Formula & medicinals: Herba Leonuri Heterophylli (*Yi Mu Cao*), 2 *liang*, Radix Angelicae Sinensis (*Dang Gui*), 1 *liang*, Hangzhou Radix Albus Paeoniae Lactiflorae (*Hang Bai Shao*), 1 *liang*, Radix Ligustici Wallichii (*Chuan Xiong*), 3 *qian*, Guangdong Radix Auklandiae Lappae (*Guang Mu Xiang*), 3 *qian*, stir-fried Fructus Citri Aurantii (*Zhi Ke*), 3 *qian*, Radix Bupleuri (*Chai Hu*), 5 *qian*, processed Rhizoma Cyperi Rotundi (*Xiang Fu*), 5 *qian*

The above medicinals were ground into fine powder and made into pills with honey. Each pill weighed 3 *qian* and one pill was taken every night with boiled water.

Course of treatment: The above medicinals were taken in the form of pills from Dec. 15, 1959 to Jan. 1960. Afterwards, due to hepatitis, these medicinals were stopped. On June 17, 1960, the hepatitis had been completely cured and [the patient] again came for examination. Her symptoms were the same as before. [Dr. Liu] continued to use the previous formula plus Fructus Rubi Chingii (*Fu Pen Zi*), 3 *qian*, and Cortex Cinnamomi Cassiae (*Rou Gui*), 5 *qian*, in order to warm the kidneys and warm the uterus. After treating for 14 whole months and having administered four doses of pills, the symptoms had gradually taken a turn for the better and her menstrual cycle was now normal and the amount of blood was moderate. Its color was red and the abdominal pain had disappeared. When [the patient] came for examination on Nov. 21, 1961, she complained that her menstruation was late by six days and had not come. There was a slight degree of nausea and vomiting and her low back was achey and slightly painful. Her pulse image was bowstring, slippery, and slightly rapid. [Therefore, Dr. Liu] used a

197

prescription to clear heat, harmonize the stomach, and stop vomiting and advised [the patient] to have a urine frog [pregnancy] test after two weeks' observation. The result was positive. On follow-up on May 29, 1962, [the patient] had been pregnant for eight months.

Commentary: This case was categorized as kidney vacuity and blood depletion with qi stagnation and blood stasis. Because the qi and blood were not sufficient, the sea of blood was not full. Therefore, menstruation was not able to descend on time each month and the volume of the menstrual blood was scanty. Kidney depletion had led to the appearance of lumbar aching and pain and profuse white vaginal discharge. Qi stagnation and blood stasis resulted in the appearance of the menstrual movement being stagnant, astringent, and not smoothly flowing. [In addition,] there were clots and menstrual pain.

First, [Dr. Liu] used the methods of nourishing the blood and harmonizing the liver, soothing the qi and transforming stasis. Within this formula, Dang Gui and Ligusticum Wallichium quicken the blood and regulate menstruation, thus making the qi and blood regular and harmonious. Leonurus and White Peony quicken the blood, regulate the menses, transform stasis and engender the new. Bupleurum, Auklandia, Aurantium, and Cyperus resolve depression and open binding, soothe the qi and move stagnation. Free flow and regulation of the qi and blood leads to the menstrual water's being able to descend periodically [alternate reading: on time]. He continued to use Cortex Cinnamomi which is an acrid, sweet, greatly hot ingredient which directly enters and supplements the life gate, warms the uterus and scatters cold. Rubus supplements the liver and kidneys. Once the qi and blood obtained regulation and stasis and binding were freed and smoothed, [the patient] was able to conceive. In this case history, medicinal pills were used. These were chosen so that there was mild but persistent action of the medicinals.

It can be seen from the treatment of the above-mentioned five cases, that the condition of infertility is comparatively complicated. Therefore, it should be treated in accordance with the disease condition *and* the pattern discrimination. In addition, cases #4 and #5, based on examination, [had] bilateral blockage of the fallopian tubes. Nevertheless, after having been treated with Chinese medicine and Chinese medicinals, they were able to conceive. This clearly shows that their fallopian tubes were already [*i.e.*, by then] free flowing and, [therefore,] the mature ovum was able to pass through the oviduct to reach the uterus. By examining the formula and medicinals, besides [medicinals] for clearing and disinhibiting dampness and heat, there were also [medicinals] which regulated and supplemented the qi and blood. [However,] their common characteristic is that they move the qi and quicken the blood, and this is certainly worth paying special attention to and further researching.[26]

---

[26] Since this book was published in China, it has become routine practice in the People's Republic to treat fallopian tube blockage with blood-quickening, stasis-transforming medicinals. These are given *per os*, *per anum*, and topically applied over the abdomen along the course of the tubes.

199

Anovulatory Menstruation: Two Cases

Case 1: Li, female, 27 years old, a simple case in the out-patient department

Date of initial examination: May 19, 1972

Major complaints: Menstruation behind schedule and menstrual movement abdominal pain for two years

Present case history: By the end of 1970, [the patient's] menstruation was behind schedule by 8-9 days. Its color was black purple and it contained clots. During the menstrual movement, there was lower abdominal aching and pain as well as lower limb pain and flaccidity. Although she had been married for more than one year, she had not conceived. Her basal body temperature [BBT] was monophasic.[27] Her Western medical diagnosis was anovulatory menstruation. Gynecological examination showed anteversion and anteflexion of her uterus with both normal size and activity.

Tongue image: Thin, white fur

Pulse image: Fine and relaxed

---

[27] When a woman ovulates, her basal body temperature rises as much as one degree Fahrenheit and remains high until 12-36 hours before the onset of ovulation. Therefore, there are hypothermal and hyperthermal phases of the basal body temperature when correlated to menstruation. The transition from hypo- to hyperthermal stage is one indication that ovulation has occurred. Therefore, if a woman's BBT is monophasic when plotted on a graph chart, this indicates that she is not ovulating.

Western medical diagnosis: Anovulatory menstruation

Chinese medical pattern discrimination: Blood vacuity and kidney depletion, lower burner cold and chilled

Treatment methods: Nourish blood and supplement the kidneys, warm the lower burner

Formula & medicinals: Radix Angelicae Sinensis (*Dang Gui*), 3 *qian*, stir-fried Radix Albus Paeoniae Lactiflorae (*Bai Shao*), 3 *qian*, Radix Ligustici Wallichii (*Chuan Xiong*), 1 *qian*, cooked Radix Rehmanniae (*Shu Di*), 4 *qian*, Fructus Rubi Chingii (*Fu Pen Zi*), 4 *qian*, Semen Cuscutae Chinensis (*Tu Si Zi*), 4 *qian*, Radix Disocoreae Oppositae (*Shan Yao*), 5 *qian*, Radix Morindae Officinalis (*Ba Ji Tian*), 3 *qian*, Semen Litchi Chinensis (*Li Zhi He*), 3 *qian*

Course of treatment: It was reported on re-examination on July 5 that, in the last 5-6 months, [the patient] had taken 20 *ji* of the above formula. On June 27, the menses had moved [*i.e.*, come] and their amount was increased. Her BBT was biphasic. This clearly demonstrated that she had ovulated. Her menstrual cycle was normal and its amount was moderate. Its color was normal and the blood clots were less. There was no abdominal pain.

Case 2: Chen, female, 29 years old, case No. 228652

Date of initial examination: March 20, 1962

Major complaints: Blocked menstruation for five months

Present case history: [The patient's] menarche had occurred when she was 19 years old. It came one time every 2-6 months. Each time the menses moved for 3-4 days. Their amount was moderate, their color was red, and there were no clots. [Menstruation] was accompanied by menstrual pain. In 1960, there had been blocked menstruation for one year. Therefore, she was hospitalized for treatment in order to [induce] a man-made cycle for 3-4 months. During treatment, her menses came like a tide, but when the medicinals were stopped, blocked menstruation returned. Basal body temperature examination had been done for three months and all were monophasic. Endometrial examination showed [abnormal] changes in the proliferative phase. The level of hormones were low and the development of the uterus was not good. She was treated continuously for half a year but the treatment effects were not consolidated and she came to this hospital. Her symptoms were occasional dizziness and headache, polyuria at night, ok eating and drinking, and normal stools.

Gynecological examination: The external genitalia were normal. The vaginal tract was open and smooth. The uterine cervix was slightly eroded. The uterine os was small and its body was anteriorly positioned. Its body was smaller than normal, but its activity was good. Bilateral adnexa were negative. Vaginal tract cell smear showed low levels of hormones and no fern-like crystalizaton in the cervical mucus.[28]

Tongue image: A red tongue tip with static macules and thin, white fur

Pulse image: Bowstring, slippery, and forceless bilaterally in the cubit

Western medical diagnosis: Anovulatory menstruation and primary amenorrhea

Chinese medical pattern discrimination: Spleen-kidney insufficiency, blood vacuity and liver effulgence, qi stagnation and blood stasis

---

[28] The mucus and saliva of women after they ovulate displays a crystalline pattern like a fern when viewed microscopically. This is another indication that ovulation has occurred.

Treatment methods: Rectify the qi and quicken the blood, level the liver and clear heat, supplement the kidneys and regulate menstruation

Formula & medicinals: Semen Pruni Persicae (*Tao Ren*), 2 *qian*, Flos Carthami Tinctorii (*Hong Hua*), 2 *qian*, Herba Lycopi Lucidi (*Ze Lan*), 3 *qian*, Herba Leonuri Heterophylli (*Yi Mu Cao*), 4 *qian*, Radix Salviae Miltiorrhizae (*Dan Shen*), 4 *qian*, Tuber Curcumae (*Yu Jin*), 3 *qian*, Radix Cyathulae (*Chuan Niu Xi*), 3 *qian*, Concha Haliotidis (*Shi Jue Ming*), 1 *liang*, Flos Chrysanthemi Morifolii (*Ju Hua*), 4 *qian*, Radix Linderae Strychnifoliae (*Wu Yao*), 2 *qian*, Placenta Hominis (*Zi He Che*), 1 *qian* (taken separately [washed down by the decoction])

Course of treatment: Mainly, the above formula was [administered] with additions and subtractions such as Radix Albus Paeoniae Lactiflorae (*Bai Shao*), Cortex Radicis Moutan (*Dan Pi*), Fructus Gardeniae Jasminoidis (*Zhi Zi*), and Radix Scutellariae Baicalensis (*Huang Qin*). This was combined with administration of De Sheng Dan (Obtaining Birth Elixir), *Xiao Yao Wan* (Rambling Pills), and *Wu Zi Yan Zong Wan* (Five Seeds Increase Progeny Pills). After over one month's treatment, menstruation came like a tide on May 1 and the menses moved for four days. The volume and the color were normal. [However,] there was menstrual movement abdominal pain. [Therefore,] the methods of regulating menstruation were continued with the preceding formula with additions and subtractions. The menses came like a tide again on Jun. 7, July 9, Aug. 10, and [again] in September at regular intervals. During treatment, endocrine function was examined and the BBT was charted for four months. These were all monophasic. Cervical mucus examination showed atypical fern-like crystallization. Vaginal secretion examination was III grade clear. Vaginal cell smear showed that the level of hormones was persistently low, 16 times in total. There was no cyclic changes in 3.5 cycles.

After treatment, the menstruation began five times. However, it was found by examination that all of these were anovulatory menstruations.

[The patient] suffered from irregular menstruation, habitual, profuse, white vaginal discharge, and insidious lower abdominal pain. These were discriminated as lower burner vacuity cold. On the 10th day of the menstrual cycle, medicinal pills for supplementing the kidneys and warming the lower [burner or source], rectifying the qi, quickening the blood, and regulating menstruation were used with the formula and medicinals as follows: Semen Citri Reticulatae (*Ju He*), 8 *qian*, Semen Litchi Chinensis (*Li Zhi He*), 1.5 *qian*, Fructus Meliae Toosendan (*Chuan Lian Zi*), 5 *qian*, Rhizoma Cyperi Rotundi (*Xiang Fu*), 5 *qian*, Semen Pruni Persicae (*Tao Ren*), 3 *qian*, Fructus Foeniculi Vugaris (*Xiao Hui Xiang*), 8 *qian*, Semen Trigonellae Foeni-graeci (*Hu Lu Ba*), 1 *liang*, Radix Morindae Officinalis (*Ba Ji Tian*), 1 *liang*, Herba Epimedii (*Yin Yang Huo*), 4 *qian*.

The above medicinals were ground into fine powder and made into pills with honey. Each pill weighed 3 *qian*, and two pills were taken orally per day. This was combined with acupuncture which was given every other day. The acupuncture points chosen were *Qi Hai* (CV 6), *Zhong Ji* (CV 3), *Guan Yuan* (CV 4), and *San Yin Jiao* (Sp 6). The last menstruation was on Nov. 30. A frog test [for confirming pregnancy] was given 45 days after cessation of menstruation. This was positive. During the pregnancy, [the patient's] condition was good. On Sept. 6, 1963, she gave birth to a baby boy, and both the mother and child were healthy.

Commentary: According to the Western medical point of view, anovulatory menstruation is caused by faulty ovarian function. The follicles form in the ovary every month, and the ovum develops well, but the mature ovum is not able to be discharged. Rather, it is reabsorbed within the ovary. Hence, only estrogen is secreted and no corpus luteum arises. There are only proliferative stage changes in the endometrium but no secretory stage [changes]. When the endometrium sheds, this creates the menstruation. However, because the time when the ovum becomes mature and [then] disappears is out of rule [*i.e.*, does not occur at the right time], the menstrual cycle is either early or late and even amenorrhea may occur. Since the mature ovum is not able to be discharged from the ovary, pregnancy cannot result.

The main clinical characteristics of anovulatory menstruation are usually delayed menstruation, blocked menstruation, and infertility. [Patients] with these symptoms usually suffer from anovulatory menstruation. Therefore, whenever [he] came across such cases, Dr. Liu usually referred them for a modern medical examination and used that as his index in their diagnosis and treatment. For instance, [he used] examination of the basal body temperature and of the endometrium. Nevertheless, he still discriminated the pattern and treated this according to basic theories of Chinese medicine.

In women, the blood is the root. When the *tian gui* arrives, the *ren mai* is free-flowing, and the *tai chong mai* is exuberant, the menses descend periodically, and, therefore, there is the possibility of having children. The *chong* is the sea of blood. If the *chong mai* is exuberant, it is able to construct and nourish the uterus, and this leads to the menstruation automatically being regulated. Therefore, delayed menstruation and blocked menstruation are, in reality, blood vacuity patterns. If there is kidney vacuity, the uterus will be cold and chilled and [thus] not able to tie up the fetus. Hence there are no children. [Therefore,] in sum, [Dr. Liu's] basic point of view is that the essence of the pathology of anovulatory menstruation is blood vacuity and kidney cold. Thus his treatment [of this condition] was to mainly nourish the blood and warm the kidneys. Nevertheless, it is essential that the pattern be discriminated according to Chinese medical theories and the disease treated in accordance with the patient's condition.

In case #1, the delayed menstruation was due to blood vacuity, while the blackish purple color, clots, and menstrual movement abdominal pain were all a lower burner vacuity cold pattern. Cold exuberance leads to blood congelation. If the blood is congealed, the vessels and passageways will not flow freely. This then leads to abdominal pain.

206

The kidneys rule the bones. If there is kidney vacuity, the marrow will be empty and the bones will lose their nourishment. Therefore, one can see lower limb soreness and flaccidity. Thus, at the time of treatment, *Si Wu Tang* (Four Materials Decoction) was the main [formula]. Rubus, Cuscuta, Dioscorea, Morinda, and Litchi supplement the kidneys and warm the kidneys.

In case #2, the condition was somewhat different. Blocked menstruation was the main symptom, but this was accompanied by dizziness, headache, vexation and agitation, and night-time sleep not replete, all blood vacuity, liver effulgence symptoms. Therefore, first [Dr. Liu] mainly rectified the qi and quickened the blood, using heavy [doses of] Persica, Carthamus, Lycopus, Leonurus, Curcuma, and Lindera to move the qi and quicken the blood, as well as Salvia, Cyathula, and Placenta to nourish the blood in order to secure the root. It was also essential to address the branch signs of blood vacuity and liver effulgence by using the medicinals Haliotis and Chrysanthemum to clear heat and level the liver. Other additions and subtractions used included Moutan, Gardenia, Scutellaria, etc. In terms of the symptoms, the menstruation was already normal when it came like a tide five times, and blocked menstruation was cured. In terms of the blood vacuity, even though the menses were already freely flowing, the basal body temperature was still monophasic and this was a clear indication of anovulation. Later, based also on the frequent urination, profuse night-time urination, insidious pain, and other such symptoms of lower burner vacuity cold, the foundation of the origin was stressed through supplementing the kidneys and warming the lower [source], but assisted by rectifying the qi, quickening the blood, and regulating menstruation. Within this formula, Fenugreek, Morinda, and Epimedium supplement the kidneys and invigorate yang. Fennel, Orange Seeds, Litchi, and Melia rectify the qi and scatter cold. Cyperus and Persica rectify the qi and quicken the blood. Based on her clinical results, [the patient] was now ovulating and was already pregnant.

Thus it is clear that stressing the foundation of blood vacuity and kidney cold accords with the objective of practice. Moreover, these two, blood vacuity and kidney cold are also closely related. From the point of view of clinical phenomena, supplementing the blood is to supplement and fill the material basis, while warming the kidneys is to promote the function of expelling the ovum.

Of the formulas and medicinals for supplementing besides *Si Wu Tang*, Old Doctor Liu was also good at using Placenta Hominis. Because it is a bloody, meaty natured ingredient, it is able to nourish the blood, supplement the kidneys, and boost detriment. Among the medicinals in the formula which warm the kidneys and invigorate yang, besides the typical medicinals, [Dr. Liu] always used Litchi because it is acrid and warm in nature and enters into the liver channel. Its function is to move the qi and scatter cold. It is recorded in the *Ben Cao Bei Yao (The Complete Essentials of the Materia Medica)* about this medicinal that it "enters the liver and kidneys, scatters stagnant qi, penetrates cold evils, and treats stomach and venter pain [as well as] women's blood and qi pain." It is Dr. Liu's opinion based on experience that, the reason why it is able to treat women's blood and qi pain may be due not only to its function of moving the qi and scattering cold but also to its ability to guide other medicinals to reach the ovaries similar to its function of guiding medicinals to the testes in the treatment of mounting [*i.e.*, hernia] pain.

Endometriosis: Two Cases

If the endometrium grows in an abnormal place outside the uterine cavity and this gives rise to pathological changes and symptoms, this is called endometriosis. The tissues of the endometrium in such abnormal locations are still affected by ovarian hormones and bleed cyclically. However, this blood has no outlet. [Therefore,] it collects and is retained in the local tissues. This results in the arising of menstrual pain and fibrosis of the peripheral tissues.

It is Old Doctor Liu's experience that this disease is caused by dead blood (static blood) congealing and binding in the uterus. This stasis stagnates circulation of the channels and vessels and viscera and bowels. The cause of the formation of static blood may be external contraction of cold and coolness, or it may be due to qi stagnation and blood stasis. If static blood collects and is retained and endures for [many] days, it may transform into heat. If dampness is habitually brewed in the body or there is qi stagnation with damp obstruction, dampness and heat may mutually bind and this may lead to the accompanying manifestations of lower burner damp heat signs. In order to treat the above, quickening the blood and transforming stasis and clearing and disinhibiting damp heat are the rulers. The formulas [Dr. Liu] used [for this] were *Di Dang Tang* (Resistance Decoction) and *Ba Zheng San* (Eight [Ingredients] Correcting Powder) with additions and subtractions. If the tendency was towards lower burner cold congelation, the methods were to quicken the blood and transform stasis, warm the channels and scatter cold. The formula [Dr. Liu] used [in that case] was *Shao Fu Zhu Yu Tang* (Lower Abdomen Dispel Stasis Decoction) with additions and subtractions. [However,] because the pathological essence of this disease is due to dead blood stasis and obstruction, the typically used medicinals for quickening the blood have difficulty dispersing and scattering it. As certain medical experts have said, "Those people in whose bodies blood has just become obstructed and who still have living qi are easy to treat, while those with obstruction which has endured [for many days] and who do not have living qi are difficult to treat." Therefore, no matter whether this disease is cold or hot, [Dr. Liu believed that] all may be treated with *Di Dang Tang* as the main formula.

Case 1: Liu, female, 37 years old, a simple case in the out-patient department

Date of initial examination: July 1, 1973

Major complaints: Severe menstrual movement abdominal pain enduring for 12 years with even heavier symptoms in the last three years

Present case history: [This patient's] menarche occurred at 15 years of age and since then she had had painful menstruation. Twelve years previously she had a difficult postpartum and her menstrual pain had gotten heavier. In Aug. 1972, the menstrual pain got even more heavy so that the bitterness during her menses was difficult to bear. Previously used pain-stopping medicinal substances had not been able to relax and resolve [this pain]. Each time during her menstruation she is not able to work at all. She habitually had lumbar pain, abdominal distention, and a profuse, white vaginal discharge. During midcycle, there was also lower abdominal aching and pain which was difficult to bear. She had not conceived for 12 years after her [last] birth. Prior gynecological examination at a hospital showed that there were many node-like things on the posterior wall of the uterus which were markedly painful to pressure. The uterine body was not movable and there were lumps on the adnexa on both sides with adhesions in the peripheral tissues. Salpingogram followed by uterine curettage did not reveal any pathological changes due to tuberculosis. [The patient's] last menses had occurred on Jun. 18 and the menses had moved for four days. The last time the menses had come, they were 5-6 days ahead of schedule. Their volume was relatively profuse, their color was purple, and they contained blood clots. [The patient] reported that there was bodily heat, a dry mouth, and dry stools.

Examination: The external genitalia and vaginal tract were normal. The uterine cervix was slightly red and there was a light degree of erosion. The uterine body was approximately normal but posteriorly positioned. Its movement was not normal. On the posterior wall, there were various sized small nodes which were markedly tender to the touch. Bilaterally, both adnexa had irregular masses ([the one] on the right side was 3.5 x 3 x 2.5cm, while [the one] on the left was 3 x 3 x 2cm), and there were adhesions in the surrounding region. These were [also] markedly painful to pressure and were immobile. Those that were on the uterine-sacral ligament were even more severely painful to pressure.

Tongue image: A dark red tongue body

Pulse image: Bowstring and slippery

Western medical diagnosis: A) Endometriosis; B) secondary infertility

Chinese medical pattern discrimination: Uterine blood stasis, lower burner damp heat

Treatment methods: Quicken the blood and transform stasis, clear and disinhibit dampness and heat

Formula & medicinals: Semen Pruni Persicae (*Tao Ren*), 2 *qian*, Radix Et Rhizoma Rhei (*Da Huang*), 1 *qian*, Hirudo (*Shui Zhi*), 1.5 *qian*, Tabanus (*Niu Meng*), 1.5 *qian*, Fructus Meliae Toosendan (*Chuan Lian Zi*), 3 *qian*, Rhizoma Corydalis Yanhusuo (*Yan Hu Suo*), 3 *qian*, Feces Trogopterori Seu Pteromi (*Wu Ling Zhi*), 3 *qian*, Resina Myrrhae (*Mo Yao*), 1 *qian*, Herba Dianthi (*Qu Mai*), 4 *qian*, Herba Polygoni Avicularis (*Bian Xu*), 4

211

qian, Caulis Akebiae Mutong (*Mu Tong*), 1 *qian*, Semen Plantaginis (*Che Qian Zi*), 3 *qian*

Course of treatment: [The patient] was re-examined on July 16, [at which time she said that,] after taking 10 *ji* of the above formula, her lumbar pain and abdominal pain had markedly decreased. However, her menstrual period abdominal region pain was still very severe. Menstruation had come like a tide on July 13 and had moved for four days. Its color was red purple and it contained clots. Its amount was somewhat profuse. [Therefore, Dr. Liu] removed Dianthus, Polygonum Avicularis, Akebia, and Plantago and added Radix Salviae Miltiorrhizae (*Dan Shen*), processed Rhizoma Cyperi Rotundi (*Xiang Fu*), and Radix Linderae Strychnifoliae (*Wu Yao*), 3 *qian* each, in order to strengthen the functions of moving the qi, quickening the blood, and transforming stasis. Because there had been diarrhea, the Rhubarb was reduced to 5 *fen*. After continued administration for 10 *ji*, the habitual lumbar pain and abdominal distention as well as the midcycle lumbar pain were all decreased. On July 31, in order to begin strengthening the quickening of the blood and transformation of stasis, scattering of binding [or nodulation] and stopping of pain [even more, Dr. Liu] removed Akebia and Plantago and added Rhizoma Sparganii (*San Leng*) and Rhizoma Curcumae Zedoariae (*E Zhu*), 3 *qian* each, and Radix Angelicae Sinensis (*Dang Gui*), 1 *liang*.

At the Aug. 18 re-examination, [the patient reported that], after taking [another] 10 *ji* of the above formula, the habitual lumbar pain and midcycle abdominal pain had disappeared. On Aug. 7, her menses had come like a tide and her blood had flowed freely and smoothly. There was only slight lower abdominal pain. The menses had moved for 3-4 days. The amount of blood and the blood clots were both less compared to previously. Internal examination [revealed] that the small nodes on the posterior wall of the uterus and the lumps on the adnexa were all smaller than previously. After taking 20 *ji* of the above formula over the three months from July 1 to Oct. 5, she was administered another 50 *ji* of Chinese medicinals. Her habitual lumbar pain and midcycle abdominal pain had disappeared and her menses had come four times (July 13-17, Aug. 7-11, Sept. 4-8, and Sept. 29-Oct. 1). Excluding a single episode of slight abdominal region pain, the other three times menstrual pain had basically disappeared. Internal examination [showed] that the small nodes on the posterior wall of her uterus had basically disappeared, the masses bilaterally on the adnexa had completely disappeared, and the peripheral adhesions had also disappeared. [Therefore, Dr. Liu] advised [the patient] to take 10-15 *ji* of the preceding formula before each menstruation in order to secure the treatment effect.

Case 2: Xi, female, 30 years old, a simple case in the out-patient department

Date of initial examination: August 29, 1974

Major complaints: Severe lower abdominal pain during the menstrual period for seven months

Present case history: There was no previous history of menstrual pain. Beginning in 1972, there had been menstrual period lower abdominal pain which was diagnosed in a hospital as endometriosis. She had been [treated] by placental extract injections for two months to no effect. Internally, she had been administered methyltestosterone for two months. She had also been treated with injections of penicillin and streptomycin. [However,] the menstrual period abdominal region pain was so severe it was difficult to bear. Before the menses, there was lower abdominal iciness and coolness. When this obtained heat, the pain decreased. Defecation sometimes caused the abdominal pain to be heavier. Each time the menses moved, she was given injections of pain-stopping medicinals which were able to relax and resolve [the pain]. The volume of the menses was sometimes profuse and sometimes scanty. Its color was dark and it contained blood clots. When many blood clots were expelled, the abdominal pain diminished. Gynecological

213

examination [revealed] that inside the body of the uterus there were node-like things.

Tongue image: A pale tongue body

Pulse image: Deep and bowstring

Western medical diagnosis: Endometriosis

Chinese medical pattern discrimination: Qi stagnation and blood stasis, cold congelation in the channels and vessels [alternate reading: in the menstrual vessels]

Treatment methods: Quicken the blood and transform stasis, warm the channels and stop pain

Formula & medicinals: Processed Rhizoma Cyperi Rotundi (*Xiang Fu*), 3 *qian*, Fructus Meliae Toosendan (*Chuan Lian Zi*), 3 *qian*, Semen Pruni Persicae (*Tao Ren*), 2 *qian*, Radix Angelicae Sinensis (*Dang Gui*), 3 *qian*, Fructus Foeniculi Vulgaris (*Xiao Hui Xiang*), 2 *qian*, Feces Trogopterori Seu Pteromi (*Wu Ling Zhi*), 3 *qian*, uncooked Pollen Typhae (*Pu Huang*), 2 *qian*, Herba Leonuri Heterophylli (*Yi Mu Cao*), 3 *qian*, Rhizoma Corydalis Yanhusuo (*Yan Hu Suo*), 3 *qian*, Radix Rubrus Paeoniae Lactiflorae (*Chi Shao*), 3 *qian*

Course of treatment: Re-examination [occurred] on Sept. 9, [at which time] 6 *ji* of this formula had been taken. On Sept. 6, the menstruation moved on time and abdominal pain was still seen. [Therefore, Dr. Liu] modified [this formula] by adding Radix Linderae Strychnifoliae (*Wu Yao*), 2 *qian*, Semen Trigonellae Foeni-graeci (*Hu Lu Ba*), 3 *qian*, Resina Myrrhae (*Mo Yao*), 1 *qian*, Semen Citri Reticulatae (*Ju He*), 3 *qian*, and Semen Litchi Chinensis (*Li Zhi He*), 3 *qian*. After giving another 15 *ji* continuously, the menses came on Oct. 5 and still there was abdominal pain. Another 12 *ji* of the above formula was administered. On Nov. 1,

214

the menstruation came and there was relatively slight abdominal pain. Therefore, over 40 *ji* of this fomula with additions and subtractions were given before there were relatively slight abdominal pains with the menstrual period and [before] not needing to take pain-stopping medicinals. However, at the time of defecation, there was still lower abdominal pain, and at normal times the lower abdomen emitted coolness. Again she received a gynecological examination. The nodes in the body of her uterus were not seen to be any smaller. Occasionally during menstruation, the abdominal region emitted coolness or there was lumbar pain. [Dr. Liu] suggested that [the patient] take the following formula continuously: Fructus Foeniculi Vulgaris (*Xiao Hui Xiang*), 3 *qian*, Semen Trigonellae Foeni-graeci (*Hu Lu Ba*), 3 *qian*, Rhizoma Corydalis Yanhusuo (*Yan Hu Suo*), 3 *qian*, Cortex Cinnamomi Cassiae (*Rou Gui*), 1.5 *qian*, Feces Trogopterori Seu Pteromi (*Wu Ling Zhi*), 3 *qian*, Semen Pruni Persicae (*Tao Ren*), 3 *qian*, Flos Carthami Tinctorii (*Hong Hua*), 2 *qian*, Resina Myrrhae (*Mo Yao*), 2 *qian*, Radix Rubrus Paeoniae Lactiflorae (*Chi Shao*), 2 *qian*, Fructus Evodiae Rutecarpae (*Wu Zhu Yu*), 2 *qian*, and blast-fried Rhizoma Zingiberis (*Pao Jiang*), 1 *qian*.

Commentary: Case #1 was categorized as uterine blood stasis with lower burner damp heat. [The patient] had menstruation ahead of schedule, purple colored [blood], and clots. [Her menses] were profuse in amount. All these are symptoms of blood heat. [She also had] severe lower abdominal pain during the menstrual period. Her tongue was dark red and her pulse was bowstring and slippery. All these were signs of blood stasis obstructing the vessels. Habitual lumbar pain and abdominal distention, profuse, white vaginal discharge,[29] and severe midcycle lower abdominal pain pertained to damp heat pouring

---

[29] Here, it is not clear if *bai dai* should be translated as white vaginal discharge or by the Western generic term of leukorrhea. Because it is associated with heat and heat can make an abnormal vaginal discharge either thick, opaque, and white or yellow, the term white here may not actually indicate the real color of the discharge.

215

downward. Treatment should, [therefore,] quicken the blood and transform stasis, clear and disinhibit dampness and heat mainly using *Di Dang Tang* assisted by ingredients to quicken the blood and rectify the qi, clear and disinhibit dampness and heat.

Within this formula, Persica quickens the blood and transforms stasis. Rhubarb is bitter and cold. It enters the blood division and transforms static blood. It clears and resolves heat deep-lying [or hidden] in the blood division. Leech and Gadfly erode dead blood and transform static blood. Corydalis, Flying Squirrel Droppings, Melia, and Myrrh quicken the blood and transform stasis, rectify the qi and stop pain. Dianthus, Polygonum Avicularis, Akebia, and Plantago clear and disinhibit lower burner damp heat.

After these medicinals, the habitual lumbar pain and abdominal distention and the severe midcycle abdominal region pain all decreased. However, the pain during the menses was still severe. [Dr. Liu, therefore,] removed Dianthus, Polygonum Avicularis, Akebia, Plantago, and the other cold, cool ingredients and added Salvia, Cyperus, Lindera, Sparganium, and Zedoaria in order to strengthen the power of moving the qi and quickening the blood. He also increased the Dang Gui to 1 *liang* in order to regulate the menses and stop pain. As a whole, this formula was [now] mainly to quicken the blood, dispel stasis, and disperse concretions assisted by moving the qi and stopping pain, clearing and disinhibiting dampness and heat. Over three months of treatment, 50 *ji* of Chinese medicinals were administered. After [taking] these medicinals, the condition of three menstrual movements was good. Not only were the symptoms better, but gynecological examination was also said to be fully satisfactory.

Case #2 was categorized as qi stagnation and blood stasis with cold congealing in the channels and vessels. [The patient] had severe abdominal pain during the menstrual movement with the lower abdomen emitting coolness. When this obtained heat, the pain subsided.

The menstrual blood was dark colored and contained clots. After clots were expelled, the abdominal pain diminished. All these were symptoms of blood stasis obstructing the network vessels. Within the above treatment, quickening the blood and transforming stasis were the rulers assisted by warming the channels and stopping pain.

Within this formula, Persica, Leonurus, and Red Peony quicken the blood and transform stasis. Dang Gui nourishes the blood and quickens the blood. *Shi Xiao San* (Loose a Smile Powder) dispels stasis and stops pain. Melia and processed Cyperus rectify the qi and stop pain. And Fennel warms the channels. Afterwards, [Dr. Liu] modified this by adding Fenugreek, Lindera, Myrrh, Orange Seeds, Litchi, and other such channel-warming, cold-scattering ingredients. On follow-up, there was still some slight abdominal pain and some emission of coolness from the lower abdomen. Internal examination showed that the nodes in the body of the uterus had not disappeared. Perhaps the power and dose of the warming and transforming materials was insufficient or the course of treatment was too short.

From the above two cases, it can preliminarily be seen that the treatment effect in the damp heat pattern was good, while the treatment effect in the vacuity cold pattern still requires further observation [or research].

Pelvic Inflammation: Nine Cases

Pelvic inflammation [a.k.a. pelvic inflammatory disease or PID] is a commonly-seen gynecological disease. This is a general term for inflammatory pathological changes of the reproductive organs within the pelvic cavity, the surrounding connective tissues of the pelvic cavity, and the peritoneum of the pelvic cavity. [This includes] adnexitis (ovaritis, salpingitis), adnexal masses, inflammation of the body of the uterus, parametritis, inflammation of the uterosacral ligament, inflammation of connective tissues surrounding the uterus, and pelvic peritonitis. All of these are called pelvic inflammation. Inflammation may occur in only a single part or may occur in a number of areas at the same time. In clinic, [this disease] is divided into the two types of acute and chronic. In Chinese medicine, it is categorized as "cold dampness", "damp heat pouring downward", "internal welling abscess", and "concretions and conglomerations." Its main symptoms are lower abdominal aching and pain, lumbar pain, profuse leukorrhea, or fever. It is mostly due to invasion of damp heat or cold dampness. This results in damp heat brewing internally or cold dampness internally engendered [which then produces] qi stagnation and blood stasis, obstruction of the *chong* and *ren*, and congelation and blockage of the lower burner.

If there is enduring brewing of damp heat or cold dampness transforming heat, one may see low-grade fever, yellow vaginal discharge, and lower abdominal aching and pain. If there is damp heat brewing toxins, one may see high fever and abdominal pain which refuses pressure. If there is cold dampness congelation and blockage, one may see lower abdominal chilly pain, lumbar aching and insidious pain, and clear, watery white vaginal discharge. If there is qi stagnation, there is coming and going [alternate reading: movable] lower abdominal pain. If there is blood stasis congelation and stagnation, one may see piercing pain or wringing pain and the pain is fixed in location. If there is damp heat which has been brewing for a prolonged time with qi and blood congelation and binding, this may produce concretion lumps and abdominal pain which refuses pressure.

Case 1: Wei, female, 25 years old, a simple case in the out-patient department

Date of initial examination: October 5, 1974

Major complaints: Lumbar and abdominal aching and pain with profuse white vaginal discharge for more than one year

Present case history: Since [the patient] had undergone premature labor in Nov. 1973, she had had pain bilaterally in her lower abdomen, lumbar pain, bodily fatigue and lack of strength, essence spirit listlessness, profuse leukorrhea which was yellow in color and sticky in consistency, and frequent, numerous urination. During the menstrual period, lower abdominal sagging and pain were more severe. Her menstrual cycle was normal, its amount was profuse, and its color was red. Her last menses had occurred on Sept. 22, 1974.

Tongue image: A red tongue body

Pulse image: Bowstring, slippery, and slightly rapid

Western medical diagnosis: Chronic pelvic inflammation

Chinese medical pattern discrimination: Damp heat pouring downward, qi stagnation and blood stasis

Treatment methods: Clear heat and disinhibit dampness, move the qi and quicken the blood

Formula & medicinals: Herba Dianthi (*Qu Mai*), 4 *qian*, Herba Polygoni Avicularis (*Bian Xu*), 4 *qian*, Caulis Akebiae Mutong (*Mu Tong*), 1 *qian*, Semen Plantaginis (*Che Qian Zi*), 3 *qian*, Rhizoma Dioscoreae Hypoglaucae (*Bi Xie*), 4 *qian*, Talcum (*Shi Kuai*), 4 *qian*, Feces Trogopterori Seu Pteromi (*Wu Ling Zhi*), 3 *qian*, Rhizoma Corydalis Yanhusuo (*Yan Hu Suo*), 3 *qian*, processed Rhizoma Cyperi Rotundi (*Xiang Fu*), 3 *qian*, Radix Bupleuri (*Chai Hu*), 1.5 *qian*, stir-fried Herba Seu Flos Schizonepetae Tenuifoliae (*Jing Jie Sui*), 1.5 *qian*

Course of treatment: On October 8, 1974, after taking these medicinals, the leukorrhea had decreased, but there was still lumbar pain and lower abdominal pain. [Dr. Liu] continued to administer 10 *ji* of the above formula. On October 23, 1974, after these medicinals, the lumbar and abdominal sagging and pain were decreased and the amount of leukorrhea was also decreased. However, there was still some insidious pain on both sides of the lower abdomen. [Dr. Liu] added Herba Taraxaci Mongolici Cum Radice (*Pu Gong Ying*), 5 *qian*, and Herba Patriniae Heterophyllae Cum Radice (*Bai Jiang Cao*), 3 *qian*, to the above formula and continued to administer this for [another] five *ji*. On October 29, the symptoms had all basically disappeared. The menstruation was seven days overdue. Urine examination for pregnancy antibodies was positive and [the woman] was already pregnant.

Case 2: Yin, female, 38 years old, a simple case in the out-patient department

Date of initial examination: March 17, 1972

Major complaints: Lower abdominal pain and profuse leukorrhea for more than one year with worsening of the symptoms in the last days

Present case history: Insidious pain on the right side of the lower abdomen had begun after a uterine curettage in 1971. This had continued until the whole lower abdomen was achy and painful. There

221

was profuse leukorrhea which was thick in consistency and slightly yellow [in color]. Gynecological examination [confirmed] a diagnosis of pelvic inflammation. [The patient] had already been treated with antibiotics, but the symptoms had not decreased. In recent days, the abdominal pain had gotten worse and was accompanied by low-grade fever (37.5°C). Blood examination [showed] white blood cells at 17,000/ml.

Tongue image: A red tongue body

Pulse image: Bowstring, slippery, and slightly rapid

Western medical diagnosis: Chronic pelvic inflammation becoming acute

Chinese medical pattern discrimination: Damp heat pouring downward, heat toxins stasis and binding

Treatment methods: Clear heat and disinhibit dampness, resolve toxins and scatter binding [or nodulation]

Formula & medicinals: Herba Dianthi (*Qu Mai*), 4 *qian*, Herba Polygoni Avicularis (*Bian Xu*), 4 *qian*, Caulis Akebiae Mutong (*Mu Tong*), 1.5 *qian*, Semen Plantaginis (*Che Qian Zi*), 5 *qian*, Herba Lycopi Lucidi (*Ze Lan*), 3 *qian*, Sclerotium Polypori Umbellati (*Zhu Ling*), 3 *qian*, Fructus Meliae Toosendan (*Chuan Lian Zi*), 3 *qian*, Flos Lonicerae Japonicae (*Yin Hua*), 1 *liang*, Cortex Radicis Moutan (*Dan Pi*), 3 *qian*, Radix Et Rhizoma Rhei (*Da Huang*), 1 *qian*, Herba Patriniae Heterophyllae Cum Radice (*Bai Jiang Cao*), 7 *qian*

Course of treatment: On March 20, after taking three *ji* of the above formula, the abdominal pain decreased and the leukorrhea diminished. Repeat blood examination [showed] that white blood cells were 9,000/ml. The above formula was administered continuously for [another] three *ji* and the symptoms relaxed and resolved. At this point, there was an effect [*i.e.*, the patient was considered cured].

Commentary: The preceding two cases were categorized as damp heat and damp toxin patterns. Case #1 tended towards damp exuberance. This is because lower abdominal pain and profuse leukorrhea which was yellow in color and sticky in consistency was accompanied by frequent urination. The pulse was bowstring, slippery, and slightly rapid, while the tongue body was red. Both of these [*i.e.*, the tongue and pulse signs] are categorized as heat signs. [Therefore,] Old Doctor Liu used the experiential formula, *Qing Re Li Shi Tang* (Clear Heat & Disinhibit Dampness Decoction) with additions and subtractions. Because damp heat was causing stasis and obstruction of the channels and vessels [alternate reading: menstrual vessels], he used Corydalis, Flying Squirrel Droppings, and Cyperus to move the qi, quicken the blood, and stop pain. Within this formula, stir-fried Schizonepeta and Bupleurum assist the coursing of qi and upbearing, scattering, and elimination of dampness, upbearing and scattering damp evils above. Dianthus, Dioscorea Hypoglauca, Polygonum Avicularis, Akebia, Plantago, and Talcum clear heat and disinhibit dampness below. One [set] upbears and one [set] downbears. This helps to move the qi and quicken the blood, course and free the flow of the channels and vessels, [thus] freeing the flow of and abducting damp heat, and [hence] addressing the root and branch simultaneously.

Case #2 originally had chronic pelvic inflammation. In recent days, the abdominal pain had gotten heavier and was accompanied by low-grade fever and elevated white blood cells. The pulse was seen to be bowstring, slippery, and slightly rapid. The tongue body was red. The pattern was [thus] categorized as damp heat brewing toxins with heat heavier than dampness. Therefore, basing [his treatment] on *Qing Re Li Shi Tang* above, [Dr. Liu] added [ingredients] to strengthen its effect of resolving toxins and scattering binding [or nodulation]. Within this formula, Lycopus and Polyporus quicken the blood, move water, and

223

disinhibit dampness. Lonicera and Patrinia clear heat, resolve toxins, and disperse welling abscesses. Melia clears heat, moves the qi, and stops pain. Moutan and Rhubarb cool the blood and quicken the blood, resolve toxins and break stasis. [Taken as] a whole, this formula clears heat, resolves toxins, and disinhibits dampness, moves the qi, quickens the blood, and scatters binding. Thus it was used in order to free the flow.

Case 3: Zhao, female, 43 years old, a simple case in the out-patient department

Date of initial examination: August 9, 1974

Major complaints: Left[-sided] lower abdominal aching and pain with recurrent onset for more than six years

Present case history: Since 1968, [the patient] had had constant left-sided lower abdominal aching and pain which was accompanied by yellow vaginal discharge. She had had approximately six bouts of acute pelvic inflammation. Each time these had started due to stomach pain and had been accompanied by nausea and vomiting. If severe, she had vomited greenish water-like bile. After half an hour, it arrived at the region of the [lower] abdomen. The pain developed from upper to lower and gradually got worse with downward sagging in the lower abdomen. When [the condition] was heavy, there was headache and dizziness (low blood pressure). When severe, there was shock. This was then followed by elevation of her body temperature to approximately 39°C. On August 21, 1973, she was incorrectly diagnosed as [suffering from] acute appendicitis and was hospitalized for exploratory surgery. This revealed an ovarian cyst from which the pussy fluids were cleared and eliminated. On June 6, 1974, again due to an acute occurrence, [the patient] went into shock and was [again] hospitalized. At that time, her blood pressure was 70/50mmHg, her white blood cells were 29,000/ml, and her neutrophils were 78%. Her temperature was 38.9°C, and she was diagnosed with acute diffuse peritonitis, suppurative pelvic inflammation, and toxic shock. During her time in the hospital, she was treated with choramphenicol, erythromycin, and gentamycin. After the acute inflammation was brought under control, she was discharged from the hospital on Jun. 22 and was continuously treated with placental tissue fluid, berberine, etc. The present symptoms were abdominal pain, dizziness, nausea, torpid intake, numb hands, and aching and pain of the abdominal region refusing pressure.

Tongue image: A red tongue body

Pulse image: Bowstring, slippery, and slightly rapid

Western medical diagnosis: A) Ovarian cyst; B) acute occurrence of chronic pelvic inflammation

Chinese medical pattern discrimination: Toxic heat accumulation and exuberance, qi and blood congealing and binding

Treatment methods: Clear heat and resolve toxins, quicken the blood and disinhibit dampness

Formula & medicinals: Flos Lonicerae Japonicae (*Yin Hua*), 5 *qian*, Fructus Forsythiae Suspensae (*Lian Qiao*), 5 *qian*, Herba Taraxaci Mongolici Cum Radice (*Pu Gong Ying*), 5 *qian*, Herba Patriniae Hetrophyllae Cum Radice (*Bai Jiang Cao*), 5 *qian*, Semen Benicasae Hispidae (*Dong Gua Zi*), 1 *liang*, Semen Phaseoli Calcarati (*Chi Dou*), 5 *qian*, Cortex Radicis Moutan (*Dan Pi*), 2 *qian*, Radix Albus Paeoniae Lactiflorae (*Bai Shao*), 2 *qian*, Resina Myrrhae (*Mo Yao*), 3 *qian*, Rhizoma Corydalis Yanhusuo (*Yan Hu Suo*), 3 *qian*, Fructus Meliae Toosendan (*Chuan Lian Zi*), 3 *qian*, Niu Huang Wan (Cow Bezoar Pills), 3 *qian* (taken separately [washed down with the decoction])

Course of treatment: On August 19, after taking six *ji* of the above formula, the abdominal pain was markedly decreased. The nausea had already stopped and intake of food was increased. However, [the patient] still had a headache. [Therefore,] Folium Mori Albi (*Sang Ye*), 3 *qian*, and Flos Chrysanthemi Morifolii (*Ju Hua*), 3 *qian*, were added to the preceding formula.

On September 2, the abdominal pain had already stopped. [However,] owing to the intake of uncooked, chilled [foods and drinks], there was dysentery with lower abdominal sagging and pain. Therefore, the following formula [was given]: uncooked Radix Albus Paeoniae Lactiflorae (*Bai Shao*), 3 *qian*, Radix Scutellariae Baicalensis (*Huang Qin*), 3 *qian*, Rhizoma Thalictri Foliosi (*Ma Wei Lian*), 3 *qian*, Radix Glycyrrhizae (*Gan Cao*), 1 *qian*, Radix Auklandiae Lappae (*Mu Xiang*), 1.5 *qian*, Pericarpium Citri Reticulatae (*Chen Pi*), 2 *qian*, Semen Plantaginis (*Che Qian Zi*), 3 *qian*, and Talcum (*Hua Shi*), 5 *qian*.

On September 19, 1974, after taking three *ji* of the above formula, the dysentery had stopped and the abdominal pain had disappeared. All the other symptoms had disappeared and repeat examination of white blood cells was normal. Based on gynecological examination, it was said that the adnexitis and ovarian cysts were basically cured.

Commentary: This case had been diagnosed by Western medicine as an ovarian cyst and had been treated surgically. Since 1968, there was constant left-sided lower abdominal aching and pain which was accompanied by yellow vaginal discharge. This clearly indicated damp heat brewing in the lower burner. This had endured for [many] days and had brewed toxins. Toxic heat then caused blockage and stagnation with heat being heavier than dampness. Heat toxins assailed the stomach and, therefore, each time, the onset was preceded by stomach venter aching and pain, nausea, and vomiting. If severe, there was even clouding reversal. This time, after the onset, [the patient] had been treated with antibiotics. These had brought the acute pelvic inflammation under control. However, there was still heat toxins and damp evils which were yet to be cleared and resolved. The qi and blood was congealed and bound and was blocking and stagnating the channels and network vessels. Therefore, there was still abdominal pain.

In terms of its pattern discrimination, Old Doctor Liu categorized this case as internal welling abscess. Therefore, the main [methods] he employed were to clear heat, resolve toxins, and disperse abscesss assisted by quickening the blood and disinhibiting dampness. Within this formula, Lonicera, Forsythia, Dandelion, and Patrinia are the main medicinals which clear heat and resolve toxins, disperse abscesses and scatter binding [or nodulation]. Semen Benincasae and Aduki Beans disperse swelling and expel pus. Moutan and Red Peony cool the blood and quicken the blood. Myrrha quickens the blood and stabilizes pain. Corydalis and Melia regulate the qi and blood and stop pain. Bezoar Pills clear heat and quicken the blood, transform stasis and stop pain. Based on his experience in treating this type of disease condition, [Dr. Liu held] that one should use large doses of heat-clearing, toxin-resolving, swelling-dispersing, and pus-expelling medicinals, while the doses of quickening and cooling the blood medicinals should be small, typically not more than 1-2 *qian*. If these are used excessively, the blood will be so quickened that suppurative toxins will be scattered widely and spread.

After taking over 10 *ji* of the formula, dysentery also arose. According to the principle of "treating the branch in acute [cases] and treating the root in chronic [cases]," the disease was cured by using *Qin Lian Shao Yao Gan Cao Tang* (Scutellaria, Coptis, Peony Root & Licorice Decoction) plus Auklandia, Orange Peel, Plantago, and Talcum in order to move the qi and harmonize the stomach, disinhibit dampness and clear heat.

Case 4: Cai, female, 35 years old, a simple case in the out-patient department

Date of initial examination: December 6, 1971

Major complaints: Lumbar pain and lower abdominal pain for more than five years with the lumbar and abdominal aching and pain having become heavier in the last five days

Present case history: Five years ago, after [the patient] had had a spontaneous miscarriage, lower abdominal pain and lumbar pain had started. Gynecological examination had diagnosed this as "pelvic inflammation." [However,] the symptoms had not been reduced even after being treated by antibiotics and physical therapy. After taking Chinese medicinals, the symptoms took a turn for the better. [The patient] was pregnant twice in 1967 and 1969 and delivered normally. Nevertheless, the symptoms of lumbar pain and lower abdominal chilly pain had not completely disappeared. Habitually, her facial complexion was yellowish white and leukorrhea was profuse, clear, and watery. There was emission of coolness from her lower abdomen. On Dec. 1, 1971, [the patient] had an artificial abortion after which the symptoms of lumbar pain and lower abdominal pain got heavier and were accompanied by vaginal tract bleeding which had lasted for five days without stopping. Repeat gynecological examination said there was left-sided adnexal thickening.

Tongue image: A dark red tongue body

Pulse image: Deep and relaxed

Western medical diagnosis: A) Chronic pelvic inflammation; B) vaginal tract bleeding after artificial abortion to be examined

Chinese medical pattern discrimination: Cold dampness congealing and gathering, static blood collecting internally

Treatment methods: Quicken the blood and transform stasis, warm the uterus and scatter cold

Formula & medicinals: Radix Angelicae Sinensis (*Dang Gui*), 3 *qian*, Radix Ligustici Wallichii (*Chuan Xiong*), 1 *qian*, Herba Lycopi Lucidi (*Ze Lan*), 1.5 *qian*, Herba Leonuri Heterophylli (*Yi Mu Cao*), 2 *qian*, Semen Pruni Persicae (*Tao Ren*), 1 *qian*, Flos Carthami Tinctorii (*Hong Hua*), 1 *qian*, mix-fried Radix Glycyrrhizae (*Gan Cao*), 1 *qian*, blast-fried Rhizoma Zingiberis (*Pao Jiang*), 1 *qian*, Fructus Foeniculi Vulgaris (*Xiao Hui Xiang*), 2 *qian*, Resina Myrrhae (*Mo Yao*), 1 *qian*

Course of treatment: On December 9, after taking three *ji* of the above formula, the vaginal bleeding had stopped, but there was still relatively slight abdominal pain. Again the methods of warming the uterus and scattering cold, moving the qi and transforming stagnation were used. The formula and medicinals were as follows: Semen Citri Reticulatae (*Ju He*), 3 *qian*, Semen Litchi Chinensis (*Li Zhi He*), 3 *qian*, Fructus Foeniculi Vulgaris (*Xiao Hui Xiang*), 3 *qian*, Semen Trigonellae Foeni-graeci (*Hu Lu Ba*), 3 *qian*, Rhizoma Corydalis Yanhusuo (*Yan Hu Suo*), 3 *qian*, Radix Angelicae Sinensis (*Dang Gui*), 3 *qian*, Fructus Meliae Toosendan (*Chuan Lian Zi*), 3 *qian*, and Fructus Citri Aurantii (*Zhi Ke*), 3 *qian*.

On Dec. 30, 1971, after taking 15 *ji* of the above formula, the lumbar and abdominal aching and pain had disappeared. In Dec. 1974, at the time of an out-patient follow-up, it was said that there was no discomfort on examination but the volume of the menstruate was relatively scanty.

Commentary: This case was categorized as a cold damp pattern. It was due to contraction of cold and coolness several years before after a spontaneous miscarriage. More recently, because of repeat contraction by cold, cool evils after an artificial abortion, cold evils had lodged in her uterus, congealing and becoming stagnant in the channels and vessels [alternate reading: the menstrual vessels]. Static blood had collected and been retained. Because static blood was not dispelled, new

229

blood did not abide [in its channels as it should], and, therefore, vaginal tract bleeding had not stopped. The channels and vessels were obstructed and stagnant and, therefore, lumbar aching and abdominal pain were seen. The lower burner had contracted cold, and, therefore, the abdomen was distended and emitted coolness. Cold and damp had poured downward, leading to profuse white vaginal discharge which was clear and watery.

Because this was a case of vaginal tract bleeding, [Dr. Liu] first used *Sheng Hua Tang* (Engendering & Transforming Decoction) plus Fennel and Myrrh to move the qi, quicken the blood, and scatter cold. When the blood obtained warmth, it flowed freely and the static blood obtained removal. The new blood was able to abide [in its channels], and therefore the bleeding automatically stopped. If cooling the blood and stopping bleeding prescriptions had been used erroneously, the blood would have become even colder, leading to even more congelation. Static blood would not have been able to be dispelled and the evils must then have been retained. Hence the bleeding would also not have been able to be stopped.

After the cessation of vaginal bleeding, the methods [used] were to heavily warm the uterus and scatter cold, assisted by moving the qi and transforming stagnation. Within this formula, Orange Seeds, Litchi, Fennel, and Fenugreek warm the uterus and scatter cold. Dang Gui, Corydalis, Melia, and Aurantium move the qi, quicken the blood, and stop pain. Once cold congelation was scattered, the blood vessels flowed freely and damp evils obtained elimination, the disease was automatically cured.

Case 5: Zhao, female, 38 years old, a simple case in the out-patient department

Date of initial examination: June 29, 1972

Major complaints: Lumbar pain, lower abdominal pain, and downward sagging in the anus which had endured already for half a year

Present case history: [The patient] had had lumbar pain, lower abdominal pain, and downward sagging of the anus for half a year. This had been diagnosed at a hospital as inflammation of the uterosacral ligament. The symptoms had not decreased after being treated by the methods of clearing heat and disinhibiting dampness or warming the uterus and scattering cold.

Tongue image: A dark red tongue body

Pulse image: Bowstring and slippery

Western medical diagnosis: Inflammation of the uterosacral ligament

Chinese medical pattern discrimination: Qi stagnation and blood stasis, channel and vessel obstruction and stagnation

Treatment methods: Move the qi and quicken the blood, free the flow of the vessels and transform stasis

Formula & medicinals: Processed Rhizoma Cyperi Rotundi (*Xiang Fu*), 3 *qian*, Radix Linderae Strychnifoliae (*Wu Yao*), 3 *qian*, Semen Pruni Persicae (*Tao Ren*), 2 *qian*, Feces Trogopterori Seu Pteromi (*Wu Ling Zhi*), 3 *qian*, Resina Myrrhae (*Mo Yao*), 1.5 *qian*, Resina Olibani (*Ru Xiang*), 1.5 *qian*, Fructus Meliae Toosendan (*Chuan Lian Zi*), 3 *qian*, Rhizoma Corydalis Yanhusuo (*Yan Hu Suo*), 3 *qian*, Radix Rubrus Paeoniae Lactiflorae (*Chi Shao*), 2 *qian*, uncooked Pollen Typhae (*Pu Huang*), 2 *qian*, Herba Dianthi (*Qu Mai*), 4 *qian*

Course of treatment: On July 4, after taking five *ji* of the above formula, the lumbar and abdominal aching and pain and the anal

231

downward sagging had basically disappeared, while the recent symptoms all had improved.

Case 6: Ma, female, 38 years old, a simple case in the out-patient department

Date of initial examination: July 7, 1972

Major complaints: Lower abdominal and anal sagging, distention, and wringing pain for four days

Present case history: On June 29, 1972, [the patient] had had an artificial abortion. On July 3, lower abdominal and anal sagging, distention, and wringing pain had begun with lumbosacral region aching and pain desiring pressure. Sagging pain and wringing pain were also felt in the anus and perineal regions. These symptoms had not been decreased after treatment with kanamycin and tetracycline. By gynecological examination, it was said that there was a node-like thing which was painful to pressure at the base of the uterus. There was [also] a small amount of coffee-colored secretion in the vaginal tract.

Tongue image: Thin, white fur with a dark tongue body

Pulse image: Bowstring and relaxed

Western medical diagnosis: Inflammation of the uterosacral ligament

Chinese medical pattern discrimination: Qi stagnation and blood stasis, vessel and channel obstruction and stagnation

Treatment methods: Move the qi and quicken the blood, transform stasis and scatter binding [or nodulation]

Formula & medicinals: Radix Angelicae Sinensis (*Dang Gui*), 3 *qian*, Radix Ligustici Wallichii (*Chuan Xiong*), 1 *qian*, Semen Pruni Persicae (*Tao Ren*), 1 *qian*, Flos Carthami Tinctorii (*Hong Hua*), 1 *qian*, Herba Lycopi Lucidi (*Ze Lan*), 1 *qian*, Herba Leonuri Heterophylli (*Yi Mu Cao*), 1 *qian*, Feces Trogopterori Seu Pteromi (*Wu Ling Zhi*), 3 *qian*, uncooked Pollen Typhae (*Pu Huang*), 2 *qian*, processed Rhizoma Cyperi Rotundi (*Xiang Fu*), 3 *qian*, Resina Olibani (*Ru Xiang*), 1 *qian*, Resina Myrrhae (*Mo Yao*), 1.5 *qian*, Rhizoma Corydalis Yanhusuo (*Yan Hu Suo*), 3 *qian*, Radix Linderae Strychnifoliae (*Wu Yao*), 2 *qian*

Course of treatment: On July 13, after taking three *ji* of these medicinals, the sagging pain and the wringing pain in the lower abdomen and anus were decreased. [However,] there was still a small amount of coffee-colored secretion in the vaginal tract. [Therefore, Dr. Liu] continued to administer the original formula. On July 7, after these medicinals, the wringing pain in the anus had already stopped. [However,] there was still a sagging, distended sensation and there was still sagging pain in the lumbosacral region with a pussy-natured vaginal discharge. The pulse was seen to be bowstring and slippery. [Therefore,] Dang Gui, Lindera, and Ligusticum Wallichium were removed from the above formula and Rhizoma Dioscoreae Hypoglaucae (*Bi Xie*) and Semen Plantaginis (*Che Qian Zi*), 3 *qian* each, and Herba Dianthi (*Qu Mai*), 4 *qian*, were added. On September 13, after administering another 11 *ji* of the above formula, the aching and pain were markedly diminished and the symptoms had basically disappeared. On follow-up more than a half year later, [the patient's] typical condition was quite good.

Commentary: Cases #5 and #6 were diagnosed by Western medicine as inflammation of the uterosacral ligament. From the point of view of their characteristic symptoms, the lower abdominal and lumbar pain was severe and fixed in location. Sometimes it was wringing pain. The tongue body tended to be dark. These were all due to qi stagnation and blood stasis. From the point of view of the combination of disease

233

discrimination and pattern discrimination, this disease is usually also accompanied by the appearance of lower burner brewing of dampness. However, the main point is qi stagnation and blood stasis.

In case #5, at the beginning, the treatment principles of clearing heat and disinhibiting dampness and of warming the uterus and scattering cold had already been used but had not been able to achieve an effect. Afterwards, [Dr. Liu] used the treatment principles of moving the qi and quickening the blood, freeing the vessels and transforming stasis, and the symptoms were able to be improved. In case #6, right from the beginning [Dr. Liu] used *Sheng Hua Tang* (Engendering & Transforming Decoction) plus *Shi Xiao San* (Loose a Smile Powder) with additions and subtractions. After a single course of treatment, the aching and pain had improved. However, there was a small amount of coffee-colored secretion from the vaginal tract. Finally, this became a pussy vaginal discharge. This clearly indicated that static blood had brewed heat and that this had combined with dampness internally. Thus damp heat and static blood wrestled and bound. [Therefore, Dr. Liu] added Dioscorea Hypoglauca, Dianthus, and Plantago to clear heat and disinhibit dampness. By simultaneously moving the qi and quickening the blood and disinhibiting dampness and clearing heat, afterwards the effect was achieved.

Case 7: Zhou, female, 32 years old, a simple case in the out-patient department

Date of initial examination: January 20, 1972

Major complaints: Lower abdominal sagging pain and profuse leukorrhea for four years

Present case history: [The patient] had been examined in a hospital due to infertility four years after getting married and a mass as large as a duck's egg which was painful to pressure was found in her pelvic cavity. She habitually had a profuse white vaginal discharge. Her menstrual cycle was normal but the amount [of the menstruate] was scanty and its color was black. Her last menstruation had occurred on Jan. 14.

Tongue image: A pale tongue body

Pulse image: Relaxed

Western medical diagnosis: Pelvic inflammatory mass

Chinese medical pattern discrimination: Qi stagnation and blood stasis

Treatment methods: Move the qi and quicken the blood

Formula & medicinals: Radix Angelicae Sinensis (*Dang Gui*), 3 *qian*, Radix Ligustici Wallichii (*Chuan Xiong*), 1 *qian*, stir-fried Radix Albus Paeoniae Lactiflorae (*Bai Shao*), 3 *qian*, Herba Leonuri Heterophylli (*Yi Mu Cao*), 3 *qian*, Radix Auklandiae Lappae (*Mu Xiang*), 1.5 *qian*, Rhizoma Cyperi Rotundi (*Xiang Fu*), 3 *qian*, Radix Bupleuri (*Chai Hu*), 1.5 *qian*, Herba Seu Flos Schizonepetae Tenuifoliae (*Jing Jie Sui*), 1.5 *qian*, Radix Linderae Strychnifoliae (*Wu Yao*), 3 *qian*

Course of treatment: On January 27, after taking three *ji* of the above formula, the leukorrhea was still profuse and the menstruation was persistent and had not stopped. Therefore, on top of the prior treatment methods as the basis, clearing heat and disinhibiting dampness were strengthened in the prescription. The formula and medicinals were as follows: Radix Scutellariae Baicalensis (*Huang Qin*), 3 *qian*, Rhizoma Thalictri Foliosi (*Ma Wei Lian*), 3 *qian*, Rhizoma Alismatis (*Ze Xie*), 3 *qian*, Semen Plantaginis (*Che Qian Zi*), 3 *qian*, Herba Dianthi (*Qu Mai*), 4 *qian*, Herba Polygoni Avicularis (*Bian Xu*), 3 *qian*, Rhizoma Dioscoreae Hypoglaucae (*Bi Xie*), 4 *qian*, Fructus Meliae Toosendan (*Chuan Lian Zi*),

235

3 *qian,* Radix Linderae Strychnifoliae (*Wu Yao*), 2 *qian,* Herba Ecliptae Prostatae (*Han Lian Zi*), 3 *qian,* and Cortex Cedrelae (*Chun Gen Bai Pi*), 3 *qian.*

On April 20, [after] a total of 16 *ji* of this formula had been taken, the leukorrhea was reduced and the lower abdominal aching and pain had disappeared. [Based on] gynecological examination at the original hospital, it was said that the inflammatory mass had completely disappeared.

Case 8: Liu, female, 16 years old, a simple case in the out-patient department

Date of initial examination: December 21, 1974

Major complaints: Lower abdominal aching and pain for more than one year

Present case history: Menarche had occurred at 14 years of age. At the very beginning of the first year, the menstrual cycle was normal, its amount was profuse, and it was painless. In the last one year, there had been lower abdominal region aching and pain. The menstrual cycle was 20-30 days and the menses moved for 6-7 days. Their amount was profuse and they contained clots. On the second and third days, there was lower abdominal colicky pain which refused pressure. Gynecological examination [showed] that the uterus was centrally placed but was somewhat small. A cystic mass could be palpated on the left side. Its surface was smooth and slippery. Its diameter was approximately 3 x 4cm and it was still movable. There was a slight degree of pressure pain. The right side was negative.

Tongue image: A pale red tongue body

Pulse image: Bowstring and slippery

Western medical diagnosis: Pelvic inflammatory mass

Chinese medical pattern discrimination: Damp heat brewing toxins, qi stagnation and blood stasis

Treatment methods: Clear heat and resolve toxins, quicken the blood and disinhibit dampness

Formula & medicinals: Flos Lonicerae Japonicae (*Yin Hua*), 5 *qian*, Fructus Forsythiae Suspensae (*Lian Qiao*), 5 *qian*, Herba Patriniae Heterophyllae Cum Radice (*Bai Jiang Cao*), 5 *qian*, Herba Taraxaci Mongolici Cum Radice (*Pu Gong Ying*), 5 *qian*, Rhizoma Corydalis Yanhusuo (*Yan Hu Suo*), 3 *qian*, Feces Trogopterori Seu Pteromi (*Wu Ling Zhi*), 3 *qian*, Fructus Meliae Toosendan (*Chuan Lian Zi*), 3 qian, Semen Phaseoli Calcarati (*Chi Xiao Dou*), 5 *qian*, Herba Dianthi (*Qu Mai*), 4 qian, Herba Polygoni Avicularis (*Bian Xu*), 4 *qian*, Semen Benincasae Hispdae (*Dong Gua Zi*), 8 *qian*, Talcum, (*Hua Shi*), 5 *qian*, Semen Plantaginis (*Che Qian Zi*), 3 *qian*

Course of treatment: On November 27, after taking five *ji* of these medicinals, the abdominal pain was decreased and the essence spirit had taken a turn for the better. [However,] there was occasional bilateral rib-side pain. [Therefore,] uncooked and processed Rhizoma Cyperi Rotundi (*Xiang Fu*), 3 *qian* each, were added to the above formula. On Dec. 6, after taking seven *ji* of the above formula, it was said [via] internal examination that the left-sided mass had already disappeared and the abdominal pain was markedly diminished.

Case 9: Zhang, female, 31 years old, a simple case in the out-patient department

Date of initial examination: January 4, 1972

Major complaints: Abdominal pain and low-grade fever for over one year

Present case history: For one year, abdominal pain had been constant. [There was also] lumbar pain and leukorrhea which had a flavor [*i.e.*, odor] and was white in color. Through examination in a hospital, it was said that there was a duck egg-size mass in the pelvic cavity with marked pressure pain. This was accompanied by low-grade fever (the temperature was between 37.3-37.5°C), heat in the centers of the hands and feet, dry mouth with thirst, and a desire to drink.

Tongue image: A red tongue body

Pulse image: Bowstring and slippery

Western medical diagnosis: Pelvic inflammatory mass

Chinese medical pattern discrimination: Yin vacuity blood heat, damp heat congelation and binding

Treatment methods: Nourish yin and clear heat, move the qi flow and scatter binding [or nodulation]

Formula & medicinals: Cortex Radicis Lycii Chinensis (*Di Gu Pi*), 3 *qian*, Herba Artemisiae Apiaceae (*Qing Hao*), 3 *qian*, Carapax Amydae Sinensis (*Bie Jia*), 7 *qian*, Semen Benincasae Hispidae (*Dong Gua Zi*), 1 *liang*, Fructus Meliae Toosendan (*Chuan Lian Zi*), 3 *qian*, Radix Linderae Strychnifoliae (*Wu Yao*), 3 *qian*, Thallus Algae (*Kun Bu*), 1 *liang*, Herba Taraxaci Mongolici Cum Radice (*Pu Gong Ying*), 5 *qian*, Herba Seu Flos Schizonepetae Tenuifoliae (*Jing Jie Sui*), 5 *qian*, Radix Bupleuri (*Chai Hu*), 1.5 *qian*

Course of treatment: On January 8, after taking four *ji* of the above formula, the body temperature returned to normal. The rest of the symptoms were the same as before. The administration of the above formula was continued with the addition of Radix Rubrus Paeoniae Lactiflorae (*Chi Shao*), 3 *qian*, and Herba Patriniae Heterophyllae Cum Radice (*Bai Jiang Cao*), 5 *qian*.

On Jan. 16, after taking eight *ji* of the above formula, the body temperature was normal. [Based on] examination at the original hospital, it was said that the pelvic mass had disappeared.

Commentary: Although cases #7, #8 and #9 all were categorized as concretion lump patterns, each had its special points. In case #7, there was habitual profuse leukorrhea and lower abdominal pain. The menstrual cycle was almost accurate [*i.e.*, normal], but the volume of blood was not much and its color was black. Examination found that there was a mass in the pelvic cavity. At the beginning of treatment, [Dr. Liu] was not able to grasp its pathological essence, and a stress was laid on moving the qi and quickening the blood. However, this was not sufficient for dealing with the damp heat congelation and accumulation. All that was used was Bupleurum and Schizonepetae to upbear yang, move the qi, and hold back dampness. Therefore, the symptoms did not appear to improve. At the second examination, in order to strengthen the prescription's clearing of heat and disinhibiting of dampness, a little Cedrela was added in order to restrain, astringe, and stop bleeding, and stress was laid on treating the damp heat evils which had congealed, gathered, and endured [for many days]. After administering these medicinals, [all] the symptoms basically disappeared and the pelvic inflammatory mass also disappeared.

In case #8, there was lower abdominal pain which refused pressure and the pulse was seen to be bowstring and slippery. This clearly indicated damp heat smoldering and enduring, thus brewing toxins. Therefore, clearing heat and resolving toxins and quickening the blood and disinhibiting dampness were equally [used]. Within this formula, Lonicera, Forsythia, Patrinia, and Dandelion clear heat, resolve toxins,

239

disperse swelling, and stop pain. Dianthus, Polygonum Avicularis, Plantago, and Talcum clear heat and disinhibit dampness. Melia, Corydalis, and Flying Squirrel Droppings move the qi and quicken the blood. Aduki Beans and Semen Benicasae quicken the blood, disinhibit dampness, and expel pus. [Dr. Liu] then added uncooked *and* processed Cyperus in order to strengthen the effect of moving the qi and stopping pain. Uncooked Cyperus is able to course and regulate the qi of the chest, rib-side, and stomach venter. Processed [Cyperus] is used to draw aside the qi of the low back and abdomen. Both of these were used to move the qi and stop pain.

In case #9, damp heat had brewed for a long time and [heat] had entered into the yin and blood. Therefore, low-grade fever, vexatious heat in the five hearts, a dry mouth with thirst, a desire to drink, and a red tongue were seen, all of which were yin vacuity, blood heat symptoms. Damp heat and yin vacuity are mutually contradictory, and the treatment of this situation is very difficult to grasp. Excessive disinhibition of dampness may damage yin blood, while excessive nourishment of yin may easily entangle evils. Therefore, taking into account [a.] the main symptoms of abdominal pain, profuse leukorrhea which was yellow in color and had an odor, and low-grade fever, [b.] the characteristics of the inflammatory mass [found through] examination of the pelvic cavity, [c.] the above thoughts about the treatment of [damp heat and yin vacuity], and [d.] the integrated body, [Dr. Liu] paid special attention to the local region and mainly used [the methods of] nourishing yin and clearing heat and moving the qi and scattering binding, assisted by resolving toxins. Therefore, Artemisia Apiacea, Carapax Amydae, and Cortex Lycii were mainly used to nourish yin and clear heat. Melia and Lindera move the qi and stop pain. Dandelion, Semen Benincasae, and Thallus Algae soften the hard and scatter nodulation, disperse swelling and expel pus. Carapax Amydae is able to assist both the nourishing of yin and the softening of the hard. Lindera, Schizonepeta, and Bupleurum move the qi, course the liver, and scatter dampness.

Old Doctor Liu used these three medicinals in combination as a medicinal group. Based on his experience, Lindera is able to move the qi. After taking it, the volume of leukorrhea may increase. Adroitly guiding action according to the circumstance, one can make damp heat follow the leukorrhea and discharge and expel it. Schizonepeta and Bupleurum harmonize the liver and course the qi. [Thus] they can upbear and scatter damp evils by making them follow qi transformation to the upper burner. [Hence,] when these three flavors and medicinals are used together, one [group of two] upbears and the other [one] downbears. By upbearing, scattering, and blocking dampness, the source of dampness is broken. By moving the qi and expelling dampness, free flow is able to function. Thus damp evils are not able to be retained. Although medicinals for disinhibiting dampness were not used, the principle of treating "dampness" was by no means to be abandoned. Thus, the contradiction between nourishing yin and disinhibiting dampness was solved quite reasonably.

In sum, [Dr. Liu] held that damp heat and cold damp are the main factors in pelvic inflammation. Damp heat congelation and gathering, cold damp congelation and gathering, and qi stagnation and blood stasis are the essential pathophysiological courses [i.e., mechanisms] of this disease. If damp heat brewing endures, toxic heat will blaze and become exuberant. Thus the signs of acute or subacute pelvic inflammation will manifest. No matter whether cold damp or damp heat, either can lead to qi stagnation and blood stasis. Therefore, treatment of damp heat or cold dampness and moving the qi, quickening the blood, and transforming stasis are the essential principles for treating this disease. Even more important is to discriminate the pattern and determine treatment according to the patient's own bodily condition.

Vaginal Tract Bleeding After Uterine Curettage Surgery: Two Cases

Case 1: Zhang, female, 29 years old, a simple case in the out-patient department

Date of initial examination: March 30, 1973

Major complaints: Vaginal tract bleeding for over 10 days

Present case history: On March 17, 1973, after uterine curettage following a spontaneous miscarriage, there was vaginal tract bleeding which dribbled and dripped without stop. The amount of the blood was sometimes profuse and sometimes scanty. Its color was pale and it contained small blood clots. This was accompanied by lumbar pain, abdominal sagging, distention, and pain, headache, tinnitus, and nausea.

Tongue image: A dark yet pale tongue body

Pulse image: Fine and relaxed

Western medical diagnosis: Vaginal tract bleeding after uterine curettage surgery, the cause to be examined

Chinese medical pattern discrimination: Blood vacuity and contraction of cold, loss of harmony of the qi and blood

Treatment methods: Quicken the blood and transform stasis, nourish the blood and harmonize the constructive

Formula & medicinals: Radix Angelicae Sinensis (*Dang Gui*), 2 *qian*, Radix Ligustici Wallichii (*Chuan Xiong*), 1 *qian*, Radix Bupleuri (*Chai Hu*), 1 *qian*, Herba Seu Flos Schizonepetae Tenuifoliae (*Jing Jie Sui*), 1 *qian*, processed Rhizoma Cyperi Rotundi (*Xiang Fu*), 2 *qian*, Feces Trogopterori Seu Pteromi (*Wu Ling Zhi*), 2 *qian*, Resina Myrrhae (*Mo Yao*), 1 *qian*, Fructus Meliae Toosendan (*Chuan Lian Zi*), 2 *qian*, Herba Leonuri Heterophylli (*Yi Mu Cao*), 1 *qian*, Herba Lycopi Lucidi (*Ze Lan*), 1 *qian*

Course of treatment: On April 6, after taking two *ji* of the above formula, the vaginal tract bleeding had already stopped and the lumbar pain, abdominal distention, dizziness, and nausea had disappeared.

Case 2: Zhang, female, 26 years old, a simple case in the out-patient department

Date of initial examination: June 13, 1973

Major complaints: Vaginal tract bleeding for over 10 days

Present case history: [The patient] had had uterine curettage surgery after a spontaneous miscarriage on May 26. After surgery, there had been vaginal tract bleeding for 17 days non-stop. The color of the blood was not fresh and it contained blood clots. This was accompanied by lower abdominal distention and pain and lumbar pain. In the last week, there had been a low-grade fever (the temperature was 37.4°C), heart vexation and tension, and yellowish red urination. Blood examination [showed] white blood cells to be 14,300/ml.

Tongue image: A dark red tongue body with slimy, yellow fur

Pulse image: Bowstring, slippery, and rapid

Western medical diagnosis: Vaginal tract bleeding after uterine curettage surgery with secondary infection

Chinese medical pattern discrimination: Damp heat pouring downward, heat damaging the blood network vessels

Treatment methods: Clear and disinhibit dampness and heat, cool the blood and stop bleeding

Formula & medicinals: Herba Dianthi (*Qu Mai*), 4 *qian*, Herba Polygoni Avicularis (*Bian Xu*), 4 *qian*, Talcum (*Hua Shi*), 5 *qian*, Semen Plantaginis (*Che Qian Cao*), 3 *qian*, Radix Scutellariae Baicalensis (*Huang Qin*), 3 *qian*, Herba Patriniae Hetrophyllae Cum Radice (*Bai Jiang Cao*), 4 *qian*, Flos Lonicerae Japonicae (*Yin Hua*), 4 *qian*, carbonized Pollen Typhae (*Pu Huang*), 3 *qian*

Course of treatment: On June 15, after taking three *ji* of the above formula, the vaginal tract bleeding had already stopped and the lumbar pain and abdominal pain were decreased. All the symptoms were eliminated after taking [another] two *ji* continuously.

Commentary: Western medicine holds that, during an abortion,[30] the villi are automatically shed, the membranes part, the blood sinuses open, and thus there is bleeding. When the fetus is stripped off and completely expelled and the uterus contracts fully, bleeding is able to cease and stop in a timely manner. After uterine curettage, any

---

[30] The words abortion or miscarriage as technical medical terms are synonymous. However, in everyday American English, abortion means an artificial abortion, while miscarriage means a spontaneous miscarriage. In Chinese, there is only the term *liu chan*, flowing birth, which is then prefaced by the words artificial or spontaneous. When not prefaced by either of these two adjectives, it is difficult to know which of these concepts the Chinese author has in mind or if they intentionally mean both. Dilation and curettage may be done for either incomplete abortion or miscarriage.

remaining or retained fetal membranes or infection may lead to the arising of vaginal tract bleeding that does not stop. Old Doctor Liu held that there are two great reasons for vaginal tract bleeding that does not stop after spontaneous miscarriage, uterine curettage after miscarriage, or after artificial abortion:

1. Static blood internally collecting, new blood not abiding

If static blood is retained and remains, it causes disharmony in the channels and network vessels and blood vessels. This causes the new blood not to abide [within the channels]. As it was said by the ancients:

> If malign blood is not ended [*i.e.*, eliminated], it is difficult for good blood to be quiet. Together these descend, enduring for days without stopping.

Typically, this manifests as relatively fresh red colored blood or purple blood clots. Mostly this is accompanied by abdominal pain with the pain fixed in location. There may also be the expulsion of large blood clots.

2. Cold lodged in the uterus obstructing the movement of the blood

As it says in the *Zhu Bing Yuan Hou Lun (Treatise on Origin & Symptoms of Various Diseases)*:

> If, after a new birth, wind coolness is contracted, wind chill may wrestle [or struggle] with the blood. This may then result in the blood not diffusing and dispersing. [Rather,] it amasses and accumulates internally and this leads in time to blood dribbling and dripping downward without end.

In the course of uterine curettage surgery, if [the patient] is affected by cold and coolness, this may result in wind chill lodging in the uterus, causing detriment and damage to the vessels of the *chong* and *ren*. The blood movement is not smoothly [or easily] flowing and static blood is retained and accumulates. The new blood is not able to abide in the channels. Therefore, the blood flows without stop. In both of the above two types of patterns, although their disease causes are different, in the end, it is static blood which causes the bleeding which does not stop. Therefore, treatment of both of the above should mainly quicken the blood and transform stasis.

If cold evils becomes depressed and endure, they may transform into heat. Cold is also able to engender dampness. [In that case,] dampness and heat may wrestle together and this may manifest as vexatious heat or fever. Heat damages the blood network vessels. The blood flows and does not stop. Its color is dark and not fresh. This is accompanied by abdominal pain, a dark red tongue, and a bowstring, slippery, and simultaneously rapid pulse. Treatment [of this] should mainly clear heat and disinhibit dampness.

Case #1 was categorized as cold lodged in the uterus with obstruction of the blood's movement. The volume of the vaginal tract bleeding was profuse, its color was pale, and it contained clots. Simultaneously, there were signs of constructive and defensive loss of harmony. Therefore, in the midst of quickening the blood and transforming stasis, [Dr. Liu] additionally used Schizonepeta and Bupleurum to regulate and harmonize, course and resolve. Within this formula, there are no warming medicinals. However, by regulating and harmonizing the constructive and defensive, cold evils are coursed and resolved.

In case #2, besides vaginal tract bleeding which would not stop, there was lower abdominal pain, low-grade fever, vexation and tension within the heart, yellow urine, and slimy, yellow tongue fur which were symptoms of dampness and heat brewing and binding. Thus dampness and heat mutually wrestled, with heat damaging the blood network vessels, forcing the blood to move frenetically. Treatment was mainly in order to clear and disinhibit heat and dampness assisted by quickening the blood. Within this formula, Dianthus, Polygonum Avicularis,

Plantago, and Talcum clear and disinhibit lower burner damp heat. Scutellaria, Lonicera, and Patrinia clear heat and resolve toxins. Carbonized Pollen Typhae quickens the blood and stops bleeding. Thus clearing and resolving and quickening the blood were used together. Without using large doses of blood-stopping medicinals, clearing of damp heat led to the bleeding's being able to be stopped.

Amenorrhea After Uterine Curettage Surgery: Two Cases

A menorrhea or blocked menstruation[31] arising after artificial abortion clinically has certain definite characteristics.[32] Old Doctor Liu held that besides the bodily constitution (postpartum), uterine curettage surgery [itself] may well be one of the external causes of blocked menstruation. From the point of view of Chinese medicine, uterine curettage surgery usually damages the kidneys and damages the blood, thus producing detriment and damage of the uterus. Due to this detriment and damage, the blood spills over and dead blood and vanquished blood become static and stagnant within the uterus. This then results in the arising of blocked menstruation whose basic patterns are kidney vacuity, blood vacuity, and blood stasis.

---

[31] *Bi jing* means blocked menstruation in Chinese medicine and is one of the traditional Chinese medical menstrual disease categories. It is called blocked menstruation in order to clearly imply that there is no menstruation because of some pathological cause as opposed to lack of menstruation post-menopausally. This term is also used to translate the modern medical English term, amenorrhea. When this term appears to be used as a Western medical concept, we have, therefore, translated it as amenorrhea. However, when it appears to be used within the conceptual framework of Chinese medicine, we have translated it as blocked menstruation. Unfortunately, this distinction is not so clear cut. However, if one only translates this term as amenorrhea, then the logic inherent in the traditional categorization of menstrual diseases is lost.

[32] As these case histories make clear, uterine curettage was used in China at the time this book was compiled not only to treat the after effects of spontaneous miscarriage and artificial abortion but as a method of abortion itself. Therefore, when one sees reference to uterine curettage in the Chinese medical literature one must be careful not to assume that the D & C was performed for the same typical reasons as in the West where vacuum extraction is the most common form of early stage abortion.

However, because of the variability of [patients'] constitutions, the result [after surgery] are not all the same. If the body's yang is habitually vacuous or there is lower burner vacuity cold, this mostly leads to the manifestation of vacuity cold symptoms. If the body is habitually healthy and strong and the *chong* and *ren* are effulgent and exuberant, post-surgically, the qi and blood may counterflow chaotically. [In that case,] the menstrual blood may not flow temporarily but may obstruct the uterus. If static blood blocking internally endures for [many] days, it may transform heat. If this occurs during the menstrual period when the *chong* and *ren* vessels are exuberant, static blood and depressive heat may obstruct and block and the menstrual blood may not be able to move downward. Rather, it counterflows and moves upward along the two vessels of the *chong* and *ren*. Mostly this manifests as symptoms of mixed vacuity and repletion. Because the liver channel networks with the yin organs [*i.e.*, the genitalia], if the *chong* and *ren* counterflow chaotically, stasis heat may penetrate upwards. This may then affect the two channels of the liver and stomach and manifest the pattern of liver heat and/or *yang ming* stomach heat. In a word, in the treatment [of this disease], the basic methods and principles are to supplement the kidneys and supplement the blood and to quicken the blood and transform stasis. [For cases] tending towards vacuity cold, there should be ingredients for warming the channels and scattering cold. [For cases] tending towards repletion mixed with simultaneous heat, there should be ingredients for clearing heat and freeing the flow of the menses, moving the qi and coursing sternly.

Case 1: Mao, female, 41 years old, a simple case in the out-patient department

Date of initial examination: August 1, 1974

Major complaints: Amenorrhea after uterine curettage surgery for more than four months

Present case history: On March 20, 1974, due to unstopping vaginal tract bleeding, [the patient] had a pregnancy antibody test which was positive. After having uterine curettage surgery [as a means of surgical abortion], there commenced amenorrhea. After being injected with progesterone, her menses moved one time on July 27. It amount was scanty. Habitually, she had constant lower abdominal emission of coolness. The symptoms seen were lumbar pain and seeing things as if through a membrane [*i.e.*, blurred vision].

Tongue image: A pale tongue body

Pulse image: Deep, fine, and forceless

Western medical diagnosis: Secondary amenorrhea after artificial abortion

Chinese medical pattern discrimination: Kidney vacuity and blood depletion, cold congelation blocked menstruation

Treatment methods: Supplement the kidneys and nourish the blood, quicken the blood and warm the channels

Formula & medicinals: Radix Angelicae Sinensis (*Dang Gui*), 3 *qian*, Radix Albus Paeoniae Lactiflorae (*Bai Shao*), 4 *qian*, Radix Ligustici Wallichii (*Chuan Xiong*), 1.5 *qian*, cooked Radix Rehmanniae (*Shu Di*), 3 *qian*, Semen Cuscutae Chinensis (*Tu Si Zi*), 3 *qian*, Fructus Lycii Chinensis (*Gou Qi Zi*), 2 *qian*, Herba Cistanchis Deserticolae (*Rou Cong Rong*), 4 *qian*, Fructus Amomi (*She Ren*), 1 *qian*, Semen Pruni Persicae (*Tao Ren*), 5 *fen*, Flos Carthami Tinctorii (*Hong Hua*), 1 *qian*, Placenta Hominis (*Zi He Che*), 3 *qian*

Course of treatment: When re-examined on August 10, it was said that the stools were loose after taking these medicinals and her whole body lacked strength. Therefore, the following modified formula was

251

administered: Radix Angelicae Sinensis (*Dang Gui*), 3 *qian*, Radix Albus Paeoniae Lactiflorae (*Bai Shao*), 3 *qian*, Radix Ligustici Wallichii (*Chuan Xiong*), 1.5 *qian*, cooked Radix Rehmanniae (*Shu Di*), 4 *qian*, Fructus Foeniculi Vulgaris (*Xiao Hui Xiang*), 3 *qian*, Semen Trigonellae Foenigraeci (*Hu Lu Ba*), 3 *qian*, Cortex Cinnamomi Cassiae (*Rou Gui*), 1 *qian*, dried Rhizoma Zingiberis (*Gan Jiang*), 5 *fen*, Fructus Amomi (*Sha Ren*), 1.5 *qian*, Placenta Hominis (*Zi He Che*), 3 *qian*, Semen Cuscutae (*Tu Si Zi*), 5 *qian*, and Flos Carthami Tincotrii (*Hong Hua*), 2 *qian*.

On August 13, after taking these medicinals, the lower abdominal emission of coolness had taken a turn for the better. Stomach intake had increased and the number of bowel movements was normal. [However,] they were still watery and there were profuse dreams during sleep. The following formula and medicinals [were administered]: Radix Angelicae Sinensis (*Dang Gui*), 3 *qian*, Radix Albus Paeoniae Lactiflorae (*Bai Shao*), 3 *qian*, Radix Ligustici Wallichii (*Chuan Xiong*), 1.5 *qian*, cooked Radix Rehmanniae (*Shu Di*), 4 *qian*, Herba Epimedii (*Xian Ling Pi*), 4 *qian*, Semen Cuscutae Chinensis (*Tu Si Zi*), 3 *qian*, Placenta Hominis (*Zi He Che*), 3 *qian*, Semen Plantaginis (*Che Qian Zi*), 3 *qian*, Fructus Rubi Chingii (*Fu Pen Zi*), 3 *qian*, Fructus Lycii Chinensis (*Gou Qi Zi*), 3 *qian*, Radix Achyranthis Bidentatae (*Niu Xi*), 5 *qian*, Herba Leonuri Heterophylli (*Yi Mu Cao*), 4 *qian*, and Fructus Amomi (*Sha Ren*), 1.5 *qian*.

On September 13, after taking these medicinals, the lower abdominal emission of coolness and lumbar pain had taken a turn for the better. Sleep was [still] a problem and there were [still] profuse dreams. [Therefore,] White Peony, cooked Rehmannia, Achyranthes, and Leonurus were removed from the above formula, and Cortex Cinnamomi Cassiae (*Rou Gui*), Semen Pruni Persicae (*Tao Ren*), Flos Carthami Tinctorii (*Hong Hua*), and Fructus Schisandrae Chinensis (*Wu Wei Zi*), 1 *qian* each, were added. Administration was continued [another] seven *ji*.

When re-examined on October 8, it was said that, after taking the above medicinals, the menses had come on October 1. The menses had moved for six days and their volume was moderate. However, sleep was a slight problem and intake was torpid. White Peony, Achyranthes, and Leonurus were removed from the above formula. Cortex Cinnamomi was changed to 1.5 *qian*. Schisandra was changed to 3 *qian*. And 4 *qian* of stir-fried Semen Zizyphi Spinosae (*Zao Ren*) were added. Administration was [then] continued in order to secure the treatment effect.

Case 2: Wang, female, a simple case in the out-patient department

Date of initial examination: July 15, 1975

Major complaints: Amenorrhea after artificial abortion for the last four months

Present case history: [The patient's] past menstrual cycle was 23-24 days. The menses moved for 6-7 days. [She had] delivered after sufficient months two times. The last delivery was six years ago. On March 24, she had had an artificial abortion. After surgery, there had been amenorrhea for nearly four months. The menstruation had moved after injecting progesterone. [The patient reported that] she felt heart vexation, tension and agitation, a dry mouth with bitter [taste], dizziness, lumbar aching, lower limb flaccidity and lack of strength, bilateral rib-side distention, and devitalized food intake. Her two excretions were self-regulated [*i.e.*, normal].

Tongue image: A dark yet pale tongue body

Pulse image: Fine and bowstring

Western medical diagnosis: Secondary amenorrhea after artificial abortion

Chinese medical pattern discrimination: Blood vacuity and blood stasis, brewing heat penetrating upward

Treatment methods: Supplement the blood and boost the kidneys, clear heat and free the flow of the menses

Formula & medicinals: Radix Angelicae Sinensis (*Dang Gui*), 3 *qian*, Radix Ligustici Wallichii (*Chuan Xiong*), 1.5 *qian*, stir-fried Radix Albus Paeoniae Lactiflorae (*Bai Shao*), 3 *qian*, cooked Radix Rehmanniae (*Shu Di*), 4 *qian*, Semen Pruni Persicae (*Tao Ren*), 1 *qian*, Flos Carthami Tinctorii (*Hong Hua*), 1 *qian*, Herba Dianthi (*Qu Mai*), 4 *qian*, Herba Polygoni Avicularis (*Bian Xu*), 4 *qian*, Caulis Akebiae Mutong (*Mu Tong*), 1 *qian*, Semen Plantaginis (*Che Qian Zi*), 3 *qian*, Radix Gentianae Scabrae (*Long Dan Cao*), 2 *qian*, Fructus Gardeniae Jasminoidis (*Zhi Zi*), 3 *qian*, Fructus Meliae Toosendan (*Chuan Lian Zi*), 3 *qian*, Fructus Trichosanthis Kirlowii (*Gua Lou*), 8 *qian*, Radix Achyranthis Bidentatae (*Niu Xi*), 3 *qian*

Course of treatment: On July 24, after taking five *ji* of the above formula, the heart vexation, tension and agitation had taken a marked turn for the better. [Therefore,] Dang Gui was removed from the above formula and 3 *qian* of Rhizoma Thalictri Foliosi (*Ma Wei Lian*) were added. On re-examination on Aug. 9, it was said that, after administering another five *ji* of the above formula, all the symptoms had improved. The menses had come on Aug. 1 and had moved for three days. Their amount was scanty and they were coffee-colored. There was still a slight sensation of rib-side distention and the left side of the face and shoulder were numb. [Therefore,] Dang Gui, Polygonum Avicularis, Akebia, Gentiana Scabra, Gardenia, and Achyranthes were removed from the above formula, and Herba Dendrobii (*Shi Hu*), 4 *qian*, Caulis Milletiae Seu Spatholobi (*Ji Xue Teng*), 5 *qian*, and Fasciculus Vascularis Luffae Cylindricae (*Si Gua Luo*), 2 *qian*, were added. Administration was continued.

On follow-up on October 9, 1975, the above medicinals had been administered continuously for 15 *ji*. On September 28, the menses had come like a tide and had moved for four days. Their amount was normal and there was no discomfort.

Commentary: In case #1, amenorrhea after uterine curettage surgery had already occurred for more than four months. On normal days [*i.e.*, regularly], there was lower abdominal emission of coolness. The symptoms seen were lumbar pain, seeing things as if through a membrane, a pale tongue body, and a deep, fine, forceless pulse. She had already received injection of progesterone. However, the amount of blood in the menstrual movement was extremely scanty. The pattern was discriminated as kidney vacuity and blood depletion, cold congelation blocked menstruation. Treatment was in order to supplement the kidneys and nourish the blood, quicken the blood and warm the channels.

The formula used was *Tao Hong Si Wu Tang* (Persica & Carthamus Four Materials Decoction) combined with *Wu Zi Yan Zong Wan* (Five Seeds Increase Progeny Pills) with additions and subtractions. To this was added Cistanches combined with Cuscuta to warm the kidneys and supplement yang, while Amomum [was added] to move the qi and open the stomach. In addition, Placenta Hominis was added. This ingredient is salty and level and simultaneously warms. It enters the kidneys, supplements the kidneys, and boosts essence blood. It rules the treatment of qi and blood dual depletion, the five taxations and seven damages, womens' scanty menstruation, and menstrual irregularities. This medicinal is a bloody, meaty natured ingredient.

Because [this patient] had lower burner vacuity cold, after administration of these medicinals, watery stools appeared and the body was without strength. This clearly showed that the power and dosage of warming the channels and invigorating yang [medicinals] was insufficient and the menses did not come like a tide in August

255

[Therefore,] to the foundation of the above formula [Dr. Liu] added Fennel, Fenugreek, Cortex Cinnamomi, and dry Ginger in order to add to and strengthen the effect of warming the channels and scattering cold. The result was that the menses became free-flowing and their amount and the date they moved returned to normal.

In case #2, there had been post-uterine curettage surgery amenorrhea for the last four months. After injecting progesterone the menses had [still] not moved. [The patient] felt heart vexation, tension and agitation, dizziness, dry mouth, and a bitter [taste] in the mouth, and her food intake was devitalized. This was due to depressive heat penetrating upward, resulting in heat brewing in the heart and stomach channels. Blood vacuity and liver depression had appeared as bilateral rib-side distention and a fine, bowstring pulse. Because of blood vacuity and static blood retained internally, there was a dark, pale tongue body. Pattern discrimination categorized this as blood vacuity and blood stasis, brewing heat penetrating above. Therefore, treatment was in order to supplement the blood and quicken the blood, clear heat and free the flow of the menses.

The formula used was [again] Tao Hong Si Wu Tang in order to supplement the blood and quicken the blood. The aim was the same as in case #1. However, it was combined with Gentiana Scabra and Akebia to clear liver heat. Dianthus, Polygonum Avicularis, and Plantago course sternly, free the flow, and disinhibit, thus making the penetrating counterflow of two vessels of the chong and ren follow their channels to descend and be downborne. Trichosanthes clears heat and moistens dryness. Melia and Achyranthes move the qi and quicken the blood and lead the menses to move downward. After administering these medicinals, the symptoms of vexatious heat improved and the menstrual blood flowed freely. Therefore, on the foundation of the original formula, Dendrobium was added to nourish stomach yin, clear heat and moisten dryness, while Milletia and Luffa [were added] to quicken the blood and free the flow of the network vessels, thus securing the treatment effect.

Abdominal Pain After Uterine Curettage Surgery: Two Cases

Case 1: Zhang, female, 44 years old, a simple case in the out-patient department

Date of initial examination: April 6, 1974

Major complaints: After having a uterine curettage two days [before], there had been severe abdominal pain for one day

Present case history: On Apr. 4, [the patient] had had uterine curettage surgery due to incomplete miscarriage. On the night of Apr. 5, severe paroxysmal pain in the lower abdomen had suddenly occurred [along with] lumbar pain. She had taken pain-stopping tablets and tetracycline, but the aching and pain had not decreased. [There was] lumbar and abdominal aching and pain. The lochia was not profuse. There was dizziness, torpid intake, lower leg flaccidity and lack of strength, and a chilly sweat when the pain [occurred]. Her facial complexion was somber white.

Tongue image: A dark yet pale tongue body

Pulse image: Bowstring and relaxed

Western medical diagnosis: A) Post incomplete miscarriage surgery; B) abdominal pain after uterine curettage surgery awaiting examination

Chinese medical pattern discrimination: Static blood internally collecting, simultaneous contraction of cold and coolness

Treatment methods: Quicken the blood and transform stasis, nourish the blood and warm the uterus

Formula & medicinals: Radix Angelicae Sinensis (*Dang Gui*), 3 *qian*, Radix Ligustici Wallicii (*Chuan Xiong*), 1 *qian*, Flos Carthami Tinctorii (*Hong Hua*), 1 *qian*, Herba Leonuri Heterophylli (*Yi Mu Cao*), 1 *qian*, Herba Lycopi Lucidi (*Ze Lan*), 1 *qian*, Semen Pruni Persicae (*Tao Ren*), 5 *fen*, mix-fried Radix Glycyrrhizae (*Gan Cao*), 5 *fen*, blast-fried Rhizoma Zingiberis (*Pao Jiang*), 5 *fen*, southern Fructus Crataegi (*Nan Shan Zha*), 2 *qian*, Pollen Typhae (*Pu Huang*), 3 *qian*, Feces Trogopterori Seu Pteromi (*Wu Ling Zhi*), 3 *qian*

Course of treatment: On April 8, after taking two *ji* of the above fomula, the abdominal pain was decreased. The flow was black in color with two blood clots. The lower abdomen still had a sagging sensation. The stools were loose and watery and resolved two times each day. [Therefore,] blast-fried Ginger was removed from the above formula and dry Rhizoma Zingiberis (*Gan Jiang*), 2 *qian*, and Rhizoma Atractylodis Macrocephalae (*Bai Zhu*), 3 *qian*, were added. Another three *ji* were administered.

On April 13, after taking these medicinals, the lochia had already disappeared. The lower abdomen was not painful and the number of bowel movements were normal. All the symptoms had relaxed and resolved.

Case 2: Li, female, 41 years old, a consultant case from another hospital

Date of consultant examination: April 22, 1975

Major complaints: After artificial abortion, severe paroxysmal pains in the lower abdomen for one week

Present case history: [The patient] had had an artificial abortion on April; 18, 1974 because early pregnancy had been complicated by rheumatic heart disease. She had been hospitalized for observation due to shock during the course of the operation. After surgery, there was fever (the body temperature was 37.3-38.2°C), dry stools, dizziness, torpid intake, lumbar pain, and vaginal tract bleeding. In the last two days, the amount of bleeding had increased (similar to the volume of menstruation). Its color was red and it contained clots. There was severe paroxysmal pain in the lower abdomen which was fixed in location.

Examination: The body temperature was 37.3°C. The pulse was 80 beats per minute. The facial complexion was typical [*i.e.*, normal]. The throat was hyperemic. Double mummur could be heard at the apex of the heart. The abdomen was soft and there was marked pressure pain of the lower abdomen. The blood pressure was 110/70mmHg. On April 4, blood examination showed the white blood cells at 7,400/ml. Neutrophils were 61%.

Tongue image: A dark tongue body with slimy, yellow fur

Pulse image: Bowstring and slippery

Western medical diagnosis: A) Abdominal pain after uterine curettage awaiting examination; B) rheumatic heart disease

Chinese medical pattern discrimination: Static blood internally bound, damp heat pouring downward

Treatment methods: Clear heat and eliminate dampness, quicken the blood and transform stasis

Formula & medicinals: Radix Angelicae Sinensis (*Dang Gui*), 4 *qian*, Caulis Akebiae Mutong (*Mu Tong*), 1 *qian*, Semen Plantaginis (*Che Qian Zi*), 3 *qian*, Talcum (*Hua Shi*), 5 *qian*, Radix Et Rhizoma Rhei (*Da Huang*),

261

1 *qian*, Herba Patriniae Hetrophyllae Cum Radice (*Bai Jiang Cao*), 5 *qian*, Herba Taraxaci Mongolici Cum Radice (*Pu Gong Ying*), 5 *qian*, Rhizoma Corydalis Yanhusuo (*Yan Hu Suo*), 3 *qian*, Feces Trogopterori Seu Pteromi (*Wu Ling Zhi*), 3 *qian*, Pollen Typhae (*Pu Huang*), 3 *qian*, Resina Myrrhae (*Mo Yao*), 2 *qian*, Semen Pruni Persicae (*Tao Ren*), 5 *fen*, Herba Leonuri Heterophylli (*Yi Mu Cao*), 1 *qian*

Course of treatment: On April 29, after taking three *ji* of the above formula, a membranous-like thing was expelled along with small clots. After this, the flow of blood decreased, the abdominal pain diminished, and the body temperature returned to normal. Administration of the above-mentioned formula was continued. When re-examined on May 2, it was said that, after taking the above medicinals, the bleeding and abdominal pain had stopped on April 30. [The patient's] body temperature had been normal for three days. [Therefore, she] was discharged from the hospital on May 2.

Commentary: Abdominal pain after artificial abortion is mostly caused by retention in the uterine cavity of villous tissues from part of the placenta or to post-surgical infection. Old Doctor Liu held that this disease is mostly seen in the following three conditions:

1. Static blood collecting internally

If a part of the placental tissues is not completely cleared and eliminated or post-surgical blood flow is not smooth [and unobstructed], this is categorized in Chinese medicine as static blood collecting in the uterus. This then results in pain. Its symptoms are pain which is fixed in location and refuses pressure, vaginal tract bleeding which is purple or black in color, and occasional accompaniment of lumbar pain. Treatment should mainly quicken the blood and transform stasis. Mostly, [Dr. Liu] chose *Sheng Hua Tang* (Engendering & Transforming Decoction) with additions and subtractions.

2. Cold lodged in the uterus

If cold and coolness are contracted during the course of surgery, this mostly appears as lower abdominal colicky pain, emission of coolness, a bluish-greenish white facial complexion, and a bowstring, tight pulse image. Treatment should mainly warm the uterus and scatter cold. [Dr. Liu] mostly chose *Wen Jing Tang* (Warm the Channels Decoction) with additions and subtractions.

3. Static blood collecting internally with simultaneous damp heat

Besides abdominal pain which refuses pressure and other such symptoms of static blood collecting internally, if due to simultaneous damp heat, mostly these will be accompanied by fever, uterine bleeding which is red in color, abdominal pain which refuses pressure, a dark tongue body with yellow fur, and a bowstring, slippery pulse. [Dr. Liu] treated this mainly with *Ba Zheng San* (Eight [Ingredients] Correcting Powder) combined with medicinal substances which clear heat and resolve toxins, quicken the blood and transform stasis.

In case #1, after uterine curettage surgery, bleeding was not profuse, but there was severe lower abdominal pain and lumbar pain. These were due to static blood internally. The somber white facial complexion and colicky pain in the abdominal region were signs of blood vacuity with simultaneous cold. Because, after miscarriage [with its loss of blood, the patient] had also had uterine curettage [with even more loss of blood], her qi and blood were vacuous and in decline. Therefore, dizziness, torpid intake, and lower leg flaccidity and lack of strength were seen. That the tongue was dark and pale was due to blood vacuity and blood stasis. A bowstring pulse governs pain and a relaxed pulse governs vacuity. Thus the pattern was discriminated as static blood congealing and stagnating with blood vacuity and simultaneous contraction of cold and coolness. Therefore, treatment of the above used the methods of quickening the blood and transforming stasis, nourishing the blood and warming the channels. *Chan Hou Sheng Hua Tang* (Postpartum Engendering & Transforming Decoction) was employed and this achieved the effect.

Case #2 was complicated by shock during the surgery. After surgery, there was severe fixed pain in the lower abdomen, vaginal tract bleeding which would not stop, and a dull tongue body, all of which were caused by the existence of static blood internally. The low-grade fever, slimy, yellow tongue fur, and bowstring, slippery pulse were signs of damp heat. [Thus] the pattern was categorized as static blood binding internally with damp heat pouring downward. Therefore, [Dr. Liu] used *Ba Zheng San* with additions and subtractions. This was mainly in order to clear heat and disinhibit dampness, assisted in small [measure] by ingredients which quicken the blood and transform stasis. After [taking] these medicinals and a membranous material was expelled, the abdominal pain was alleviated and the vaginal tract bleeding stopped. The pain and bitterness [*i.e.*, suffering] of a second uterine curettage was thus avoided.

In both of the above two cases, there was severe abdominal region pain after uterine curettage, and the basic pathophysiology in both was due to static blood collecting internally. However, in case #1, there was simultaneous vacuity cold, while in case #2, there was simultaneous damp heat, and it was necessary to minutely discriminate these.

Chronic Fibrous Hyperplastic Breast Disease: Three Cases

Chronic fibrous hyperplastic breast disease is a commonly-seen disease in women.[33] The cause of this disease is related to loss of regulation of the function of the ovaries. In terms of its present clinical condition, it is mostly seen in adolescent and menopausal women. Either constantly or during the second half [of the menstrual cycle] there are numerous large and small, round-shaped, hard nodules within the breasts on both sides. Their edges are clearly distinguishable and they do not adhere to the surrounding tissues. [Patients] commonly feel piercing pain in their breasts or distended pain. This becomes relatively more pronounced during the premenstruum. At times, a scanty, yellowish green, palm fiber colored, or bloody liquid may flow from within the nipples.

Based on its clinical characteristics, [this disease] is categorized in our national medicine [*i.e.,* Chinese medicine] as "breast nodes", "breast elusive mass", and "breast kernel." This disease's momentum is relaxed, and it lingers and endures for [many] days [*i.e.,* years]. Mostly, it is due to qi and blood insufficiency, liver depression and blood stagnation, and liver-stomach channel vessel stasis and obstruction with congelation and binding of the qi and blood. Because the qi in the *chong mai* is congested during the premenstruum, it may become stagnant, blocked,

---

[33] In English, this is more usually referred to a fibrocystic breast disease (FBD). However, many Western doctors are now coming to the conclusion that this is not a "disease" per se. Rather, it is a symptom of aging in some women. However, this does not address the fact that A) it may be uncomfortable, B) not all women develop fibrocystic breasts as they age, and C) there is an increased incidence of breast cancer in women with a history of fibrocystic breasts. In Chinese medicine, fibrocystic breasts are considered pathological and Chinese medicine does routinely attempt to treat this condition, it being a common one in the modern Chinese medical literature.

and not freely flowing. Therefore, breast distention and pain increase and get heavier [during the premenstruum]. During the menstrual movement, the *chong mai* qi is discharged. Therefore, the pain decreases [with the onset of menstruation]. In addition, if liver-stomach channel vessel stasis and obstruction endure and brew heat, heat may damage the network vessels of the breasts. This then leads to a coffee-colored (bloody) secretion flowing and spilling. [Likewise,] liver-stomach channel and vessel stasis and obstruction may lead to loss of harmony of the liver and stomach. If the liver qi loses its orderly reaching and the stomach loses its harmony and downbearing, this leads to the spleen's movement losing its fortification. If the spleen becomes vacuous and the damp becomes exuberant, then yellowish water will flow from the nipples.

Therefore, treatment of the above should mainly regulate and supplement the qi and blood, soothe depression and transform stagnation. If heat is seen to damage the network vessels of the breasts, this should be assisted by clearing heat and cooling the blood. If damp signs are marked, this should be assisted by fortifying the spleen and eliminating dampness.

Case 1: Li, female, 26 years old, a simple case in the out-patient department

Date of initial examination: September 2, 1974

Major complaints: Premenstrual breast distention and pain for more than two years

Present case history: For more than two years, there had been breast distention and pain. The menstruation was ahead of schedule and its volume was scanty. Its color was pinkish, and the menses moved for [only] two days. There was abdominal pain during the menstrual period, lumbar pain, whole body lack of strength, torpid intake, and breast distention and pain. Scattered throughout both breasts were numerous small, hard, nodules which were aching and painful to pressure. Two weeks before menstruation, this aching and pain would get heavier and she was not able to press or push [against the breasts]. After the menses moved, the breast distention and pain gradually disappeared until next time during the premenstruum when they got worse again. [The patient's] last menstruation had come on Aug. 15, 1974. There was habitual vexation and agitation and easy anger and her emotions were not well.

Tongue image: A pale tongue body

Pulse image: Deep and relaxed

Western medical diagnosis: Chronic fibrous hyperplastic breast disease

Chinese medical pattern discrimination: Qi and blood insufficiency, liver depression and blood stagnation

Formula & medicinals: Uncooked Radix Astragali Membranacei (*Huang Qi*), 5 *qian*, Radix Angelicae Sinensis (*Dang Gui*), 3 *qian*, Radix Ligustici Wallichii (*Chuan Xiong*), 1.5 *qian*, Radix Polygalae Tenuifoliae (*Yuan Zhi*), 3 *qian*, Rhizoma Polygonati (*Huang Jing*), 4 *qian*, Radix Glycyrrhizae (*Gan Cao*), 2 *qian*, Radix Albus Paeoniae Lactiflorae (*Bai Shao*), 3 *qian*

Course of treatment: On September 9, after taking seven *ji* of the above formula, the premenstrual bilateral breast aching and pain was decreased. There was still bodily lassitude, lack of strength, lumbar pain, and abdominal pain. Administration of seven *ji* [more] was continued, [after which] her symptoms basically were alleviated.

Case 2: Wei, female, 39 years old, a simple case in the out-patient department

Date of initial examination: August 31, 1974

Major complaints: A coffee-colored secretion from her nipples for more than one year

Present case history: Beginning in the previous October, [the patient] had had premenstrual breast distention and pain. On one side there was a constant flow of a coffee-colored, bloody secretion from the nipple. Previous pathological examination had excluded cancer. The diagnosis was chronic fibrous hyperplastic breast disease. The stools were sometimes watery and there was profuse leukorrhea which was yellow in color and had a flavor [*i.e.*, an odor].

Tongue image: A dark red tongue body with thin, white tongue fur

Pulse image: Fine and slippery

Western medical diagnosis: Chronic fibrous hyperplastic breast disease

Chinese medical pattern discrimination: Blood heat mixed with dampness, heat damaging the breast network vessels

Treatment methods: Clear heat and disinhibit dampness assisted by cooling the blood

Formula & medicinals: Rhizoma Imperatae Cylindricae (*Bai Mao Gen*), 1.5 *liang*, Nodus Rhizomatis Nelumbinis Nuciferae (*Ou Jie*), 1.5 *liang*, Cortex Radicis Moutan (*Dan Pi*), 3 *qian*, carbonized Radix Et Rhizoma Rhei (*Chuan Jun*), 1 *qian*, Rhizoma Coptidis Chinensis (*Huang Lian*), 1.5 *qian*, Radix Scutellariae Baicalensis (*Huang Qin*), 3 *qian*, Herba Dianthi (*Qu Mai*), 4 *qian*, Herba Polygoni Avicularis (*Bian Xu*), 4 *qian*, Semen Plantaginis (*Che Qian Zi*), 3 *qian*, Sclerotium Poriae Cocos (*Fu Ling*), 3 *qian*

Course of treatment: On September 13, after taking six *ji* of the above formula, the coffee-colored secretion flowing from the nipple had already stopped and the premenstrual symptoms had taken a turn for the better. Administration of the above formula was continued in order to secure the treatment effect.

Case 3: Zhang, female, 26 years old, a simple case in the out-patient department

Date of initial examination: July 4, 1972

Major complaints: Yellow water flowing from the nipples for half a year already

Present case history: For the last half year, there had been premenstrual breast distention and pain. On one side, yellow water constantly flowed from the nipple. This was accompanied by shortness of breath, bodily lassitude, lack of strength, diminished intake of food, and loose stools. Prior pathological examination had shown no cancer cells.

Tongue image: A dark yet pale tongue body with teeth prints [along its edges]

Pulse image: Fine and slippery

Western medical diagnosis: Chronic fibrous hyperplastic breast disease

Chinese medical pattern discrimination: Spleen vacuity with damp exuberance, liver depression not soothed [alternate reading: liver depression and discomfort]

Treatment methods: Fortify the spleen and soothe the liver, boost the qi and eliminate dampness

Formula & medicinals: Sclerotium Poriae Cocos (*Fu Ling*), 3 *qian*, Rhizoma Atractylodis Macrocephalae (*Bai Zhu*), 5 *qian*, Herba Seu Flos Schizonepetae Tenuifoliae (*Jing Jie Sui*), 1.5 *qian*, Radix Bupleuri (*Chai Hu*), 1.5 *qian*, Radix Dioscoreae Oppositae (*Shan Yao*), 5 *qian*, Radix Codonopsitis Pilosulae (*Dang Shen*), 5 *qian*, Semen Euryalis Ferocis (*Qian Shi*), 8 *qian*, Semen Gingkonis Bilobae (*Bai Guo*), 3 *qian*, Fructus Amomi (*Sha Ren*), 2 *qian*

Course of treatment: On July 10, after taking six *ji* of the above formula, there already was no yellow water flowing from the nipple and all the symptoms were decreased. Administration of the above formula was continued in order to secure the treatment effect.

Commentary: The main symptoms in the above three cases were breast distention and pain, hard nodules, and the flowing of a bloody (or watery) secretion from the nipples. Case #1 was categorized as qi and blood insufficiency, liver depression and blood stagnation. Treatment was in order to boost the qi and nourish the blood, soothe the liver and transform stagnation. Within the formula, Dang Gui, Ligusticum Wallichium, and White Peony nourish the blood, quicken the blood, and transform stasis and stagnation. Uncooked Astragalus supplements the qi and boosts the spleen. Polygonatum nourishes yin. When combined with Astragalus and Dang Gui, these supplement both the qi and blood. Peony combined with Licorice relaxes tension and stops pain. As for Polygala, it is usually used in clinical practice to quiet the spirit and boost the intelligence. In the *Ben Cao Zheng Yi (Correct Meaning of the Materia Medica)*, it is recorded that when it "is used for cold congelation and stagnation and damp phlegm entering the network vessels giving rise to symptoms of welling abscesses and swelling, its effect is most rapid." In the *Ben Cao Cong Xin (Newly Compiled Materia Medica)* it says it is "good at sweeping [away] phlegm."

Old Doctor Liu's experience is that the combination of the three [medicinals of] Astragalus, Polygonatum, and Polygala has the action of boosting the qi and supplementing the spleen, soothing depression, transforming phlegm, and scattering binding [or nodulation]. He used [this combination] to treat breast lumps categorized as qi and blood vacuity with cold congelation and qi stagnation, phlegm pits gathering and binding with relatively good effect. If aching and pain is relatively heavy, one can add Radix Bupleuri (*Chai Hu*). If there is depressive heat, one can add Spica Prunellae Vulgaris (*Xia Ku Cao*).

In case #2, besides breast distention and pain, there was a bloody secretion from the nipple and simultaneous diarrhea and profuse yellow vaginal discharge, all damp heat signs and symptoms. Damp heat had damaged the breast network vessels and forced blood to exit. Therefore, the methods were to clear heat, disinhibit dampness, and cool the blood. Within the formula, Scutellaria clears liver heat, while Coptis clears stomach heat. Imperata, Nodus Nelumbinis, and Moutan clear heat from the blood in order to stop bleeding. Rhubarb clears heat and transforms stasis. When stir-fried and carbonized, it is also able to stop bleeding. Scutellaria, Coptis, and Rhubarb form *San Huang Tang* (Three Yellows Decoction). The ancient medical expert, Tang Rong-chuan, used *San Huang Tang* to treat *yang ming* bleeding by making full use of its action of clearing *yang ming* heat and stopping bleeding. Dianthus, Polygonum Avicularis, and Plantago clear heat and disinhibit dampness. Poria blandly seeps and disinhibits dampness. After [taking] these medicinals, damp heat in the blood division was cleared and the blood movement returned to the channels. Thus the bloody secretion from the nipple automatically stopped.

In case #3, the main symptom was yellow water flowing from the nipple. There was also premenstrual breast distention and pain. In combination with the other symptoms, such as bodily lassitude, lack of strength, shortness of breath, scanty intake, and loose stools, these were categorized as spleen vacuity with damp exuberance, liver depression not soothed. Treatment was by the methods of supplementing the qi and fortifying the spleen, eliminating dampness and soothing depression,

271

using *Wan Dai Tang* (End Vaginal Discharge Decoction) with additions and subtractions.

Within this formula, Codonopsis and Dioscorea supplement the spleen. Poria and Atractylodes fortify the spleen and eliminate dampness. Amomum arouses the spleen and opens the stomach. Bupleurum and Schizonepeta upbear yang and eliminate dampness at the same time as soothing the liver and resolving depression. Euryales and Gingko restrain, constrain, secure, and astringe. In this case, although yellow water flowing from the nipple was the main symptom and not leukorrhea, it matches the indications of *Wan Dai Tang* in terms of disease causes and pathophysiology. Both of these [*i.e.,* the yellow water flowing from the nipples and vaginal discharge] may be categorized as spleen vacuity and damp exuberance, liver depression not soothed.

After [taking the prescribed] medicinals, the treatment effect was obtained [in all these cases]. In terms of the above three cases, they were all categorized as a single disease in Western medicine. However, the main symptoms they manifest were not the same. In Chinese medicine, their patterns were, [therefore,] differently discriminated. [However,] by using different formulas and methods, the same treatment effect was achieved. This fully illustrates that the same disease may be treated differently. [34]

---

[34] This is an allusion to one of the most important statements in Traditional Chinese Medicine (TCM) as a specific style of medicine. The statement is, "Same disease, different treatments; different diseases, same treatment." The implication of this statement is that different *patterns* of a single disease will receive different treatments, while different named diseases which exhibit the same *patterns* will receive the same treatment. This means that, in TCM as a specific style of medicine, treatment is primarily based on pattern discrimination, not on disease diagnosis. As the reader will recognize, this is a point that Old Doctor Liu or his students reiterate a number of times in this book.

Climacteric Syndrome: Four Cases

Climacteric syndrome [a.k.a. perimenopausal syndrome], excluding menstrual abnormalities (such as frequent menstruation, sparse menstruation, menstruation [sometimes] early, [sometimes] late, [coming at] no fixed schedule, and flooding and leaking) has varying degrees of generalized symptoms, such as dizziness, headache, heart palpitations, heart vexation and easy anger, vexatious heat in the five hearts, tidal heat and agitated sweating [*i.e.*, hot flashes], insomnia with profuse dreams, lumbar soreness and lower leg flaccidity, edema, loose stools, lassitude, fatigue, and lack of strength, etc., etc. The above-mentioned symptoms usually appear irregularly [meaning not every woman has all of these or any of them all the time] and they may last 2-3 years. "The Treatise on Former Ancient Heavenly Simplicity" in the *Su Wen (Simple Questions)* says, "At seven [times] seven the *ren mai* is vacuous, the *tai chong mai* is declining and scanty, and the *tian gui* is exhausted." This clearly says that approximately 49 years of age in women is correctly a period of transition when the *chong* and *ren* vessel function gradually declines and organic body's yin and yang balance loses its regulation.

Old Doctor Liu held that this disease can be divided into the two patterns of yin vacuity with liver effulgence and spleen-kidney insufficiency. The former is usually vacuity within which is mixed repletion. The latter is a pure vacuity pattern. The yin vacuity with liver effulgence pattern is relatively more frequently seen and mainly manifests as dizziness, headache, heart vexation, tension and agitation, chest fullness, rib-side distention, profuse dreams, scanty sleep, a dry mouth, heat in the hands, feet, and heart [alternate reading: heat in the centers of the hands and feet], tinnitus, heart palpitations, tidal heat and sweating (if severe, high blood pressure), a red tongue tip, and a bowstring, fine, rapid pulse. Treatment of the above mostly uses the methods of enriching yin and leveling [or calming] the liver, for which [Dr. Liu] commonly used the experiential formula, *Qing Xuan Ping Gan Tang* (Clear Vertigo & Level the Liver Decoction).

The spleen-kidney insufficiency pattern mostly manifests as menstruation [sometimes] early, [sometimes] late, [coming at] no fixed schedule, sometimes profuse and sometimes scanty menstruation, possible dribbling and dripping without stop or no movement for several months, dizziness, vertigo, lumbar pain, cold limbs, scanty intake, lack of strength, a bland [taste in the] mouth, edema, loose stools, copious night-time urination, a pale tongue body with thin, white fur, and a deep, fine, forceless pulse. Treatment of the above mostly uses the methods of fortifying the spleen and supplementing the kidneys, for which [Dr. Liu] commonly used the following formula and medicinals: Radix Dioscoreae Oppositae (*Shan Yao*), Semen Nelumbinis Nuciferae (*Lian Zi*), Semen Cuscutae Chinensis (*Tu Si Zi*), Radix Dipsaci (*Chuan Duan*), cooked Radix Rehmanniae (*Shu Di*), Fructus Rubi Chingii (*Fu Pen Zi*), Rhizoma Atractylodis Macrocephalae (*Bai Zhu*), Sclerotium Poriae Cocos (*Fu Ling*), Herba Epimedii (*Xian Ling Pi*), Rhizoma Curculiginis Orchioidis (*Xian Mao*), etc.

If spleen vacuity is more marked, besides the above mentioned symptoms, whole body edema and menstrual dribbling and dripping without cease will be seen. [In that case,] one may use *Gui Pi Tang* (Restore the Spleen Decoction) plus Radix Ledebouriellae Divaricatae (*Fang Feng*) and Radix Et Rhizoma Notopterygii (*Qiang Hao*). If there is great flooding and leaking [*i.e.*, heavy uterine bleeding], one may add Radix Astragali Membranacei (*Huang Qi*), carbonized Fibra Stipulae Trachycarpi (*Zong Lu*), carbonized Cacumen Biotae Orientalis (*Ce Bai*), and Gelatinum Corii Asini (*E Jiao*). If the menstruation is blocked and stopped or delayed by [many] days with manifestations of vexation, tension, agitation, and sweating, a red tongue, and a bowstring, slippery pulse, one may use the experiential formula, *Gua Shi Tang* (Trichosanthes & Dendrobium Decoction), to treat this.

Case 1: Shu, female, 48 years old, a simple case in the out-patient department

Date of initial examination: March 22, 1972

Major complaints: Dizziness and headache for half a year

Present case history: Each menstrual period, [the patient] had dizziness and headache [so bad] she could not stand up, nausea, thoughts for chilled drinks, stomach venter distention and oppression, dry stools, and yellow urine. Her menstrual cycle was normal. Her blood pressure was 170/100mmHg.

Tongue image: Dark red

Pulse image: Bowstring and relaxed

Western medical diagnosis: Climacteric syndrome

Chinese medical pattern discrimination: Yin vacuity and liver effulgence

Treatment methods: Nourish yin, clear heat, and level [or calm] the liver

Formula & medicinals: Folium Mori Albi (*Sang Ye*), 3 *qian*, Flos Chrysanthemi Morifolii (*Ju Hua*), 3 *qian*, Radix Scutellariae Baicalensis (*Huang Qin*), 3 *qian*, Fructus Ligustri Lucidi (*Nu Zhen Zi*), 3 *qian*, Herba Ecliptae Prostratae (*Han Lian Cao*), 3 *qian*, Tuber Ophiopogonis Japonici (*Mai Dong*), 3 *qian*, uncooked Radix Rehmanniae (*Sheng Di*), 3 *qian*, Radix Albus Paeoniae Lactiflorae (*Bai Shao*), 3 *qian*, Radix Achyranthis Bidentatae (*Niu Xi*), 4 *qian*, Fructus Trichosanthis Kirlowii (*Gua Lou*), 1 *liang*

Course of treatment: On Mar. 27, after taking three *ji* of the above formula, the menses moved and the above-mentioned symptoms disappeared. The blood pressure was 132/80mmHg. Administration of [another] three *ji* was continued in order to secure the treatment effect.

Case 2: Cao, female, 49 years old, a simple case in the out-patient department

Date of initial examination: March 22, 1974

Major complaints: Dizziness, head distention, heart vexation, agitation, and perspiration for more than two years

Present case history: For the last two years, whenever her menses came, she had dizziness, head distention, heart fluster [*i.e.*, palpitations], shortness of breath, heart vexation, agitation, and perspiration, and numbness of her right upper extremities. This was accompanied by menstruation ahead of schedule which was profuse in amount, red in color, and contained large blood clots. Examination [showed] her blood pressure was 180/120mmHg. Internal examination [revealed] that her uterus was as large as an eight week pregnancy.

Tongue image: Dark red

Pulse image: Bowstring and slippery

Western medical diagnosis: A) Climacteric syndrome; B) uterine myoma

Chinese medical pattern discrimination: Yin vacuity and liver effulgence, brewing heat in the blood division

Treatment methods: Nourish yin and clear heat, cool the blood and level [or calm] the liver

Formula & medicinals: Folium Mori Albi (*Sang Ye*), 3 *qian*, Flos Chrysanthemi Morifolii (*Ju Hua*), 3 *qian*, Radix Scutellariae Baicalensis (*Huang Qin*), 3 *qian*, uncooked Radix Rehmanniae (*Sheng Di*), 4 *qian*, Radix Albus Paeoniae Lactiflorae (*Bai Shao*), 4 *qian*, Tuber Ophiopogonis Japonici (*Mai Dong*), 3 *qian*, Fructus Ligustri Lucidi (*Nu Zhen Zi*), 3 *qian*, Herba Ecliptae Prostratae (*Han Lian Cao*), 3 *qian*, uncooked Concha Ostreae (*Mu Li*), 1 *liang*, uncooked Dens Draconis (*Long Chi*), 1 *liang*, Gelatinum Corii Asini (*E Jiao*), 5 *qian*

Course of treatment: On April 19, 1974, after taking over 20 *ji* of the above formula, the symptoms had taken a turn for the better. The menstrual period was 3-4 days early. The volume of blood was decreased by one third. Blood pressure was 160/90mmHg. [Dr. Liu] advised [the patient] to add *Qin Xin Wan* (Scutellaria Heart Pills), 3 *qian*, each day, in order to secure the treatment effects.

Case 3: Fu, female, 48 years old, a simple case in the out-patient department

Date of initial examination: April 3, 1974

Major complaints: Dizziness and head distention with early menstruation for two years already

Present case history: In the last two years, [the patient] had been having headache and head distention, heart vexation, tension and agitation, and lower leg flaccidity. Her menstruation was early, moving two times each month. After becoming overtaxed, her menses movement endured for days, sometimes for as long as 18 days. Her last menstruation had occurred on March 15. She habitually had profuse leukorrhea. Her blood pressure was 170-160/110-100mmHg. Her hematochrome was 9.2g.

Tongue image: Dark red

Pulse image: Bowstring and slippery

Western medical diagnosis: Climacteric syndrome

Chinese medical pattern discrimination: Yin vacuity and liver effulgence

Treatment methods: Nourish yin, clear heat, and level [or calm] the liver

Formula & medicinals: Folium Mori Albi (*Sang Ye*), 3 *qian*, Flos Chrysanthemi Morifolii (*Ju Hua*), 3 *qian*, Radix Scutellariae Baicalensis (*Huang Qin*), 3 *qian*, Radix Angelicae Sinensis (*Dang Gui*), 1.5 *qian*, Radix Ligustici Wallichii (*Chuan Xiong*), 1.5 *qian*, cooked Radix Rehmanniae (*Shu Di*), 4 *qian*, Tuber Asparagi Cochinensis (*Tian Men Dong*) and Tuber Ophiopogonis Japonici (*Mai Men Dong*), 3 *qian* each, Herba Dianthi (*Qu Mai*), 4 *qian*, Rhizoma Dioscoreae Hypoglaucae (*Bi Xie*), 4 *qian*, Semen Plantaginis (*Che Qian Zi*), 3 *qian*

Course of treatment: On April 10, after taking seven *ji* of these medicinals, all symptoms were decreased. The menstruation came like a tide on April 21 (6 days late). The menstruation moved for seven days, and its volume was slightly decreased. [Therefore, Dr. Liu] removed the Plantago, Dianthus, and Dioscorea Hypoglauca and added Cortex Cedrelae (*Chun Gen Bai Pi*) and calcined Concha Ostreae (*Mu Li*) to the above formula.

On April 24 ,after taking 14 *ji* of the above formula, the dizziness had disappeared and the swelling in the lower legs had decreased. The leukorrhea was diminished and re-examination of the hematochrome was 10g. Administration of the above formula was continued to increase and strengthen the power of supplementing yin blood. The formula and medicinals were as follows: Radix Angelicae Sinensis (*Dang Gui*), 3 *qian*, uncooked Radix Rehmanniae (*Sheng Di*), 4 *qian*, Radix Albus Paeoniae

Lactiflorae (*Bai Shao*), 5 *qian*, Radix Ligustici Wallichii (*Chuan Xiong*), 1.5 *qian*, Fructus Ligustri Lucidi (*Nu Zhen Zi*), 4 *qian*, Herba Ecliptae Prostratae (*Han Lian Cao*), 3 *qian*, Cortex Cedrelae (*Chun Gen Bai Pi*), 3 *qian*, and calcined Concha Ostreae (*Mu Li*), 1 *liang*.

On May 20, after taking 26 *ji* of the above formula, re-examination of the hematochrome was 11g. The blood pressure was 130-110/90mmHg. The lower limbs were slightly swollen. [Dr. Liu] advised [the patient] to add *Qin Xin Wan* (Scutellaria Heart Pills), 3 *qian* per day, in order to secure the treatment effect.

Commentary: The previous cases were all categorized as yin vacuity with liver effulgence. All had dizziness, headache, and high blood pressure. And all were treated with the methods and principles of nourishing yin, clearing heat, and leveling the liver. However, because their symptoms were not the same, additions and subtractions of the medicinals used were also not the same.

In case #1, besides the menstrual period dizziness, headache, high blood pressure, dark red tongue, and bowstring, relaxed pulse, there was simultaneous nausea, venter [*i.e.*, epigastric] oppression, thought for chilled drinks, dry stools, and yellow urine. These clearly indicated internal brewing of heat. Therefore, besides using nourishing yin, clearing heat, and leveling the liver medicinal substances, [Dr. Liu] added Trichosanthes to harmonize the stomach and broaden the center, clear heat and moisten the stools.

In case #2, there was simultaneously seen heart fluster, shortness of breath, heart vexation, agitation and perspiration, and other such heart yin insufficiency symptoms. The menstruation ahead of schedule which was profuse in amount and fresh red in color and which contained large blood clots were symptoms of yin vacuity with blood heat. At the time of treatment, [Dr. Liu, therefore,] added uncooked Dragon's Teeth and Oyster Shell to settle the liver and quiet the spirit. He also removed

Achyranthes and added Donkey Skin Glue. Combined with Oyster Shell, these nourish yin, cool the blood, and stop bleeding.

In case #3, there was simultaneously seen profuse leukorrhea, lower leg flaccidity, menstrual movement which endured for days, and other such signs of damp heat. In treating the above, at the same time as nourishing yin, clearing heat, and leveling the liver, [Dr. Liu] added Asparagus and Ophiopogon to nourish heart yin and Dianthus, Dioscorea Hypoglauca, and Plantago to clear heat and disinhibit dampness. Afterwards, he also added Cedrela and calcined Oyster Shell in order to secure and astringe the *chong* and *ren*.

Case 4: Zhu, female, 46 years old

Date of initial examination: March 13, 1974

Major complaints: Whole body edema and pain for one year

Present case history: In the last year, before and after menstruation, there was whole body [*i.e.*, generalized] edema, lack of strength, and body pain. Her menstruation was ahead of schedule, its amount was profuse, and its color was pale. There was insomnia, profuse dreams, chest oppression, shortness of breath, heart fluster, heart jumping, no flavor for food taken in, and dry stools.

Tongue image: A pale tongue body with slimy, white fur

Pulse image: Slippery and slightly rapid, forceless when taken deep[35]

---

[35] If a pulse becomes weaker with the application of heavier pressure, this is a floating pulse. In this case, due to blood vacuity and dampness spilling over into the space between the muscles and skin, the pulse is floating, not the deep, forceless pulse most textbooks give for spleen-kidney yang vacuity. This is an important point underscoring the difference between textbook signs and symptoms and real-life cases whose patterns are typically mixed and, therefore, whose symptoms are also modified.

Western medical diagnosis: Climacteric syndrome

Chinese medical pattern discrimination: Spleen-kidney insufficiency, blood vacuity and damp obstruction

Treatment methods: Supplement the qi and nourish the blood, fortify the spleen and eliminate dampness

Formula & medicinals: Radix Astragali Membranacei (*Huang Qi*), 5 *qian*, Radix Angelicae Sinensis (*Dang Gui*), 3 *qian*, Rhizoma Atractylodis Macrocephalae (*Bai Zhu*), 4 *qian*, Sclerotium Poriae Cocos (*Fu Ling*), 4 *qian*, Arillus Euphoriae Longanae (*Gui Yuan Rou*), 5 *qian*, Radix Polygalae Tenuifoliae (*Yuan Zhi*), 3 *qian*, Radix Et Rhizoma Notopterygii (*Qiang Huo*), 1.5 *qian*, Radix Ledebouriellae Divaricatae (*Fang Feng*), 1.5 *qian*, stir-fried Semen Zizyphi Spinosae (*Zao Ren*), 3 *qian*

Course of treatment: On March 26, after taking three *ji* of the above medicinals, the edema was decreased and the heart fluster, shortness of breath, and other symptoms were seen to be slight. Still, [however,] the stools were dry. [Therefore,] the above formula was assisted by warming the kidneys and moistening dryness prescriptions [*i.e.*, medicinals]. The formula and medicinals were as follows: Radix Astragali Membranacei (*Huang Qi*), 5 *qian*, Radix Angelicae Sinensis (*Dang Gui*), 3 *qian*, Rhizoma Atractylodis Macrocephalae (*Bai Zhu*), 4 *qian*, Sclerotium Poriae Cocos (*Fu Ling*), 4 *qian*, Arillus Euphoriae Longanae (*Gui Yuan Rou*), 5 *qian*, Radix Polygalae Tenuifoliae (*Yuan Zhi*), 3 *qian*, Herba Cistanchis Deserticolae (*Rou Cong Rong*), 5 *qian*, Semen Cannabis Sativae (*Huo Ma Ren*), 2 *qian*, and Caulis Milettiae Seu Spatholobi (*Ji Xue Teng*), 1 *liang*.

After taking a total of 13 *ji* of these medicinals, all the symptoms had taken a turn for the better. On April 14, the menses came. Their color was normal and their amount was slightly less than the previous time.

The edema and lack of strength had already disappeared. [Thus] all the symptoms had improved.

Commentary: This case was different from the previous three cases. It was categorized as spleen-kidney insufficiency, the spleen not moving and transforming water dampness. Before and after the menstrual period, [the patient] had whole body edema, lack of strength, and body pain due to spleen yang vacuity not able to warm and transform water dampness. This then resulted in damp qi obstructing the channels and network vessels. Because the spleen was not fortified and moving, intake of food was without flavor and the stools were dry. Because the spleen was not restraining the blood and the *chong* and *ren* were insecure [or not securing], menstruation was ahead of schedule. Its pale color and profuse amount as well as the chest oppression, shortness of breath, heart palpitations, night-time sleep not quiet, pale tongue with slimy, white fur, and a slippery, slightly rapid, forceless pulse were all categorized as signs of heart blood insufficiency, qi and blood dual debility, and damp evils obstructing the network vessels. Treatment was mainly with the formula *Gui Pi Tang* (Restore the Spleen Decoction) [with] Cistanches and Cannabis to warm yang and moisten dryness. Taken as a whole, this formula supplements the qi and nourishes the blood, warms the channels and eliminates dampness, thus treating the root.

BOOK THREE
EXPERIENTIAL FORMULAS

Below are 16 experiential formulas commonly used by Old Doctor Liu. Each is accompanied by the formula's composition, functions, and indications as well as comments taken from the source text. These comments are only a synopsis of the most important points made in the source text and are not a translation per se.

An Chong Tiao Jing Tang
(Quiet the *Chong* & Regulate Menstruation Decoction)

Composition: Radix Dioscoreae Oppositae (*Shan Yao*), 5 *qian*, Rhizoma Atractylodis Macrocephalae (*Bai Zhu*), 3 *qian*, mix-fried Radix Glycyrrhizae (*Gan Cao*), 2 *qian*, Semen Nelumbinis Nuciferae (*Shi Lian*), 3 *qian*, Radix Dipsaci (*Chuan Xu Duan*), 3 *qian*, cooked Radix Rehmanniae (*Shu Di*), 4 *qian*, Cortex Cedrelae (*Chun Gen Bai Pi*), 3 *qian*, uncooked Concha Ostreae (*Mu Li*), 1 *liang*, Os Sepiae Seu Sepiellae (*Wu Zei Gu*), 4 *qian*

Functions: Evenly supplements the spleen and kidneys, regulates menstruation and secures the *chong*

Main indications: Spleen-kidney insufficiency mixed with vacuity heat resulting in the arising of menstruation ahead of schedule, menstruation arriving [too] frequently, or light degree uterine bleeding

Commentary: Menstruation ahead of schedule, menstruation arriving [too] frequently, and light degree uterine bleeding may all be divided into vacuity and repletion. For the vacuity pattern, typically one mostly uses Radix Panacis Ginseng (*Ren Shen*) and Radix Astragali

Membranacei (*Huang Qi*) to supplement the spleen and Cortex Cinnamomi Cassiae (*Rou Gui*), Radix Lateralis Praeparatus Aconiti Carmichaeli (*Fu Zi*), Cornu Cervi Parvum (*Lu Rong*), and Gelatinum Cornu Cervi (*Lu Jiao*) to supplement the kidneys. And this is suitable when treating pure vacuity patterns. However, it is Old Doctor Liu's clinical experience that, in most patients, this disease is categorized as vacuity within which is mixed repletion. Especially in adolescent girls, amongst the vacuity signs are mixed heat signs. For instance, although there may be spleen-kidney insufficiency symptoms such as a fine pulse, a sallow yellow facial complexion, lassitude and fatigue, and lack of strength in the four limbs, there may also be a black colored menstruate containing clots.

In such cases, if one recklessly uses Ginseng, Astragalus, Cinnamon, and Aconite, this will lead to heat being boosted and blazing internally and the menstruation will come even earlier and the volume of the blood will be increased. On the other hand, if, seeing such heat signs, one overuses bitter, cold medicinals such as Radix Scutellariae Baicalensis (*Huang Qin*) and Rhizoma Coptidis (*Huang Lian*), this may damage the righteous and make the spleen and kidneys even more vacuous. Hence, in this type of condition, one cannot use too much warm supplementation nor use too much bitter and cold.

This formula is mainly composed of three groups of medicinals—those that supplement the spleen, those that supplement the kidneys, and those that clear heat, secure and astringe. Dioscorea, Atractylodes, and mix-fried Licorice supplement the spleen. Dipsacus and cooked Rehmannia supplement the kidneys. And Semen Nelumbinis, Cedrela, uncooked Oyster Shell, and Cuttlefish Bone clear heat, secure and astringe. Thus this formula evenly supplements the spleen and the kidneys, yet is supplementing without being drying. It clears heat, secures and astringes, yet it also does not damage the righteous.

In sum, this formula evenly supplements the spleen and kidneys. If the spleen qi is full, it is able to restrain the blood. If the kidney qi is sufficient, it is able to close and treasure. In addition, it clears heat, constrains and astringes, clearing and supplementing simultaneously and treating root and branch at the same time. When qi and blood are regulated and harmonized, the menstrual water is automatically quieted. Therefore, [Dr. Liu] fixed its name as Quiet the *Chong* & Regulate Menstruation Decoction.

Gua Shi Tang
(Trichosanthes & Dendrobium Decoction)

Composition: Fructus Trichosanthis Kirlowii (*Gua Lou*), 5 *qian*, Herba Dendrobii (*Shi Hu*), 4 *qian*, Radix Scrophulariae Ningpoensis (*Xuan Shen*), 3 *qian*, Tuber Ophiopogonis Japonici (*Mai Dong*), 3 *qian*, uncooked Radix Rehmanniae (*Sheng Di*), 4 *qian*, Herba Dianthi (*Qu Mai*), 4 *qian*, Semen Plantaginis (*Che Qian Zi*), 3 *qian*, Herba Leonuri Heterophylli (*Yi Mu Cao*), 4 *qian*, Rhizoma Thalictri Foliosi (*Ma Wei Lian*), 2 *qian*, Radix Achyranthis Bidentatae (*Niu Xi*), 4 *qian*

Functions: Enriches yin and clears heat, loosens the chest and harmonizes the stomach, quickens the blood and frees the flow of the channels [or menses]

Main indications: Yin vacuity and stomach heat leading to the arising of sparse emission of menstruation, delayed menstruation, and blood dried up blocked menstruation

Commentary: This formula mainly treats stomach heat which has burned and damaged fluids and humors and thus led to sparse emission of menstruation [*i.e.*, infrequent menstruation], delayed menstruation, and essence blood desiccation and exhaustion blocked menstruation [*i.e.*, amenorrhea]. Typically, in this type of patient, there is habitual overexuberance of yang qi with liver heat counterflowing upward. This results in dry heat striking the stomach which then burns and damages fluids and humors. Because the *yang ming* channel should have a lot of qi and a lot of blood and because it is subordinate to the two vessels of the *chong* and *ren* below, as long as *yang ming* fluids are full and repelete, the *chong* and *ren* essence and blood are full and exuberant and the menstruation is able to descend periodically [alternate reading: be precipitated on time]. If dry heat in the *yang ming* is excessively exuberant and fluids and humors become desiccated and exhausted, they are not able to be transformed into the menstruate. If light, there will be sparse emission of menstruation and delayed menstruation. If heavy, there will be blocked menstruation which does not arrive for years.

In terms of the main points in clinical practice, there is blocked menstruation, but there are no signs of qi and blood dual vacuity. Contrarily, what one sees is a dry mouth, dry tongue, heart and chest vexation and oppression, tension and agitation, and profuse dreams. If severe, there is heat emitted from the center of the chest and vexatious heat in the five hearts. The pulse is bowstring, slippery, deep, and forceless or slippery and rapid, all signs of yin vacuity and blood dryness.

The ancients used *San He Tang* (Three [Formulas] Combined Decoction, *i.e., Si Wu Tang,* Four Materials Decoction, *Tiao Wei Cheng Qi Tang,* Regulate the Stomach & Order the Qi Decoction, and *Liang Ge San,* Cool the Diaphragm Powder) to treat this disease. However, Old Doctor Liu noticed that patients with this condition do not necessarily have dry stools. Since this disease is a chronic one, many *ji* are usually necessary in order to treat it. If *San He Tang* is used for a long period of time, the Radix Et Rhizoma Rhei (*Da Huang*) and Mirabilitum (*Yuan Ming Fen*), which are bitter, cold, draining, and precipitating ingredients, may easily consume and damage fluids and humors.

Instead, the main ingredients in this formula are Trichosanthes and Dendrobium. Trichosanthes is sweet and cold and moistens dryness, loosens the chest and disinhibits the qi. Dendrobium is sweet and bland and slightly cold. It boosts the stomach and engenders fluids, enriches yin and eliminates heat. Together, they have the effect of loosening the chest and moistening the intestines, disinhibiting the qi and harmonizing the stomach. In addition, Scrophularia and Ophiopogon nourish yin and increase fluids. Since the origin of this disease is yin vacuity and blood dryness, uncooked Rehmannia is used from *Si Wu Tang* (Four Materials Decoction) in order to enrich yin and engender the blood. Radix Angelicae Sinensis (*Dang Gui*) and Radix Ligustici Wallichii (*Chuan Xiong*) are omitted because they are warm and drying. Dianthus and Plantago quicken the blood and free the flow of the channels [or menses]. Leonurus, which tends to be cold, frees the menses and quickens the blood but is also able to engender fluids and humors. Thalactrum (or Fructus Gardeniae Jasminoidis, *Zhi Zi*) clears stomach heat. When heat is removed, the fluids and humors are able to be engendered. Achyranthes leads the blood to move downward, with an aim to making the menstrual blood arrive.

In sum, this formula as a whole enriches yin and clears heat, loosens the chest and harmonizes the stomach at the same time as it quickens the blood and frees the flow of the menses. Because the nature of these medicinals is level and harmonious, they can be given for a long period. In clinical practice, if dry, bound stools are seen, then one can use *San He Tang*. If *yang ming* dry repletion has already been resolved, then one can still use this formula in order to afterwards continue treatment.

Si Er Wu He Tang
(Four, Two, Five Combined Decoction)

Composition: Radix Angelicae Sinensis (*Dang Gui*), 3 *qian*, Radix Albus Paeoniae Lactiflorae (*Bai Shao*), 3 *qian*, Radix Ligustici Wallichii (*Chuan*

Xiong), 1 *qian*, cooked Radix Rehmanniae (*Shu Di*), 4 *qian*, Fructus Rubi Chingii (*Fu Pen Zi*), 3 *qian*, Semen Cuscutae Chinensis (*Tu Si Zi*), 3 *qian*, Fructus Schisandrae Chinensis (*Wu Wei Zi*), 3 *qian*, Semen Plantaginis (*Che Qian Zi*), 3 *qian*, Radix Achyranthis Bidentatae (*Niu Xi*), 4 *qian*, Fructus Lycii Chinensis (*Gou Qi Zi*), 5 *qian*, Rhizoma Curculiginis Orchioidis (*Xian Mao*), 3 *qian*, Herba Epimedii (*Xian Ling Pi*), 4 *qian*

Functions: Nourishes the blood and boosts yin, supplements the kidneys and engenders essence

Main indications: Blood vacuity and kidney debility leading to the arising of blocked menstruation or Sheehan's syndrome

Commentary: This formula treats blood vacuity and kidney debility leading to the arising of blocked menstruation or great bleeding postpartum leading to the arising of Sheehan's syndrome. In patients with this type of disease, the manifestations are essence spirit listlessness, shedding of axillary and pubic hair, atrophy of the reproductive organs, blocked menstruation, decreased sexual desire, scanty vaginal tract secretions, breast atrophy, and other such symptoms. In terms of their Chinese medical characteristics, these symptoms all arise because of great postpartum bleeding damaging the kidneys and damaging the blood. Because the kidneys store the essence, they govern growth, development [*i.e.*, maturation], and the function of reproduction. If the kidney qi is vacuous then the hair is shed and sexual desire is decreased. If kidney yin is vacuous, then kidney essence will be decreased and scanty. Thus the menses become blocked and stop and vaginal tract secretions are decreased and scanty. If the kidneys are vacuous, the governing vessel will be empty and vacuous and [thus] not able to moisten and nourish the brain marrow. Therefore, the power of memory is diminished and there is essence spirit listlessness.

This formula uses *Wu Zi Yan Zong Wan* (Five Seeds Increase Progeny Pills) to supplement the kidney qi. Within it, Cuscuta is bitter and level [*i.e.*, its temperature is even or neutral]. It supplements the kidneys and boosts the essence and marrow. Rubus is sweet and sour and slightly warm. It secures the kidneys and astringes essence. Lycium is sweet and sour and transforms yin. It is able to supplement kidney yin. Schisandra has all five flavors. [Therefore,] it enters the five viscera and greatly supplements the qi of the five viscera. Because it enters the kidneys, it also strengthens [this formula's] power to supplement the kidneys. Plantago's nature is cold and has the effect of descending, downbearing, and disinhibiting the portals. It is able to discharge turbidity from the kidneys, supplement kidney yin, and engender essence and fluids. The combination of Curculigo and Epimedium is in order to supplement the kidneys and strengthen yang. *Wu Zi* (Five Seeds) are combined with *Er Xian* (Two Immortals) with an aim to supplement kidney yang as well as supplement kidney yin. Supplementing kidney yang is able to beat the drum [*i.e.*, arouse] the kidney qi, while supplementing kidney yin is able to increase the essence and fluids. When kidney qi is full and replete, kidney essence is also plentiful and full. Thus the hair may grow and lengthen and vaginal tract secretions increase and are profuse. Sexual desire increases, and the menses return. [Dr. Liu's] clinical observation is that this promotes the function of the ovaries. When the kidney qi and essence and fluids are full and sufficient, the governing vessel is full and exuberant. [Therefore,] the brain marrow is moistened and nourished. When the brain is fortified, then the power of the memory increases and the power of the essence is full and abundant.

In addition, the combination of *Si Wu Tang* (Four Materials Decoction) has the effect of increasing the nourishing of blood and boosting of yin. Also adding Achyranthes enables the supplementing of the kidneys *and* freeing the flow of the channels [or menses]. The function of this formula is to supplement and not free the flow. When the kidney qi is full and the kidney essence is sufficient, then the menstrual water has a source and the menses automatically return.

If postpartum there is an extreme degree of qi and blood vacuity weakness, one may also add Radix Panacis Ginseng (*Ren Shen*) and Radix Astragali Membranacei (*Huang Qi*) in order to supplement the qi. This is then called *Shen Qi Si Er Wu He Fang* (Ginseng & Astragalus Four, Two Five Combined Formula). The method of supplementing the qi then increases and strengthens the effect of supplementing the blood, and thus the qi and blood are also able at the same time to strengthen the function of supplementing the kidneys.

Liang Xue Zhi Nu Tang
(Cool the Blood & Stop Spontaneous Ejection of Blood Decoction)

Composition: Radix Gentianae Scabrae (*Long Dan Cao*), 3 *qian*, Radix Scutellariae Baicalensis (*Huang Qin*), 3 *qian*, Fructus Gardeniae Jasminoidis (*Zhi Zi*), 3 *qian*, Cortex Radicis Moutan (*Dan Pi*), 3 *qian*, uncooked Radix Rehmanniae (*Sheng Di*), 5 *qian*, Nodus Rhizomatis Nelumbinis Nuciferae (*Ou Jie*), 1 *liang*, Rhizoma Imperatae Cylindricae (*Bai Mao Gen*), 1 *liang*, Radix Et Rhizoma Rhei (*Da Huang*), 5 *fen*, Radix Achyranthis Bidentatae (*Niu Xi*), 4 *qian*

Functions: Clears heat and levels [or calms] the liver,[36] cools the blood and downbears counterflow

Main indications: Liver heat upward counterflow with the blood following the qi upward, resulting in the arising of spontaneous ejection of blood [*i.e.*, nosebleed] and shifted menstruation

---

[36] Wiseman gives "calms the liver " for the Chinese, *ping gan*. Although this does mean to calm hyperactivity of the liver, the Chinese character also conveys a spatial sense as well. The character *ping* shows and means something level or flat. Therefore, leveling the liver not only means to calm liver hyperactivity but also to restrain yang from ascending upward. Therefore, we prefer to use the term level in order to retain the spatial implications of this treatment principle.

Commentary: One or two days before, during the menstrual period itself, or after menstruation, one may see spontaneous ejection of blood. If severe, there may be spitting [*i.e.*, vomiting] of blood. This is called shifted menstruation or counterflow movement menstruation. Mainly this is due to liver yang hyperactivity and exuberance with blood heat counterflowing upward. If liver yang is hyperactive and exuberant and the *chong* qi is comparatively exuberant, while the sea of blood is full and exuberant, heat may force the blood to follow the *chong* qi to counterflow upward and it is not able to obtain downward movement. Therefore, the amount of the menstruate may be scanty, the menstrual movement may not be smoothly flowing, or there may be blocked menstruation and no movement. Contrarily, there is spontaneous ejection of blood and spitting of blood.

[In that case,] Old Doctor Liu chose Gentiana, Scutellaria, and Gardenia, the ruling [or main] medicinals in *Long Dan Xie Gan Tang* (Gentiana Drain the Liver Decoction) for clearing upper burner heat. The combination of Moutan and uncooked Rehmannia clears heat and cools the blood. Nodus Nelumbinis and Imperata clear blood heat and stop spitting and spontaneous ejection of blood. In addition, he also used five *fen* of Rhubarb, not a large dose, to enter the blood division, move the blood, and break the blood. Rhubard not only drains heat from the blood but, when combined with Achyranthes, it is also able to move the blood downward, thus wonderously taking the firewood from under the cauldron. [Taken as] a whole, this formula clears heat and levels the liver, cools the blood and downbears counterflow. Not only may spitting and spontaneous ejection of blood stop, the menstrual blood becomes self-regulated.

Qing Xuan Ping Gan Tang
(Clear Vertigo & Level the Liver Decoction)

Composition: Radix Angelicae Sinensis (*Dang Gui*), 3 *qian*, Radix Ligustici Wallichii (*Chuan Xiong*), 1.5 *qian*, Radix Albus Paeoniae Lactiflorae (*Bai Shao*), 4 *qian*, uncooked Radix Rehmanniae (*Sheng Di*), 4 *qian*, Folium Mori Albi (*Sang Ye*), 3 *qian*, Flos Chrysanthemi Morifolii (*Ju Hua*), 3 *qian*, Radix Scutellariae Baicalensis (*Huang Qin*), 3 *qian*, Fructus Ligustri Lucidi (*Nu Zhen Zi*), 3 *qian*, Herba Ecliptae Prostratae (*Han Lian Cao*), 3 *qian*, Flos Carthami Tinctorii (*Hong Hua*), 3 *qian*, Radix Achyranthis Bidentatae (*Niu Xi*), 3 *qian*

Functions: Enriches yin and nourishes the liver, clears heat and levels the liver, quickens the blood and regulates menstruation

Main indications: Women's climacteric syndrome and premenstrual tension categorized as liver-kidney yin vacuity with liver yang hyperactivity and exuberance with dizziness, headache (possible high blood pressure), and vexation and agitation

Commentary: In climacteric syndrome and premenstrual tension one may often see headache, dizziness, vexation and tension and easy anger, sleep that is not replete, and all sorts of confused and chaotic dreams. If severe, there may be fullness and oppression within the chest, a red facial complexion, red ears, tidal heat, and sweating, with a bowstring, large, forceful pulse (one may also possibly see hypertension). In Chinese medicine, this pattern is mostly discriminated as liver-kidney yin vacuity with ascendant hyperactivity of liver yang. The fact that these symptoms usually occur during the climacteric or premenstrually is closely related to loss of regulation in the function of the *chong* and *ren*. They occur premenstrually because liver heat counterflows upward with blood following heat upward. It is also possible for internal binding of menstrual blood to boost liver yang more severely. Therefore, at the time of treatment, one should enrich and supplement kidney yin, clear heat and level the liver, nourish the blood, quicken the blood, and regulate menstruation.

Within this formula, Dang Gui, Ligusticum Wallichium, White Peony, uncooked Rehmannia, Carthamus, and Achyranthes nourish the blood and quicken the blood as well as lead the blood to move downward and thus regulate the menses. Ligustrum Lucidum and Eclipta enrich and supplement the liver and kidneys in order to bank the root. Scutellaria clears liver heat. Mulberry Leaves and Chrysanthemum Flowers clear heat and level the liver in order to treat the branch. If heat was heavy, [Dr. Liu] removed the Dang Gui and Ligusticum Wallichium and added Rhizoma Thalictri Foliosi (*Ma Wei Lian*), 3 *qian*. If there was liver yang hyperactivity, [Dr. Liu] added Dens Draconis (*Long Chi*), 1 *liang*. This formula addresses root and branch simultaneously. It supplements the kidneys but without making stagnation more. It clears liver heat without damaging the righteous. One of its special characteristics is the heavy amount of Achyranthes it uses in order to lead the blood to move downward combined with Scutellaria, Mulberry Leaves, and Chrysanthemum Flowers which clear above and lead downward. In clinical practice, [this formula] not only is able to improve the symptoms but, in those with high blood pressure, its effect of lowering the pressure is relatively pronounced.

Qing Gan Li Shi Tang
(Clear the Liver & Disinhibit Dampness Decoction)

Composition: Herba Dianthi (*Qu Mai*), 4 *qian*, Herba Polygoni Avicularis (*Bian Xu*), 4 *qian*, Caulis Akebiae Mutong (*Mu Tong*), 1 *qian*, Semen Plantaginis (*Che Qian Zi*), 3 *qian*, Radix Scutellariae Baicalensis (*Huang Qin*), 3 *qian*, Radix Achyranthis Bidentatae (*Niu Xi*), 3 *qian*, Cortex Radicis Moutan (*Dan Pi*), 3 *qian*, Fructus Meliae Toosendan (*Chuan Lian Zi*), 3 *qian*, Radix Bupleuri (*Chai Hu*), 1.5 *qian*, Herba Seu Flos Schizonepetae Tenuifoliae (*Jing Jie Sui*), 1.5 *qian*

Functions: Clears the liver and disinhibits dampness, upbears yang and eliminates dampness, quickens the blood and stops vaginal discharge

Main indications: Liver channel damp heat or heat entering the blood division leading to the arising of red and white vaginal discharge or midcycle bleeding, pelvic inflammation leading to the arising of uterine bleeding, or menstrual dribbling and dripping without stop

Commentary: For the treatment of red and white vaginal discharge, midcycle bleeding, and endometritis resulting in the arising of uterine bleeding, it is typically the custom to use *Wan Dai Tang* (End Vaginal Discharge Decoction) or *Qing Gan Zhi Lin Tang* (Clear the Liver & Stop Dribbling Decoction). *Wan Dai Tang* mainly treats white vaginal discharge due to yin cold mixed with dampness. It is, [therefore,] difficult to get a satisfactory effect [with this formula] for red vaginal discharge. The dosage of disinhibiting dampness medicinals in *Qing Gan Zhi Lin Tang* is comparatively slight. [Therefore,] its treatment effect is relaxed and slow. Based on his clinical experience, Old Doctor Liu held that this type of disease is very closely related to liver channel damp heat damaging the blood division. This is because the liver channel encircles the yin [*i.e.*, reproductive] organs and reaches the lower abdomen. This type of disease is located in the yin organs and lower abdominal region. The onset of this disease is mostly nothing other than lower burner cold and dampness which has endured for [many] days transforming into heat or lower burner damp heat. Heat then damages the blood division. The main manifestations of this are:

1. Red vaginal discharge

Because of heat damaging the blood division, there is vaginal tract bloody secretions or white vaginal discharge containing threads [or streaks] of blood. This is called red and white vaginal discharge and is mostly accompanied by lumbar aching, lower leg flaccidity, lack of strength, a bowstring, slippery pulse, and a red tongue tip.

2. Midcycle bleeding

Each time, in between two menstruations, there is vaginal tract bleeding which is scanty in amount and may last for 3-5 days. There may also be one-sided lower abdominal aching and pain. This may be due to chronic inflammation of the ovaries leading to the arising of ovulatory bleeding. In Chinese medicine, this clearly shows that damp heat has damaged the blood network vessels.

3. Pelvic inflammation

This may lead to the arising of uterine bleeding. This is due to damp heat brewing and accumulating in the lower burner. Thus heat evils enter the blood division and damage the blood network vessels. Its characteristics are that the amount of blood is scanty and not smoothly flowing or it may dribble and drip without stop. This is accompanied by lower abdominal pain, lumbar pain, and other such symptoms.

This formula's functions are to clear heat and disinhibit dampness, upbear yang and eliminate dampness, quicken the blood and regulate menstruation. Within it, Scutellaria, bitter and cold, enters the blood division, cools the blood and clears the liver. Dianthus, Polygonum Avicularis, Akebia, and Plantago, bitter and cold, clear heat and disinhibit dampness. Bupleurum, Schizonepeta, and Melia are able to harmonize the liver, upbear yang, and eliminate dampness. They also course and resolve heat within the blood. Moutan and Achyranthes quicken the blood and regulate the menses. When used together, they clear heat deep-lying [or hidden] within the blood and abduct damp heat in the blood division to be exited externally. [Thus,] this formula's special characteristics are that it clears heat and disinhibits dampness without damaging the righteous, while it upbears yang and scatters dampness without assisting heat. This is because, amongst the heat-clearing medicinals, Old Doctor Liu did not use Gentiana but rather Scutellaria as the ruler. The former is so excessively bitter and cold that

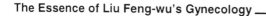

it easily damages the righteous, while Scutellaria's bitterness and cold enter the blood division and cool the blood and clear liver heat without damaging the righteous.

An Wei Yin
(Quiet the Stomach Drink)

Composition: Herba Agastachis Seu Pogostemi (*Huo Xiang*), 3 *qian*, Caulis Perillae Frutescentis (*Su Gen*), 2 *qian*, Cortex Magnoliae Officinalis (*Chuan Hou Po*), 2 *qian*, Fructus Amomi (*Sha Ren*), 2 *qian*, Caulis Bambusae In Taeniis (*Zhu Ru*), 3 *qian*, Rhizoma Pinelliae Ternatae (*Ban Xia*), 3 *qian*, Pericarpium Citri Reticulatae (*Chen Pi*), 3 *qian*, Sclerotium Poriae Cocos (*Fu Ling*), 3 *qian*, uncooked Succus Zingiberis (*Jiang Zhi*), 20 drops

Functions: Harmonizes the stomach, downbears counterflow, and stops vomiting

Main indications: Stomach vacuity and loss of its qi's harmony and downbearing leading to the arising of nausea during pregnancy

Commentary: Malign obstruction during pregnancy refers to nausea and vomiting which do not stop occurring during the first part [*i.e.,* trimester] of pregnancy due to fetal qi counterflowing upward. Typically, this is mostly due to habitual stomach vacuity. Thus the stomach qi is not able to move downward. Contrarily, it follows counterflowing qi to penetrate [or thrust] upward, thus resulting in nausea and vomiting with food and drink not descending. If mild, it may cure itself in several days. If heavy, there may be vomiting. If severe, not even a drop of water may descend.

This formula is mainly suitable for habitual stomach qi vacuity weakness resulting in malign obstruction [*i.e.,* nausea and vomiting]

during pregnancy. Within this formula, bitter, cold ingredients are not used. Rather, acrid, aromatic medicinals which harmonize the stomach are used simultaneously with those which downbear counterflow and stop spitting [*i.e.,* vomiting]. Once the stomach qi is level and harmonious and counterflow qi is descended and downborne, spitting stops and the fetus is quiet. Old Doctor Liu based this formula on *Huo Xiang Zheng Qi San* (Agastaches Correct the Qi Powder) and *Ju Pi Zhu Ru Tang* (Orange Peel & Caulis Bambusae Decoction) and gradually modified these with additions and subtractions until he eventually had this stable [*i.e.,* set] experiential formula.

Within this formula, Agastaches and Caulis Perillae, acrid, warm, penetrating, and aromatic, rectify the qi and harmonize the stomach as well as eliminate dampness. Magnolia loosens the center and downbears the qi, harmonizes the stomach and stops spitting. Poria seeps dampness and boosts the stomach. Amomum and Orange Peel, acrid and aromatic, rectify the qi and harmonize the stomach. Caulis Bambusae, acrid and cool, harmonizes the stomach, downbears counterflow, and stops vomiting. Uncooked Ginger Juice, whose flavor is [also] acrid, rectifies the qi and harmonizes the stomach as well as stops spitting. And Pinellia, acrid, bitter, and slightly warm, dries dampness and transforms phlegm, harmonizes the stomach and downbears counterflow.

Most of the medicinals in this formula have the effect of rectifying the qi and harmonizing the stomach, downbearing counterflow and stopping vomiting. [However,] among these, the efficacy of Ginger Juice and Pinellia is particularly pronounced. Uncooked Ginger is a sage-like medicinal for stopping vomiting. Its flavor is acrid and it governs opening and it governs moistening. It is neither cold nor hot, and it should not be entered in prescriptions which are boiling. Instead, it should be added [just before] administration in order to conserve its medicinal nature. Because acridity is scattering and vomiting is qi counterflow which is not scattered, this medicinal moves yang and scatters the qi. Therefore, it is able to stop vomiting. Its mashed juice is used to mainly treat vomiting counterflow and inability to descend food. It scatters vexation and oppression and opens the stomach qi. Its effect is also fast-acting.

Pinellia is acrid, bitter, and slightly warm. It enters the *yang ming* stomach channel. Because there is no doubt to its acridity, scattering, warming, and drying, its effect of downbearing counterflow and stopping vomiting is marked. It may be used for many types of vomiting. However, it says in the *Ben Cao Gang Mu (The Comprehensive Outline of Materia Medica)* that Pinellia may fell the fetus [*i.e.,* make the fetus fall] and is, [therefore,] prohibited during pregnancy. [Hence,] it should be used cautiously during pregnancy. However, based on his many years of clinical experience, Old Doctor Liu used Pinellia to treat malign obstruction during pregnancy and never saw falling fetus [*i.e.,* a miscarriage]. Rather, its treatment efficacy is extremely good. Although Pinellia is one of the medicinals which should be used cautiously during pregnancy, based on the saying, "If one is diseased, ward off that disease," when used in this formula, Pinellia is able to downbear counterflow and stop vomiting and does not cause fallen fetus. This may be said to be one of the special characteristics of this formula.

Qing Re An Tai Yin
(Clear Heat & Quiet the Fetus Drink)

Composition: Radix Dioscoreae Oppositae (*Shan Yao*), 5 *qian*, Semen Nelumbinis Nuciferae (*Shi Lian*), 3 *qian*, Radix Scutellariae Baicalensis (*Huang Qin*), 3 *qian*, Rhizoma Coptidis Chinensis (*Chuan Lian*), 1 *qian* (or Rhizoma Thalictri Foliosi, *Ma Wei Lian*, 3 *qian*), Cortex Cedrelae (*Chun Gen Bai Pi*), 3 *qian*, carbonized Cacumen Biotae Orientalis (*Ce Bai*), 3 *qian*, Gelatinum Corii Asini (*E Jiao*), 5 *qian* (dissolved)

Functions: Fortifies the spleen and supplements the kidneys, clears heat and quiets the fetus, stops bleeding and stabilizes pain

Main indications: Fetal leakage and precipitation of blood during the initial stage of pregnancy, lumbar aching, and abdominal pain categorized as fetal heat

Commentary: Fetal leakage is the same as threatened miscarriage in Western medicine. This disease is divided into vacuity and repletion [types]. The vacuity pattern should be supplemented with formulas such as *Tai Shan Pan Shi Yin* (Mt. Tai Bedrock Drink). This formula treats fetal leakage categorized as a heat pattern. During the initial stage of pregnancy, due to the gathering of blood in order to nourish the fetus, one mostly sees patients with yin vacuity and yang qi tending to be overwhelming. Yang exuberance leads to heat. Below, this harasses the sea of blood and forces the blood to move frenetically. This then results in fetal leakage and precipitation of blood, lumbar aching, and abdominal pain.

In the *Ben Cao Bei Yao (The Complete Essentials of the Materia Medica)*, it says that Rhizoma Atractylodis Macrocephalae (*Bai Zhu*) and Radix Scutellariae Baicalensis (*Huang Qin*) are sage-like medicinals for quieting the fetus. This is because Atratylodes is able to fortify the spleen. When the spleen is fortified, it is able to restrain the blood. Scutellaria is bitter and cold and is able to clear fetal heat. [However,] it is Old Doctor Liu's experience that Atractylodes tends to be warming and drying. Since pregnant [women] are mostly yin vacuous with blood heat, he used Dioscorea instead of Atractylodes. Its flavor is sweet and its nature [*i.e.*, its temperature] is even [or neutral]. It fortifies the spleen and supplements the kidneys. It supplements but is not heating. Semen Nelumbinis' nature and flavor are slightly bitter and cold. It is able to fortify the spleen and supplement the kidneys, enrich and nourish yin fluids. Scutellaria and Coptis clear heat and quiet the fetus. Cedrela's flavor is bitter and it is astringent and cold. It constrains, astringes, and stops bleeding. Cacumen Biotae is bitter and astringent and slightly cold. It cools the blood and stops bleeding. When stir-fried [till] carbonized, it is also able to constrain, restrain, and stop bleeding. Donkey Skin Glue is categorized as sweet and even. Old Doctor Liu's experience is that this medicinal is sweet and slightly cold. Therefore, it has the functions of clearing heat and cooling the blood, boosting yin and quieting the fetus. Because Donkey Skin Glue's nature is also sticky and slimy, it is able to congeal and secure the blood network vessels in order to stop bleeding. Therefore, it can quiet the fetus and stabilize pain in those who are pregnant.

The ancients used *Jiao Ai Tang* (Donkey Skin Glue & Mugwort Decoction) to treat precipitation of blood during pregnancy. [However,] because Folium Artemisiae Arygii (*Ai Ye*) tends to be warm, [Dr. Liu] did not use it. Instead, he used Scutellaria and Coptis to clear fetal heat and quiet the fetus. In sum, this formula fortifies the spleen and supplements the kidneys, supplements but does not heat, clears heat but does not damage the righteous. It constrains, astringes, and stops bleeding and it quiets the fetus.

Bu Shen Gu Tai San
(Supplement the Kidneys & Secure the Fetus Powder)

Composition: Ramulus Loranthi Seu Visci (*Sang Ji Sheng*), 1.5 *liang*, Radix Dipsaci (*Chuan Xu Duan*), 1.5 *liang*, Gelatinum Corii Asini (*E Jiao*), 1.5 *liang*, Semen Cuscutae Chinensis (*Tu Si Zi*), 1.5 *liang*, Cortex Cedrelae (*Chun Gen Bai Pi*), 5 *qian*. Grind these into fine powder and take 3 *qian* each time, one time each day on days 1, 2, 3, 11, 12, 13, 21, 22, and 23.

Functions: Supplements the kidneys and quiets the fetus

Main indications: Habitual miscarriage categorized as kidney vacuity

Commentary: Old Doctor Liu held that habitual miscarriage is mostly categorized as kidney vacuity. If the kidneys are vacuous, the *chong* and *ren* will be insecure [or not securing]. The *chong* is the sea of blood, while the *ren* rules the uterus and fetus. If the kidneys are vacuous, then the fetus loses its nourishment and [the kidneys] are not able to tie up the fetus. This results in flowing birth [or miscarriage]. The main manifestations of this are lumbar region aching and pain and lower abdominal downward sagging during pregnancy. If severe, there may be vaginal tract precipitation of blood, dizziness, tinnitus, aching and flacidity in the two lower legs, a history of many slippery fetuses [*i.e.,* miscarriages], a pale tongue with white, glossy fur, and a deep, weak pulse in the cubit [position].

Old Doctor Liu reflected on the fact that, for this type of miscarriage, the effect of *Shou Tai Wan* (Long-life Fetus Pills) is not completely satisfactory. Therefore, he gradually developed this formula. He began with *Shou Tai Wan* but felt that the dose when administered in pill form was too small. Therefore, he switched from a pill prescription to a powdered prescription. Compared to the pills, the dosage is greater. Then, to the original formula as a base, he added Cedrela and Donkey Skin Glue in order to strengthen the effect of cooling the blood and stopping bleeding. [Dr. Liu] also developed a very specific method for administering this formula. These medicinals are given every 10 days for three days. During pregnancy there is mostly fetal heat. [However,] habitual miscarriage is also due to kidney vacuity not tying up the fetus. When treated with the above [formula,] fetal heat is appropriately cleared, while the kidneys are appropriately supplemented.

Within this formula, Loranthus and Dipsacus enrich and supplement the liver and kidneys, boost the kidneys and quiet the fetus. Donkey Skin Glue cools the blood, secures, astringes, and stops bleeding. It is also able to nourish the blood and quiet the fetus. Cuscuta is acrid and sweet and is even slightly warm. It supplements kidney yang but is also able to boost kidney yin. It is warm but not drying and supplementing but not stagnating. The above-mentioned four medicinals all make up the supplementing and boosting prescription [of *Shou Tai Wan*]. To these, [Dr. Liu] added Cedrela. It was chosen because its nature is cold and for its ability to cool the blood and secure, astringe, and stop bleeding. If there is already bleeding, it can stop that bleeding. If there is not yet bleeding, it can prevent bleeding.

In terms of the proportions of the dosages of the above medicinals, the supplementing and boosting flavors are all 1.5 *liang* each for a total of 6 *liang*. The heat-clearing, securing and astringing prescription [*i.e.*, ingredient] is only 5 *qian*. Therefore, the ruling action of supplementing the kidneys treats the root, while the prescription for clearing heat and securing and astringing is the assistant for treating the branch. Thus [this formula] is a root treatment assisted by a branch treatment. In terms of how this formula is administered, its on again, off again method of taking does not cause excessive supplementation and boosting to increase and add to fetal heat. These changes of Dr. Liu's in the dosage, method of administration, and ingredients of *Shou Tai Wan* have resulted in a higher rate of treatment efficacy.

Jie Du Tong Mai Tang
(Resolve Toxins & Free the Flow of the Vessels Decoction)

Composition: Semen Pruni Persicae (*Tao Ren*), 3 *qian*, Radix Et Rhizoma Rhei (*Da Huang*), 2 *qian*, Hirudo (*Shui Zhi*), 2 *qian*, Tabanus (*Meng Chong*), 2 *qian*, Caulis Lonicerae Japoncae (*Yin Teng*), 1 *liang*, uncooked Gypsum Fibrosum (*Shi Gao*), 8 *qian*, Cortex Radicis Moutan (*Dan Pi*), 2 *qian*, Fructus Forsythiae Suspensae (*Lian Qiao*), 5 *qian*, Fructus Gardeniae Jasminoidis (*Zhi Zi*), 3 *qian*, Radix Scutellariae Baicalensis (*Huang Qin*), 3 *qian*, Rhizoma Corydalis Yanhusuo (*Yan Hu Suo*), 2 *qian*, Radix Rubrus Paeoniae Lactiflorae (*Chi Shao*), 2 *qian*

Functions: Quickens the blood and transforms stasis, clears heat and resolves toxins, frees the flow of the vessels and stops pain

Main indications: Acute postpartum thrombophlebitis

Commentary: Old Doctor Liu held that acute postpartum thrombophlebitis is due to cold dampness obstructing the network vessels with a lochia that does not descend. [Therefore,] toxic evils counterflow into the channels and vessels and the qi and blood become congested and stagnant. The blood vessels become blocked and enduring depression transforms into heat. This type of static blood is categorized as dead blood and the typical blood-quickening medicinals are not able to scatter it. Therefore, [Dr. Liu] took *Di Dang Tang* (Resistance Decoction) as the ruler. Then, based on the special characteristics of this disease, he added flavors [*i.e.*, ingredients] to produce this formula.

Within *Di Dang Tang*, Leech and Gadfly are the ruling medicinals. Leeches are salty, bitter, and even [or neutral]. In the *Ben Cao Jing Bai Zhong Lu (Materia Medica Classic Hundreds of Types Records)* it is said:

If a person's body has static blood recently obstructing and they still have living qi, they are easy to treat. If obstruction has endured and this has led to no living qi, this is difficult to treat. If blood has already left its channels and the righteous qi has nowhere to home in the whole [body], then putting in light medicinals will be repelled and will not be accepted, while excessively harsh medicinals are also able to damage without vanquishing the blood. Therefore, treatment is extremely difficult. Leeches like to feed on human blood and their nature is also slow and relaxed. Being slow and relaxed leads to the engenderment of blood not being damaged. They have a tendency towards entering hard accumulations and easily break [these]. Their power may be used to attack enduring accumulations of stagnation. Thus they disinhibit without causing calamity.

Gadfly is also a type of insect. It is bitter and slightly cold. In the *Ben Cao Chong Yuan (Lofty Source Materia Medica)*, it says:

> Gadfly is a blood-sucking insect. Its nature also likes to stir. Therefore, it governs the dispelling of static blood and accumulations of blood. It frees the flow and disinhibits the blood vessels and nine portals.[37]

Therefore, both of these enter the blood division, transform static blood, and erode away [or corrode] dead blood. Old Doctor Liu basically held this same point of view. In addition, Persica quickens the blood and transforms stasis. Rhubarb is bitter and cold and enters the blood division. It clears and resolves toxic heat in the blood division. Red Peony and Moutan clear heat and cool the blood, quicken the blood and break the blood.

Since this disease is related to damp toxins and heat evils causing stasis in and obstructing the blood vessels, then mostly what is seen is high fever and limb aching and pain. Therefore, [Dr. Liu] added Gypsum, Forsythia, Gardenia, and Scutellaria to clear heat, resolve toxins, and scatter binding [or nodulation]. Caulis Lonicerae is not only able to clear heat and resolve toxins, but also has the effect of freeing the flow of the blood vessels and quickening the network vessels. In addition, he also used the flavor with a even nature, Corydalis, to move the qi, quicken the blood, and stop pain.

Based on the pathological essence of acute postpartum thrombophlebitis, one should clear and resolve toxins and also quicken the blood and free the flow of the vessels, with clearing being the main [principle]. If one were to clear without freeing the flow, then heat toxins would not be able to be resolved. If one were to free the flow without clearing, then the obstruction of heat toxins combined with static blood would not be

---

[37] The nine portals are the two eyes, two ears, two nostrils, mouth, anus, and urethra in men and vaginal meatus and urethra as a single portal or orifice in women.

able to be moved. Therefore, while clearing there is [also] freeing the flow. Thus damp toxins and heat evils obtain clearing and resolution and static blood and dead blood obtain quickening and scattering. However, within this formula for quickening the blood and transforming stasis, there are not many medicinals whose force is harsh since this would only spread toxic evils and scatter them further. Therefore, there is only a single flavor to move the qi and stop pain in order that freeing the flow of qi slightly assists the movement of the blood.

Qing Re Chu Bi Tang
(Clear Heat & Eliminate Impediment Decoction)

Composition: Caulis Lonicerae Japonicae (*Jin Yin Teng*), 1 *liang*, Radix Clematidis Chinensis (*Wei Ling Xian*), 3 *qian*, Caulis Sinomenii Acuti (*Qing Feng Teng*), 5 *qian*, Caulis Piperis Futokadsurae (*Hai Feng Teng*), 5 *qian*, Caulis Trachelospermi Jasminoidis (*Luo Shi Teng*), 5 *qian*, Radix Stephaniae Tetrandrae (*Fang Ji*), 3 *qian*, Ramulus Mori Albi (*Sang Zhi*), 1 *liang*, Caulis Schizophragmae (*Zhui Di Feng*), 3 *qian*

Functions: Clears heat and scatters dampness, courses wind and quickens the network vessels

Main indications: Postpartum body pain, redness, swelling, and burning pain of the joints, etc.

Commentary: Due to postpartum qi and blood dual vacuity, the constructive and defensive may lose their harmony. Thus the defensive exterior's power to resist evils is lowered. [Evils] may then lodge [in the body] and one may easily contract wind cold. Therefore, one may often see postpartum joint aching and pain or whole body aching and pain. Typically, one commonly uses the methods of supplementing the qi and nourishing the blood, warming and scattering wind cold to treat this.

The medicinals used [in that case] are mostly acrid and warm. For instance, Radix Angelicae Sinensis (*Dang Gui*), Radix Ligustici Wallichii (*Chuan Xiong*), Radix Albus Paeoniae Lactiflorae (*Bai Shao*), and cooked Radix Rehmanniae (*Shu Di*) may be used to nourish the blood. Radix Gentianae Macrophyllae (*Qin Jiao*), Radix Ledebouriellae Divaricatae (*Fang Feng*), Radix Angelicae Pubescentis (*Du Huo*), and Ramulus Loranthi Seu Visci (*Sang Ji Sheng*) may be used to scatter wind and quicken the network vessels.

The use of such formulas and methods to treat blood vacuity wind, cold, damp impediment is reliably effective. However, their use [in the treatment of] wind, damp, heat impediment is not good. It was Old Doctor Liu's clinical experience that, if there is habitual bodily [*i.e.*, constitutional] damp exuberance and contraction of wind cold, this extremely easily transforms heat and internally within the body damp evils bind and unite. This then manifests as damp heat obstructing the network vessels which then pours into the joints causing heat impediment. If one contrarily uses acrid, warming ingredients [in such a case] one will strengthen heat. If one excessively uses supplementing and boosting prescriptions, this easily causes attachment to the evils. Only if one is able to use heat-clearing, dampness-eliminating, wind-coursing, network-quickening medicinal substances and formulas will one be able to see an effect.

This formula is mainly composed of two large types of medicinals—those which clear heat and dispel dampness and those which course wind and quicken the network vessels. Within this formula, Caulis Lonicerae, Stephania, and Ramulus Mori clear heat, eliminate dampness, and dispel wind. Clematis, Sinomenium, Piper Futokadsura, Trachelospermum, and Schizophragma scatter wind, quicken the network vessels, and eliminate dampness. The special characteristic of this formula is that it clears heat, eliminates dampness, scatters wind, and quickens the network vessels without damaging the righteous. Within the heat-clearing, dampness-eliminating medicinals, Caulis

Lonicerae is acrid and cool and scatters heat. It is also able to clear heat evils within the channels and network vessels and blood vessels. Within the wind-scattering, network-quickening, dampness-eliminating medicinals, Clematis is the main medicinal for dispelling wind. Its nature is that it is good at moving. It is able to free the flow of the 12 channels. It is acrid and so it is able to scatter evils. Therefore, it is a ruler [i.e., main ingredient] for wind. It is [also] salty and so it is able to discharge water. Therefore, it is a ruler for dampness. Because the power of these two medicinals to clear heat, eliminate dampness, and scatter wind is outstanding, they are the ruling medicinals in this formula. [Dr. Liu] then used Sinomenium, Piper Futokadsura, and Trachelospermum to strengthen the action of scattering wind and quickening the network vessels. Stephania ia bitter, acrid, and cold and moves in the spaces between the channels and network vessels and the bones and joints. It is able to disperse water swelling between the bones and joints.

Postpartum, one typically sees mostly vacuity. Mostly one encounters postpartum impediment condition within a vacuity pattern. However, if there is habitual bodily damp exuberance and also contraction of wind cold, wind, cold, and damp evils will brew and become depressed and transform into heat. Thus cold impediment may transform into heat impediment. After cold dampness has transformed into heat, the main manifestations will be body pain or bodily heat [i.e., generalized fever], redness, swelling, burning, and pain of the joints with inhibited motion, vexation and oppression, a dry mouth with thirst, a slippery pulse, and yellow tongue fur. In such cases, it was Dr. Liu's experience that evil repletion is more important than the righteous vacuity. Instead of following the saying, "Postpartum one should supplement," for this condition, he mainly dispelled evils. Once evils are dispelled, the righteous can recover automatically.

Qing Re Jie Du Tang
(Clear Heat & Resolve Toxins Decoction)

Composition: Fructus Forsythiae Suspensae (*Lian Qiao*), 5 *qian*, Flos Lonicerae Japonicae (*Yin Hua*), 5 *qian*, Herba Taraxaci Mongolici Cum Radice (*Pu Gong Ying*), 5 *qian*, Herba Violae Yedoensis Cum Radice (*Zi Hua Di Ding*), 5 *qian*, Radix Scutellariae Baicalensis (*Huang Qin*), 3 *qian*, Herba Dianthi (*Qu Mai*), 4 *qian*, Herba Polygoni Avicularis (*Bian Xu*), 4 *qian*, Semen Plantaginis (*Che Qian Zi*), 3 *qian*, Cortex Radicis Moutan (*Dan Pi*), 3 *qian*, Radix Rubrus Paeoniae Lactiflorae (*Chi Shao*), 2 *qian*, Cortex Radicis Lycii Chinensis (*Di Gu Pi*), 3 *qian*, Semen Benincasae Hispidae (*Dong Gua Zi*), 1 *liang*

Functions: Clears heat and resolves toxins, disinhibits dampness and quickens the blood, disperses swelling and stops pain

Main indications: Acute pelvic inflammation categorized as damp toxic heat pattern

Commentary: Acute pelvic inflammation is mostly categorized as toxic heat congestion and exuberance with damp heat pouring downward and qi and blood stasis and stagnation. Due to toxic heat congesting and being exuberant, besides the affected area being red, swollen, hot, and painful, there are the manifestations of high fever, dry mouth, reddish urine, bound stools, and other such disease images of whole body heat disease. Also because of damp heat pouring downward, one may see frequent urination. If damp heat fumes upward, there will be essence spirit listlessness and somnolence [literally, addiction to sleep]. Besides the high fever, the extreme pain in the lower abdomen which refuses pressure is the main symptom.

Old Doctor Liu held that acute pelvic inflammation should be categorized in Chinese medicine as internal welling abscess. Because toxic heat is congested and exuberant, damp heat is pouring downward, and there is qi and blood stasis and stagnation, one should mainly use Chinese medicinals which clear heat and resolve toxins assisted by disinhibiting dampness, cooling the blood, and quickening the blood. Within this formula, [therefore,] Forsythia, which is bitter and slightly cold, clears heat and resolves toxins, disperses welling abscesses and scatters binding [or nodulation]. Lonicera, acrid, bitter, and cold, clears heat and resolves toxins, disperses welling abscesses and swelling. Viola, bitter, acrid, and cold, clears heat and resolves toxins, disperses welling abscesses and swelling. It favors the treatment of clove sore toxins. Scutellaria, bitter and cold, clears heat and dries dampness. Cortex Lycii, sweet and cold, clears heat, cools the blood, and recedes [or abates] fever by expelling heat from the qi division. Cortex Lycii is usually used for yin vacuity fever. However, it has been found through experience that this medicinal can also treat replete pattern fever. When using it to treat yin vacuity fever, it should be combined with Herba Artemisiae Apiaceae (*Qing Hao*). When used for replete heat, it is not necessary to combine these. Dianthus, Polygonum Avicularis, and Plantago clear heat and disinhibit dampness. Semen Benincasae seeps dampness and expels pus, disperses swelling and stops pain. These are assisted by Red Peony and Moutan which clear heat and cool the blood, quicken the blood and transform stasis. [Taken as] a whole, this formula heavily clears heat and resolves toxins at the same time as it is able to disinhibit dampness, quicken the blood, transform stasis, and stop pain.

Jie Du Nei Xiao Tang
(Resolve Toxins & Internally Disperse Decoction)

Composition: Fructus Forsythiae Suspensae (*Lian Qiao*), 1 *liang*, Flos Lonicerae Japonicae (*Jin Yin Hua*), 1 *liang*, Herba Taraxaci Mongolici Cum Radice (*Pu Gong Ying*), 1 *liang*, Herba Patriniae Heterophyllae Cum Radice (*Bai Jiang Cao*), 1 *liang*, Semen Benincasae Hispidae (*Dong Gua Zi*), 1 *liang*, Radix Rubrus Paeoniae Lactiflorae (*Chi Shao*), 2 *qian*, Cortex

Radicis Moutan (*Dan Pi*), 2 *qian*, Radix Et Rhizoma Rhei (*Chuan Jun*), 1 *qian*, Semen Phaseoli Calcarati (*Chi Xiao Dou*), 3 *qian*, Nodus Radicis Glycyrrhizae (*Gan Cao Jie*), 2 *qian*, Bulbus Fritillariae (*Tu Bei Mu*), 3 *qian*, *Niu Huang Wan* (Cow Bezoar Pills), 3 *qian* (taken in two divided doses)

Functions: Clears heat and resolves toxins, quickens the blood and transforms stasis, disperses swelling and stops pain

Main indications: Pelvic suppurative swellings categorized as heat toxins congestion and gathering

Commentary: Pelvic suppurative swellings are due to heat toxins internally brewing with rotten flesh fuming the blood. Based on the region in which they are found, suppurative swellings are categorized as internal welling abscesses. Therefore, this formula uses heavy doses of Forsythia, Lonicera, Dandelion, and Patrinia to clear heat, resolve toxins, and disperse swelling. Moutan and Red Peony clear heat, cool the blood, and stop bleeding. Rhubarb quickens the blood, breaks stasis, and also clears heat and resolves toxins. All three of these are able to eliminate vanquished blood and engender new blood [alternate reading: eliminate vanquished blood so that new blood may be engendered], disperse swelling and expel pus. Semen Benincasae and Aduki Beans enter the blood division, clear heat, disperse swelling, and expel pus. Licorice Nodes and Fritillaria clear heat, resolve toxins, and disperse swelling. In addition, the combination of *Niu Huang Wan* is in order to increase and strengthen the effect of quickening the blood, dispersing swelling, clearing heat, and stopping pain.

The special characteristics of this formula are that its composition is a combination of heat-clearing, toxin-resolving medicinals with blood-cooling medicinals. Although it mainly clearss heat and resolves toxins, this is assisted by cooling the blood and quickening the blood. Heat-clearing and toxin-resolving is for the toxic heat blazing and exuberance. Cooling the blood is for the qi and blood congestion and stagnation.

Therefore, the combination of clearing and resolving and quickening the blood are most suitable. However, it is necessay that clearing heat and resolving toxins be based upon cooling the blood and quickening the blood. For quickening the blood medicinals, one is not able to use acrid, warm [medicinals] which would strengthen heat, such as Radix Angelicae Sinensis (*Dang Gui*), Radix Ligustici Wallichii (*Chuan Xiong*), Semen Pruni Persicae (*Tao Ren*), Flos Carthami Tinctorii (*Hong Hua*), etc. If one erroneously uses acrid, warm, blood-quickening medicinals, this can lead to toxic heat being spread and scattered. Therefore, one must use Moutan and Red Peony which tend to be bitter and cold, blood-cooling, blood-quickening medicinals. Using a heavy dose of these is also not appropriate. An excessively large [amount] may also spread and scatter toxic heat. This is based on [Dr. Liu's] clinical experience.

The additional use of *Niu Huang Wan* is also chosen with the intention of clearing heat and resolving toxins, quickening the blood and stopping pain. Within this [formula], although Resina Olibani (*Ru Xiang*) and Resina Myrrhae (*Mo Yao*) are blood-quickening medicinals, Frankincense and Myrrh enter the channels and scurry into the network vessels,[38] move through the qi division and free the flow of static blood, and move the qi within the blood extremely rapidly. They quicken the blood without strengthening heat. [However,] Myrrh does have the disadvantage of spreading and scattering toxic heat. Secretio Moschi Moschiferi (*She Xiang*) is even more powerful at moving through and scurrying. It is able to move through the qi division, moving the channels of the whole body. Within this [formula], Cow Bezoar is also greatly cold and clears heat. Hence there is freeing the flow within clearing and clearing within freeing the flow. Thus it may be said that [this formula] is an essential medicinal for treating yang welling

---

[38] The verb to scurry, *cuan*, may seem like a peculiar choice of words in a medical context. It is often used to describe rats scurrying away in all directions. The implication here is that only certain medicinals enter the small network vessels and can wend their way through these cracks and crevices of the body the same way that rats and insects can wend their way through the cracks and crevices of the world.

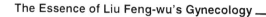

abscesses and sores and combining it with the basic formula is most appropriate.

Qing Re Li Shi Tang
(Clear Heat & Disinhibit Dampness Decoction)

Composition: Herba Dianthi (*Qu Mai*), 4 *qian*, Herba Polygoni Avicularis (*Bian Xu*), 4 *qian*, Caulis Akebiae Mutong (*Mu Tong*), 1 *qian*, Semen Plantaginis (*Che Qian Zi*), 3 *qian*, Talcum (*Hua Shi*), 4 *qian*, Rhizoma Corydalis Yanhusuo (*Yan Hu Suo*), 3 *qian*, Fructus Forsythiae Suspensae (*Lian Qiao*), 5 *qian*, Herba Taraxaci Mongolici Cum Radice (*Pu Gong Ying*), 5 *qian*

Functions: Clears heat and disinhibits dampness, moves the qi and quickens the blood, transforms stasis and stops pain

Main indications: Chronic pelvic inflammation categorized as damp heat pouring downward

Commentary: In terms of Chinese medical pattern discrimination, chronic pelvic inflammation has the two types of cold and heat. This formula is suitable for use with damp heat pouring downward with qi and blood depression and binding. In clinic, the main manifestations [of this] are lumbar pain and abdominal pain which refuses pressure accompanied by low-grade fever, yellow, thick vaginal discharge, and occasional frequent urination. In his clinical practice, Old Doctor Liu found that the effect of the typically used dampness-seeping medicinal substances was not all that good. Very early on he began using *Ba Zheng San* (Eight [Ingredients] Correcting Powder) to treat this and achieved certain [or definite] effects. However, in this type of pelvic inflammation, the disease condition is relaxed and slow and its disease course is relatively long. Therefore, effects cannot be achieved in a short period of time. Within *Ba Zheng San*, Radix Et Rhizoma Rhei (*Da Huang*) is bitter and cold and drains and precipitates. Its prolonged use is, therefore, not appropriate. Although Fructus Gardeniae Jasminoidis (*Zhi Zi*) clears heat, for the disease condition of internal brewing of heat toxins, it is not as effective as Forsythia and Dandelion. The heat-clearing effect of Medulla Junci Effusi (*Deng Cao*), bland in flavor, is not good. Therefore, as a result of step-by-step groping, [Dr. Liu] eventually removed Rhubarb, Gardenia, and Juncus and retained Dianthus, Polygonum Avicularis, Akebia, Talcum, and Plantago as the main medicinals within the original formula for their ability to clear and abduct damp heat and move it downward as well as their ability to quicken the blood and transform stasis. These are assisted by Forsythia and Dandelion which clear heat, resolve toxins, and scatter binding [or nodulation]. Through long clinical observation of this formula, [Dr. Liu found it] to be not only suitable for damp heat pelvic inflammation but for all gynecological conditions with damp heat pouring downward and simultaneous heat toxins.

Nuan Gong Ding Tong Tang
(Warm the Uterus & Stabilize Pain Decoction)

Composition: Semen Citri Reticulatae (*Ju He*), 3 *qian*, Semen Litchi Chinensis (*Li Zhi He*), 3 *qian*, Fructus Foeniculi Vulgaris (*Xiao Hui Xiang*), 3 *qian*, Semen Trigonellae Foeni-graeci (*Hu Lu Ba*), 3 *qian*, Rhizoma Corydalis Yanhusuo (*Yan Hu Suo*), 3 *qian*, Feces Trogopterori Seu Pteromi (*Wu Ling Zhi*), 3 *qian*, Fructus Meliae Toosendan (*Chuan Lian Zi*), 3 *qian*, processed Rhizoma Cyperi Rotundi (*Xiang Fu*), 3 *qian*, Radix Linderae Strychnifoliae (*Wu Yao*), 3 *qian*

Functions: Courses and scatters cold and dampness, warms the uterus, moves the qi and quickens the blood, transforms stasis and stops pain

313

Main indications: Chronic pelvic inflammation categorized as lower burner cold and dampness, qi and blood congelation and binding. It may also be used for chilly uterus infertility.

Commentary: The two most commonly seen types of pelvic inflammation are damp heat pouring downward and lower burner cold and dampness. This formula is an experiential formula for treating cold damp type pelvic inflammation. Its main symptoms are lumbar pain, lower abdominal emission of coolness, insidious pain, clear, watery leukorrhea, and fear of cold and desire for warmth. It was Old Doctor Liu's observation that the location of the aching and pain in this type of pelvic inflammation and the cold stagnating in the liver vessel [type] of cold mounting are quite similar. Therefore, formulas and medicinals pertaining to the treatment of cold mounting are suitable for those with cold damp pelvic inflammation. In chronic pelvic inflammation, the onset of the disease is relatively relaxed and slow. [However,] the heating medicinals and supplementing medicines (such as Cortex Cinnamomi Cassiae, *Rou Gui*, Rhizoma Atractylodis, *Cang Zhu*, and Cortex Magnoliae Officinalis, *Hou Po*) used to treat cold mounting are not appropriate for prolonged administration.

Therefore, through a combination of disease discrimination and pattern discrimination, [Dr. Liu] drew upon *Ju He Wan* (Orange Seed Pills) in his treatment of cold dampness enduring and brewing in the lower burner with qi and blood congelation and stagnation, and, based on the principles of warming the channels and scattering cold, moving the qi and quickening the blood, and transforming stasis and stabilizing pain, developed this formula. Within it, Orange Seeds, Litchi, Fennel, and Fenugreek warm the channels and scatter cold in order to eliminate lower burner cold and dampness. Processed Cyperus, Melia, Lindera, Corydalis, and Flying Squirrel Droppings move the qi and quicken the blood, transform stasis and stabilize pain. This formula warms the channels and scatters cold. [However,] its special characteristic is that it warms without drying. Among the channel-warming, cold-scattering medicinal substances, [Dr. Liu] did not use Cinnamon. [Rather,] he used Orange Seeds and Litchi. Among these, Orange Seeds are acrid, bitter, and warm. They enter the liver channel and move bound qi within the liver channel. Thus they treat cold mounting and bilateral lower abdominal swelling and pain. Litchi is acrid and warm and [also] enters the liver channel. It moves bound qi and stabilizes pain in both sides of the lower abdomen (including the testes in men and the ovaries and fallopian tubes in women). It is a blood division medicinal of the liver channel and moves cold qi within the blood. It is an essential medicinal for treating cold mounting and swelling and pain of the testes. These are assisted by Fenugreek and Fennel which warm the lower burner and dispel cold and dampness. Thus they increase and strengthen the effect of warming the channels and scattering cold, moving the qi and stabilizing pain. Cyperus is acrid and aromatic and tends towards warm. When used uncooked, it moves to the chest and rib-sides. When used processed, it moves to the lower abdomen, inguinal regions, low back, and knees. It enters the qi division and moves the blood within the qi. Therefore, it is able to quicken the blood. Corydalis is bitter and even and enters the blood division. It quickens the blood and transforms stasis. It moves the qi within the blood. When these two medicinals are combined together, one enters the qi division and the other enters the blood division. Thus this combination mutually assists each other in moving the qi and quickening the blood, transforming stasis and stopping pain. The combination of Melia, Flying Squirrel Droppings, and Lindera is in order to increase and strengthen the effect of moving the qi and quickening the blood. In terms of the flavor [i.e., ingredient] Lindera, it is [Dr. Liu's] experience that its nature is acrid, scattering, warming and flow-freeing. Therefore, it is able to scatter cold and quicken the blood, rectify the qi and stop pain. It is also able to expel and discharge water dampness which has collected and gathered. In terms of cold dampness leading to the arising of white vaginal discharge, it also may be used to treat what is free-flowing [i.e., the

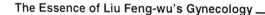

leukorrhea] by freeing the flow.[39] [In other words, Lindera] provides a way out for leukorrhea. Once dampness is dispelled, abnormal vaginal discharge stops.

Shu Qi Ding Tong Tang
(Course the Qi & Stabilize Pain Decoction)

Composition: Processed Rhizoma Cyperi Rotundi (*Xiang Fu*), 3 *qian*, Fructus Meliae Toosendan (*Chuan Lian Zi*), 3 *qian*, Rhizoma Corydalis Yanhusuo (*Yan Hu Suo*), 3 *qian*, Feces Trogopterori Seu Pteromi (*Wu Ling Zhi*), 3 *qian*, Resina Myrrhae (*Mo Yao*), 1 *qian*, Fructus Citri Aurantii (*Zhi Ke*), 1.5 *qian*, Radix Auklandiae Lappae (*Mu Xiang*), 1.5 *qian*, Radix Angelicae Sinensis (*Dang Gui*), 3 *qian*, Radix Linderae Strychnifoliae (*Wu Yao*), 3 *qian*

Functions: Moves the qi and quickens the blood, transforms stasis and stops pain

Main indications: Chronic pelvic inflammation and low back and abdominal aching and pain categorized as qi stagnation and blood stasis

---

[39] In general, Chinese medicine is based on the principle of providing the equal opposite factor to bring something within the body back into balance. Thus cold is warmed and heat is cooled. Dryness is moistened and dampness is dried, seeped, transformed, or otherwise eliminated. Here, however, Lindera is used to treat something that is already flowing when it should not. Dampness is flowing downward abnormally, but Lindera's action is to promote the movement of qi and, therefore, fluids and humors. This is based on the principle of freeing the flow of what already is freely flowing, since actually what appears to be freely flowing is nothing other than an evil accumulation which has gathered, at least in part, due to the qi's not moving and transforming it. Thus, in fact, there is nothing contradictory about this treatment principle. What looks like flow is not free flow but the abnormal spilling over of something which has stopped flowing normally.

Commentary: This formula is suitable for chronic pelvic inflammation (qi stagnation and blood stasis pattern) leading to the arising of lumbar and abdominal aching and pain. It is also possible that those with this disease may have cold and heat which is difficult to divide and discriminate and lumbar pain and abdominal pain are their main symptoms. If cold dampness is erroneously treated by overuse of acrid, warming ingredients, it will not unite with the disease mechanism. If treatment is erroneously based on damp heat, and bitter, cold, drying dampness ingredients are overused, contrarily, this will make the qi and blood congealed and stagnant and will not obtain smooth and free flow. Seizing the main symptoms, Old Doctor Liu composed this formula from medicinal substances whose medicinal nature is even and steady, neither cold nor hot and which mainly move the qi, quicken the blood, course and free the flow. Although the dosages are not large, the power of the medicinals is concentrated together. Thus qi stagnation obtains free flow, blood stasis obtains scattering, qi and blood flow freely and smoothly, and aching and pain are automatically resolved.

Within this formula, Cyperus, Melia, Corydalis, Flying Squirrel Droppings, Myrrh, and Lindera move the qi, quicken the blood, and stop pain. Aurantium and Auklandia rectify the qi. And Dang Gui nourishes the blood. [Taken as] a whole, this formula's combined effect is to move the qi and quicken the blood, transform stasis and stop pain.

General Index

stomach vacuity, habitual 296
stomach venter distention and oppression 275
stools, dry 25, 163, 172, 181, 182, 211, 261, 275, 279, 280, 286
stools, dry, bound 287
stools, loose 9, 116, 143, 144, 191-193, 269, 271, 273, 274
stools, premenstrual bloody 133
strength, lack of 95, 98, 99, 116, 140, 158, 160, 165, 166, 187, 188, 220, 253, 259, 263, 266, 267, 269, 271, 273, 274, 280, 282, 284, 294
strength, lack of, before menstruation 140
strength, whole body lack of 266
streptomycin 213
Su Wen 13, 15, 17, 25, 28, 46, 91, 93, 118, 122, 273
sweat, chilly 259
sweating 19, 68, 69, 83, 128, 143, 165, 178, 273, 274, 292
sweating, agitated 273
sweating, vacuity 165

T

tachycardia 141
Tang Rong-chuan 271
taxation 21, 23, 112, 116, 124
testicular or vaginal area swelling and pain 25
tetany reversal 26
tetany wind 25, 31
tetracycline 232, 258
The Complete Essentials of the Materia Medica 208, 299
thirst, dry mouth and 149, 238, 240, 307
thirst, oral 25, 65, 142
throat, itchy 27
throat, parched 25
tian gui 15, 37, 122-124, 126, 206, 273
tidal heat 273, 292
tinnitus 243, 273, 301
torpid intake 9, 69, 83, 127, 163, 172, 191, 225, 259, 261, 263, 266
toxemia during pregnancy 87, 88
toxic heat 3, 50, 225, 226, 241, 304, 308, 310, 311
Treatise on Damage [Due to] Cold 63, 105-108, 112

Treatise on the Origins & Symptoms of Various Diseases 91
tremors 25, 26
tremors and contractions 25, 26
triple burner 18

U

upbearing 3-6, 8-12, 25, 27, 29, 60, 103, 109, 111, 115-118, 126, 130, 155, 167, 223, 241
upbearing and downbearing 3, 5, 12, 29
upward counterflow 5, 24, 95, 128, 290
urinary tract infection 95
urination, frequent 14, 194, 195, 207, 223, 308, 312
urination, frequent, numerous 193, 220
urination, reddish 25
urination, short, yellow 68
urination, yellowish red 244
urine, yellow 182, 247, 275, 279
uterine bleeding 67, 93, 94, 96, 121, 163, 164, 166, 169-173, 263, 283, 294, 295
uterine bleeding, functional 67, 121, 163, 164, 166, 169-173
uterine cervix was slightly eroded 203
uterine chill infertility 51
uterine contractions 180, 181
uterine curettage 78, 80, 82, 83, 85-87, 163, 168, 173, 210, 221, 243-246, 249-251, 255, 256, 259, 261, 263, 264
uterine curettage, abdominal pain after 259, 261
uterine curettage, electric 83
uterine mouth, polyps on the 98
uterine myomas ix, 50, 91, 92, 97, 113
uterine-sacral ligament 211
uterus 15, 23, 32, 36, 37, 40, 49, 51, 61-63, 65, 67, 80, 84, 87, 90, 91, 94, 98, 100, 147, 150, 151, 154, 181, 185-187, 189, 191-193, 196-199, 201, 203, 206, 209, 210, 212-215, 217, 219, 229-232, 234, 236, 245-247, 249, 250, 260, 262, 263, 276, 301, 313, 314
uterus, anteversion and anteflexion of 201
uterus, cold and chilled 186
uterus, cold lodged in the 51, 191, 246, 247, 263
uterus, inflammation of the body of the 219

OTHER BOOKS ON CHINESE MEDICINE AVAILABLE FROM:
BLUE POPPY PRESS
5441 Western, Suite 2, Boulder, CO 80301
For ordering 1-800-487-9296 PH. 303\447-8372 FAX 303\245-8362
Email: info@bluepoppy.com Website: www.bluepoppy.com

ACUPOINT POCKET REFERENCE by Bob Flaws
ISBN 0-936185-93-7
ISBN 978-0-936185-93-4

ACUPUNCTURE & IVF by Lifang Liang
ISBN 0-891845-24-1
ISBN 978-0-891845-24-6

ACUPUNCTURE FOR STROKE REHABILITATION
Three Decades of Information from China
by Hoy Ping Yee Chan, et al.
ISBN 1-891845-35-7
ISBN 978-1-891845-35-2

ACUPUNCTURE PHYSICAL MEDICINE: An
Acupuncture Touchpoint Approach to the Treatment
of Chronic Pain, Fatigue, and Stress Disorders
by Mark Seem
ISBN 1-891845-13-6
ISBN 978-1-891845-13-0

AGING & BLOOD STASIS: A New Approach to TCM
Geriatrics by Yan De-xin
ISBN 0-936185-63-6
ISBN 978-0-936185-63-7

A NEW AMERICAN ACUPUNTURE By Mark Seem
ISBN 0-936185-44-9
ISBN 978-0-936185-44-6

BETTER BREAST HEALTH NATURALLY
with CHINESE MEDICINE
by Honora Lee Wolfe & Bob Flaws
ISBN 0-936185-90-2
ISBN 978-0-936185-90-3

BIOMEDICINE: A Textbook for Practitioners of
Acupuncture and Oriental Medicine
by Bruce H. Robinson, MD
ISBN 1-891845-38-1
ISBN 978-1-891845-38-3

THE BOOK OF JOOK:
Chinese Medicinal Porridges
by B. Flaws
ISBN 0-936185-60-6
ISBN 978-0-936185-60-0

CHANNEL DIVERGENCES
Deeper Pathways of the Web
by Miki Shima and Charles Chase
ISBN 1-891845-15-2
ISBN 978-1-891845-15-4

CHINESE MEDICAL OBSTETRICS
by Bob Flaws
ISBN 1-891845-30-6
ISBN 978-1-891845-30-7

CHINESE MEDICAL PALMISTRY:
Your Health in Your Hand
by Zong Xiao-fan & Gary Liscum
ISBN 0-936185-64-3
ISBN 978-0-936185-64-4

CHINESE MEDICAL PSYCHIATRY
A Textbook and Clinical Manual
by Bob Flaws and James Lake, MD
ISBN 1-845891-17-9
ISBN 978-1-845891-17-8

CHINESE MEDICINAL TEAS: Simple, Proven, Folk
Formulas for Common Diseases & Promoting Health
by Zong Xiao-fan & Gary Liscum
ISBN 0-936185-76-7
ISBN 978-0-936185-76-7

CHINESE MEDICINAL WINES & ELIXIRS
by Bob Flaws
ISBN 0-936185-58-9
ISBN 978-0-936185-58-3

CHINESE MEDICINE & HEALTHY WEIGHT
MANAGEMENT: An Evidence-based Integrated
Approach by Juliette Aiyana, L. Ac.
ISBN 1-891845-44-6
ISBN 978-1-891845-44-4

CHINESE PEDIATRIC MASSAGE THERAPY: A
Parent's & Practitioner's Guide to the Prevention &
Treatment of Childhood Illness
by Fan Ya-li
ISBN 0-936185-54-6
ISBN 978-0-936185-54-5

CHINESE SELF-MASSAGE THERAPY:
The Easy Way to Health
by Fan Ya-li
ISBN 0-936185-74-0
ISBN 978-0-936185-74-3

THE CLASSIC OF DIFFICULTIES:
A Translation of the Nan Jing
translation by Bob Flaws
ISBN 1-891845-07-1
ISBN 978-1-891845-07-9

A COMPENDIUM OF CHINESE MEDICAL
MENSTRUAL DISEASES
by Bob Flaws
ISBN 1-891845-31-4
ISBN 978-1-891845-31-4

CONTROLLING DIABETES NATURALLY WITH
CHINESE MEDICINE
by Lynn Kuchinski
ISBN 0-936185-06-3
ISBN 978-0-936185-06-2

CURING ARTHRITIS NATURALLY WITH
CHINESE MEDICINE
by Douglas Frank & Bob Flaws
ISBN 0-936185-87-2
ISBN 978-0-936185-87-3

CURING DEPRESSION NATURALLY WITH
CHINESE MEDICINE
by Rosa Schnyer & Bob Flaws
ISBN 0-936185-94-5
ISBN 978-0-936185-94-1

INTEGRATED PHARMACOLOGY: Combining Modern
Pharmacology with Chinese Medicine
by Dr. Greg Sperber with Bob Flaws
ISBN 1-891845-41-1
ISBN 978-0-936185-41-3

INTRODUCTION TO THE USE OF
PROCESSED CHINESE MEDICINALS
by Philippe Sionneau
ISBN 0-936185-62-7
ISBN 978-0-936185-62-0

KEEPING YOUR CHILD HEALTHY WITH
CHINESE MEDICINE
by Bob Flaws
ISBN 0-936185-71-6
ISBN 978-0-936185-71-2

THE LAKESIDE MASTER'S STUDY OF THE PULSE
by Li Shi-zhen, trans. by Bob Flaws
ISBN 1-891845-01-2
ISBN 978-1-891845-01-7

MANAGING MENOPAUSE NATURALLY WITH
CHINESE MEDICINE
by Honora Lee Wolfe
ISBN 0-936185-98-8
ISBN 978-0-936185-98-9

MASTER HUA'S CLASSIC OF THE
CENTRAL VISCERA
by Hua Tuo, trans. by Yang Shou-zhong
ISBN 0-936185-43-0
ISBN 978-0-936185-43-9

THE MEDICAL I CHING: Oracle of the
Healer Within
by Miki Shima
ISBN 0-936185-38-4
ISBN 978-0-936185-38-5

MENOPAIUSE & CHINESE MEDICINE
by Bob Flaws
ISBN 1-891845-40-3
ISBN 978-1-891845-40-6

MOXIBUSTION: The Power of Mugwort Fire
by Lorraine Wilcox
ISBN 1-891845-46-2
ISBN 978-1-891845-46-8

TEST PREP WORKBOOK FOR THE NCCAOM BIO-
MEDICINE MODULE: Exam Preparation & Study
Guide
by Zhong Bai-song
ISBN 1-891845-34-9
ISBN 978-1-891845-34-5

POINTS FOR PROFIT: The Essential Guide to
Practice Success for Acupuncturists 3rd Edition
by Honora Wolfe, Eric Strand & Marilyn Allen
ISBN 1-891845-25-X
ISBN 978-1-891845-25-3

PRINCIPLES OF CHINESE MEDICAL ANDROLOGY:
An Integrated Approach to Male Reproductive and
Urological Health by Bob Damone
ISBN 1-891845-45-4
ISBN 978-1-891845-45-1

PRINCE WEN HUI's COOK: Chinese Dietary Therapy
By Bob Flaws & Honora Wolfe
ISBN 0-912111-05-4
ISBN 978-0-912111-05-6

THE PULSE CLASSIC:
A Translation of the Mai Jing
by Wang Shu-he, trans. by Yang Shou-zhong
ISBN 0-936185-75-9
ISBN 978-0-936185-75-0

THE SECRET OF CHINESE PULSE DIAGNOSIS
by Bob Flaws
ISBN 0-936185-67-8
ISBN 978-0-936185-67-5

SECRET SHAOLIN FORMULAS for the Treatment of
External Injury
by De Chan, trans. by Zhang Ting-liang & Bob Flaws
ISBN 0-936185-08-2
ISBN 978-0-936185-08-8

STATEMENTS OF FACT IN TRADITIONAL
CHINESE MEDICINE   Revised & Expanded
by Bob Flaws
ISBN 0-936185-52-X
ISBN 978-0-936185-52-1

STICKING TO THE POINT 1:
A Rational Methodology for the Step by Step
Formulation & Administration of an Acupuncture
Treatment
by Bob Flaws
ISBN 0-936185-17-1
ISBN 978-0-936185-17-0

STICKING TO THE POINT 2:
A Study of Acupuncture & Moxibustion Formulas
and Strategies
by Bob Flaws
ISBN 0-936185-97-X
ISBN 978-0-936185-97-2

A STUDY OF DAOIST ACUPUNCTURE &
MOXIBUSTION
by Liu Zheng-cai
ISBN 1-891845-08-X
ISBN 978-1-891845-08-6

THE SUCCESSFUL CHINESE HERBALIST
by Bob Flaws and Honora Lee Wolfe
ISBN 1-891845-29-2
ISBN 978-1-891845-29-1

THE SYSTEMATIC CLASSIC OF ACUPUNCTURE
& MOXIBUSTION
A translation of the Jia Yi Jing
by Huang-fu Mi, trans. by Yang Shou-zhong &
Charles Chace
ISBN 0-936185-29-5
ISBN 978-0-936185-29-3

THE TAO OF HEALTHY EATING ACCORDING TO
CHINESE MEDICINE
by Bob Flaws
ISBN 0-936185-92-9
ISBN 978-0-936185-92-7

TEACH YOURSELF TO READ MODERN
MEDICAL CHINESE
by Bob Flaws
ISBN 0-936185-99-6
ISBN 978-0-936185-99-6

TEST PREP WORKBOOK FOR BASIC TCM THEORY
by Zhong Bai-song
ISBN 1-891845-43-8
ISBN 978-1-891845-43-7

TREATING PEDIATRIC BED-WETTING WITH
ACUPUNCTURE & CHINESE MEDICINE
by Robert Helmer
ISBN 1-891845-33-0
ISBN 978-1-891845-33-8

TREATISE on the SPLEEN & STOMACH: A
Translation and annotation of Li Dong-yuan's
Pi Wei Lun
by Bob Flaws
ISBN 0-936185-41-4
ISBN 978-0-936185-41-5

THE TREATMENT OF CARDIOVASCULAR
DISEASES WITH CHINESE MEDICINE
by Simon Becker, Bob Flaws &
Robert Casañas, MD
ISBN 1-891845-27-6
ISBN 978-1-891845-27-7

THE TREATMENT OF DIABETES MELLITUS WITH
CHINESE MEDICINE
by Bob Flaws, Lynn Kuchinski &
Robert Casañas, M.D.
ISBN 1-891845-21-7
ISBN 978-1-891845-21-5

THE TREATMENT OF DISEASE IN TCM, Vol. 1:
Diseases of the Head & Face, Including Mental &
Emotional Disorders
by Philippe Sionneau & Lü Gang
ISBN 0-936185-69-4
ISBN 978-0-936185-69-9

THE TREATMENT OF DISEASE IN TCM, Vol. II:
Diseases of the Eyes, Ears, Nose, & Throat
by Sionneau & Lü
ISBN 0-936185-73-2
ISBN 978-0-936185-73-6

THE TREATMENT OF DISEASE IN TCM, Vol. III:
Diseases of the Mouth, Lips, Tongue, Teeth & Gums
by Sionneau & Lü
ISBN 0-936185-79-1
ISBN 978-0-936185-79-8

THE TREATMENT OF DISEASE IN TCM, Vol IV:
Diseases of the Neck, Shoulders, Back, & Limbs
by Philippe Sionneau & Lü Gang
ISBN 0-936185-89-9
ISBN 978-0-936185-89-7

THE TREATMENT OF DISEASE IN TCM, Vol V:
Diseases of the Chest & Abdomen
by Philippe Sionneau & Lü Gang
ISBN 1-891845-02-0
ISBN 978-1-891845-02-4

THE TREATMENT OF DISEASE IN TCM, Vol VI:
Diseases of the Urogential System & Proctology
by Philippe Sionneau & Lü Gang
ISBN 1-891845-05-5
ISBN 978-1-891845-05-5

THE TREATMENT OF DISEASE IN TCM, Vol VII:
General Symptoms
by Philippe Sionneau & Lü Gang
ISBN 1-891845-14-4
ISBN 978-1-891845-14-7

THE TREATMENT OF EXTERNAL DISEASES
WITH ACUPUNCTURE & MOXIBUSTION
by Yan Cui-lan and Zhu Yun-long, trans. by Yang Shou-zhong
ISBN 0-936185-80-5
ISBN 978-0-936185-80-4

THE TREATMENT OF MODERN WESTERN
MEDICAL DISEASES WITH CHINESE MEDICINE
by Bob Flaws & Philippe Sionneau
ISBN 1-891845-20-9
ISBN 978-1-891845-20-8

UNDERSTANDING THE DIFFICULT PATIENT: A
Guide for Practitioners of Oriental Medicine
by Nancy Bilello, RN, L.ac.
ISBN 1-891845-32-2
ISBN 978-1-891845-32-1

YI LIN GAI CUO (Correcting the Errors in the Forest
of Medicine)
by Wang Qing-ren
ISBN 1-891845-39-X
ISBN 978-1-891845-39-0

70 ESSENTIAL CHINESE HERBAL FORMULAS
by Bob Flaws
ISBN 0-936185-59-7
ISBN 978-0-936185-59-0

160 ESSENTIAL CHINESE READY-MADE
MEDICINES
by Bob Flaws
ISBN 1-891945-12-8
ISBN 978-1-891945-12-3

630 QUESTIONS & ANSWERS ABOUT CHINESE
HERBAL MEDICINE:
A Workbook & Study Guide
by Bob Flaws
ISBN 1-891845-04-7
ISBN 978-1-891845-04-8

260 ESSENTIAL CHINESE MEDICINALS
by Bob Flaws
ISBN 1-891845-03-9
ISBN 978-1-891845-03-1

750 QUESTIONS & ANSWERS ABOUT
ACUPUNCTURE
Exam Preparation & Study Guide
by Fred Jennes
ISBN 1-891845-22-5
ISBN 978-1-891845-22-2